Gender, Health, and Popular Culture

Gender, Health, and Popular Culture

Historical Perspectives

Edited by Cheryl Krasnick Warsh

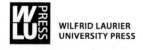

WILFRID LAURIER
UNIVERSITY PRESS

Wilfrid Laurier University Press acknowledges the financial support of the Government of Canada through its Canada Book Fund for its publishing activities.

Library and Archives Canada Cataloguing in Publication

  Gender, health, and popular culture : historical perspectives / Cheryl Krasnick Warsh, editor.

Includes index.
Issued also in electronic formats.
ISBN 978-1-55458-217-4

1. Human body—Social aspects—History. 2. Body image—Social aspects—History. 3. Women—Health and hygiene—Sociological aspects. 4. Health—Social aspects—History. I. Warsh, Cheryl Lynn Krasnick, [date]

GN298.G45 2011   306.461   C2010-905610-8

Electronic formats.
ISBN 978-1-55458-248-8 (PDF), ISBN 978-1-55458-253-2 (EPUB)

1. Human body—Social aspects—History. 2. Body image—Social aspects—History. 3. Women—Health and hygiene—Sociological aspects. 4. Health—Social aspects—History. I. Warsh, Cheryl Lynn Krasnick, [date]

GN298.G45 2011a   306.461   C2010-905611-6

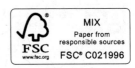

MIX
Paper from
responsible sources
FSC® C021996

Contents

II: Popular Representations of the Body in Sickness and Health

Introduction

Cheryl Krasnick Warsh

Health is a gendered concept in Western cultures.[1] The healthy man is strong, assertive, tolerant, moderate in his appetites, hard-working, adventurous, responsible, and wise. The healthy woman is attractive, youthful-looking, self-sacrificing, empathetic, consciously limiting her appetites, hard-working, careful, mindful of the needs of her loved ones and others in her social orbit, and constantly seeking the wise advice of others to improve the appearance and health of herself and her family. This advice—wise or otherwise—has been liberally offered for at least 150 years by traditional sources like older family members and friends, professional channels such as physicians and other "experts," and newer venues, including newspapers, advertisements, magazines, exhibits, lectures, websites, and other mass media.

This collection investigates the presentation and reception of gendered concepts of health from two perspectives. In both perspectives, concepts of health and gender are viewed through the lens of popular culture. The first section concerns the transmission of health information to women for their own consumption and in their customary role as family healers. This information was usually offered by public health officials, physicians, governments, and other authority figures, but also by corporations and advertisers to sell products as well as to promote healthy lifestyles. The second section is more theoretical in nature: gendered concepts of health were transmitted through visual representations of the ideal female and male bodies. These ideal bodies reflected dominant socio-economic and geopolitical ideologies: they were overwhelmingly white, young, slim, prosperous, and free of disabilities. The prevailing discourse, therefore, assumed a racialized whiteness, and the Others, if cited at all, were presented in opposition to and confirmation of the dominant/healthy ideal. A persistent bombardment of similar images through a variety of media—fine art, advertising, movies, billboards, television, and magazines—resulted in the absorption of universal standards of beauty and health, and in generalized desires to achieve them.

Both sections have been influenced by the theoretical perspectives that have fallen under the rubric of cultural studies, perspectives that have, since the 1980s, cast a giant shadow not only upon literary studies, sociology and cultural anthropology, and social history but also upon the study of women and gender, and, more recently, the study of the socio-cultural and historical determinants of health. As will be shown in these chapters, expert advice concerning health is proffered within an ideological framework. Ideology is a concept that has been employed in explaining the maintenance of power relations beyond class. Feminist theorists describe patriarchal ideology as a tool in the concealment and distortion of gender relations. Studies in popular culture outline various "ideological forms," such as television programming, fiction, or popular music, as texts that "always present a particular image of the world."[2]

Two influential definitions of ideology stress the way in which we unconsciously experience it. Roland Barthes considered "myth" (ideology) to operate at "the level of connotations ... that texts and practices carry." Barthes's insight, which is especially relevant to these chapters, was that myth is "the attempt to make universal and legitimate what is in fact partial and particular: an attempt to pass off that which is cultural (i.e. humanly made) as something which is natural (i.e. just existing)."[3] Post-structural theorists, such as Ernesto Laclau and Jacques Derrida, introduced the concept of discourse;[4] all texts and actions are seen by post-structuralists as not having inherent meaning but a meaning that is "articulated" within a certain set of circumstances and power relationships. Derrida emphasizes the power relationships that underlie binary oppositions such as black and white, sickness and health, female and male, in that these oppositions are never equal but reflect the domination of one over the other.[5] Finally, the work of Michel Foucault has been extremely influential in interpretations of how the production, transmission, and acceptance of knowledge—through courts, medical schools, academic institutions, and the media—is subject to the operation of power structures. Within the context of these chapters, medical discourses concerning what is "healthful" behaviour for women and men are underwritten by what is considered "acceptable" behaviour. Sexuality and reproduction are highlighted because, as Foucault noted, the Victorian discourse over sexuality re-invented sexuality as a construct with its binary oppositions of what constitutes male and female, normal and abnormal sexual expression, and created the corresponding regulatory experts and agencies, such as asylums and reformatories, to deal with the transgressors.[6]

To be beautiful is to be healthy: this is an axiom of Western cultures. "Health and Beauty" remains a popular section in newspapers and magazines, a section that is mostly female-oriented. Yet the achievement of the latter is often at the cost of the former. Throughout the nineteenth and twentieth centuries, and continuing today, standards of beauty that were difficult, if not impossible, for most women to adhere to have left many uncomfortable, debilitated, deformed, or even dead from the attempt. Victorian women avoided protein and laced their corsets tightly to fit into their gowns; twenties "flappers" smoked cigarettes to wear their short, tight frocks; women in the Cold War era used tranquilizers, amphetamines, and hormones to keep themselves perky and attractive; and women at the turn of the twenty-first century go under the surgeon's knife to permanently change perceived physical flaws. While the healthy male has been somewhat associated with physical appearance—that is, the muscular physique—the image has never been as extreme as for the female. The body-builder, with muscles distended by the overuse of anabolic steroids, is today more a figure of grotesque comedy (note the cartoon characters of professional wrestling) than a figure of beauty like Charles Atlas fifty years ago. Yet the ever-thinner woman remains the standard for female beauty and health.

An early example of the sale of gendered health is the patent medicine advertisement. While many early concoctions were sold to both men and women, the most popular, Lydia E. Pinkham's Vegetable Compound for Female Complaints, was the first to use saturation marketing to promote sales.[7] In the late-nineteenth and early-twentieth centuries, Lydia Pinkham's face and name were plastered on barns and hung from banners on the sides of bridges, and they dotted daily newspapers throughout North America. The Vegetable Compound was sold not only as relief for physical complaints, such as "nerves" and menstrual disorders, but as a solution to marital strife and other interpersonal difficulties arising from the physical disorders. The success of Pinkham marketing was the model for other health advertisers in the decades to come. The laxative Fletcher's Castoria, for instance, was marketed in the 1930s and 1940s as a product for good mothering, as ignorant mothers may not have known that their children's misbehaviour was due to stomach problems.[8] In both examples, the pharmaceutical products were advertised as supports for women's gendered roles as good wives and mothers as well as for their medicinal qualities.

The sale of commercial products ranging from mouthwash for the "disease" of halitosis, to menstrual products that maintained "daintiness," to amphetamines to reduce weight, to hormone replacements to retain "youthfulness," continued in the same vein throughout the twentieth century. Health was equated with the retention of sexual attractiveness and could be achieved through the purchase of the correct products. Other goods such as advice manuals, nutritional supplements and baby foods were marketed as the best guarantors for healthy outcomes to pregnancy and for the growth of vigorous children.

The chapters in this collection, while ranging in terms of subject and temporal and geographical focus, engage the intersection of gender, health, and popular culture through two broad, often interconnected themes. The first concerns how health information has been transmitted—whether through popular and professional nineteenth-century health journals, twentieth-century advertisements and television programming, or government informational pamphlets and screening programmes—as well as the content of that information and how it has been interpreted and consumed by its recipients. The content of the health information included patriarchal tenets regarding women's behaviour as experienced through reproductive choices and sexual practices. The second theme, more overtly theoretical in nature, relates to popular representations of the body in sickness and health, and illustrates how portraits of the body have supported as well as contradicted changing concepts of gender, race, and beauty. The concept of the body as a contested space requiring discipline and order permeates all of the chapters in section two, as the "natural," unchanging definitions of femininity, masculinity, and indeed death itself are challenged by economic transformation, medical technologies, and disease.[9]

I: The Transmission of Health Information

In "Confined: Constructions of Childbirth in Popular and Elite Medical Culture in Late Nineteenth-Century Australia," Lisa Featherstone examines both popular and elite medical writings to determine what expecting women learned from domestic manuals and what their physicians practised, based upon their medical texts. She concludes that the elite manuals focused upon pathology while the popular books avoided it. Similar comparisons may be made today between the emphasis upon pathology or complications in medical journals and its de-emphasis or avoidance in bestsellers such as *What to Expect When You're Expecting*. On the other hand, Featherstone notes that the nineteenth-century popular manuals also medicalized the home birth environment through emphasis upon tools, hygiene, and implements necessary for rendering the home as hospital-like as possible. The growing literature on medical history from Australia, New Zealand, and other settler societies expands the traditional focus upon the Anglo-American world to illustrate the influence of European medicine upon its colonies and the cross-fertilization of professional advancement. Like other European colonies, however, the professional advice was for the benefit of the settlers rather than the indigenous peoples.

In "Eating for Two: Shaping Mothers' Figures and Babies' Futures in Modern American Culture," Lisa Foreman Cody continues the focus on maternal and infant health by examining how American women in the twentieth century have been bombarded with ever-changing advice concerning proper prenatal care, weight gain, and nutrition. While the advice has allowed pregnant women to take a more active and "scientific" role in their own prenatal care, it has also placed an increasing burden of responsibility upon them with respect to successful outcomes.

Sharra Vostral shifts the focus to reproductive education for young girls in "Advice to Adolescents: Menstrual Health and Menstrual Education Films, 1946–1982." In her account of menstrual hygiene education in American schools in the twentieth century, she concludes that the campaigns taught young women societal expectations concerning femininity and the importance of regulating the body through the use of sanitary napkins. The sanitary napkin, through its successful concealment of menstruation from others, dislodged menstruation from sexual maturity and re-inscribed it into adolescence, thereby allowing young ladies to still pass as girls. In this respect, a product problematic for its association with sexual expression was marketed by its manufacturers and introduced by school nurses as a technology that could hide sexual availability, to the relief of anxious parents.

Like Vostral's chapter, Heather Molyneux's "Controlling Conception: Images of Women, Safety, Sexuality, and the Pill in the Sixties" illustrates attempts to introduce a new technology—in this case, the birth control pill—without overturning traditional values such as the prevention of female promiscuity and teenaged sexuality. Molyneux examines advertisements in the *Canadian Medical Association Journal* for the pill in the years of its inception and concludes that the advertisers emphasized the eugenics legacy of population control, rather than sexual freedom, to defuse anxieties about a sexual revolution and the involuntary support of such a revolution by conservative physicians who prescribed the pill.

Another pillar of late-twentieth-century female sexual expression was access to safe abortion, and in "All Aboard? Canadian Women's Abortion Tourism, 1960–1980," Christabelle Sethna discusses abortion from an international perspective. Abortion tourism was (and is) the consequence of an unequal distribution of legal abortion services, as well as improvements in international travel. Whether in New York, Montreal, or the United Kingdom, abortion tourism continues a pattern of privileging those in possession of economic, social, and psychological resources that allow access to safe abortions. Yet even the privileged women can face officious regulations and judgments from medical and bureaucratic elites in foreign countries.

The chapters by Featherstone, Cody, Vostral, and Molyneaux all discuss "advice" and treatment offered by male medical elites and corporate institutions to educate, regulate, and ultimately "fix" the reproductive functions of women and in so doing, regulate and control their movements and behaviour. This regulation is most clearly seen in Sethna's discussion of abortion tourism, demonstrating that while abortion has been sanctioned by the Canadian Parliament and legal elite, the medical elite retains control of accessibility, thereby shifting control of reproductive choices from one male/state elite to another.

Kirsten Gardner, in "Controlling Cervical Cancer from Screening to Vaccinations: An American Perspective," and Mandy Hadenko, in "The Challenge of Developing and Publicizing Cervical Cancer Screening Programs: A Canadian Perspective," discuss the challenges of initiating and maintaining mass screening programs that are highly effective in terms of early diagnosis and treatment, yet are avoided by women fearful of a negative outcome. Both authors conclude that such mass initiatives require government funding, cooperation with health providers, and a focus on rural and ethnic communities. The flip side of the popular and commercial denial and sublimation of the female genitalia recounted by Vostral is the deadly consequences of venereal diseases and cervical and uterine cancers. This reluctance on the part of women to seek medical attention for "embarrassing" disorders relating to the breast, uterus, or cervix echoes ancient patriarchal notions of women as property to be passed along unblemished and unviolated. While the Pap smear is a "simple test" for a curable cancer, the procedure itself precludes widespread voluntary use. It entails a woman lying prone on an examining table, her genitals uncovered to strangers who will invade her most private parts with a swab, after which she must wait for other strangers to determine whether she has been sexually promiscuous or engaged in unsafe sexual practices and then whether she shall suffer the ultimate consequence for her transgressions—possible death by cancer. Given this scenario, it should have been evident to public health and government officials why pamphlets and newsletters would be insufficient to convince the great majority of women to undergo the procedure voluntarily. The new HPV vaccine, which at the time of writing is being brought into middle and high schools in some Canadian provinces and American states, has the advantage, as do all vaccines, of being an easy instrument of compulsion. Contemporary criticism of mass vaccination with HPV again provides the clash of competing discourses: the public health imperatives of the state versus control of the sexual expression of young women. However, it should be expected that—unless unforeseen, serious side effects become evident after mass vaccinations—the public health imperative will prevail.

II: Popular Representations of the Body in Sickness and Health

The chapters in section II discuss the body—both male and female—as contested space requiring regulation and differentiation in wide-ranging temporal contexts. In "Hideous Monsters before the Eye: Delirium Tremens and Manhood in Antebellum Philadelphia," Ric Caric interprets the accounts of delirium tremens in temperance and other writings in the antebellum period as reflections of male anxieties in a period of economic transformations. Those suffering from delirium tremens recounted similar experiences, such as loss of control, hallucinations of wild animals devouring the self, and generalized fears. The loss of control arising from alcoholism often was accompanied by loss of income and family. This sense of failure was seen as a feminization of the self in terms of a pre-industrial model of manhood. Caric argues that the reconfiguration of manhood, through evangelical techniques of self-degradation and rebirth, and exemplified in groups such as the Sons of Temperance, was a transition from traditional to modern conceptions of masculinity.

The feminist cultural theorist Judith Williamson noted that in contemporary popular culture, the female body is on display for the male gaze. This is evident in the chapters by Annette Burfoot, Jenny Ellison, and Christina Burr.[10] In "From La Bambola to a Toronto Striptease: Drawing out Public Consent to Gender Differentiation with Anatomical Material," Annette Burfoot investigates anatomical displays from the early modern European period to the present popular and controversial "Body Worlds" exhibition. She finds that these exposures of the body were and are gendered and racialized, and are represented as both sacred and profane, even though they were created as objectively scientific teaching aids. The extreme voyeurism of anatomical displays has become a staple of early twenty-first-century television, with the popularity of the CSI franchise and other programming where bodies are literally ripped apart to learn the "truths" about violent death.

In "Let Me Hear Your Body Talk: Aerobics for Fat Women Only, 1981–1985," Jenny Ellison examines the Large as Life fitness classes and support groups that originated in Vancouver, Canada. She argues against the presumption that popular culture automatically shapes women's subjective experiences in a negative fashion, taking issue with the view that aerobics—because of the emphasis upon skinny, ultra-fit women wearing revealing, tight clothing— is an exploitative example of female display rather than legitimate exercise. Rather, she finds that fitness classes run by and for fat women can be liberating and supportive experiences, and can provide evidence that wellness is not only a privilege for the thin. This adventure in "fat liberation" may well be an artifact of the 1980s, however. Present-day North American preoccupations with obesity are firmly ensconced in negativity, as reflected in television reality shows that use humiliation as a motivating force for weight loss and in public health pronouncements that marginalize the obese as unattractive health risks overloading health care systems. These scenarios provide no space for being fit and fat.

In counterpoint is Christina Burr's "'The Closest Thing to Perfect': Celebrity and the Body Politics of Jamie Lee Curtis," which investigates the film actress's public confrontations with her own body issues. Curtis, like virtually all female film stars, was a model for display. Her progression from icon of athletic perfection, as presented in the film *Perfect*, to her unretouched, middle-aged near-nude photograph in *More* magazine is considered within the context of feminine anxiety over the perfect body as perpetuated in the media. Both Ellison and Burr discuss events in the 1980s, setting the pursuit of the perfect female form within the framework of the Reagan era of personal acquisitiveness and individualism.

Also in the 1980s, the perception of the male body as contested space and as object of display was most apparent with respect to the first generation of AIDS victims in gay communities. In "Every Generation Has Its War: Representations of Gay Men with AIDS and Their Parents in the United States, 1983–1993," Heather Murray examines newspaper articles, autobiographies, and public health pamphlets to interpret how families confronted and dealt with their sons' illnesses and deaths in the early years of the AIDS epidemic. Much of this confrontation had to do with public recognition and/or acceptance of their sons' homosexuality. While many of the afflicted had left their family of origin, perhaps for years, because of the unacceptability of their gay lifestyle, they returned home to die. Their family members' poignant accounts, while sometimes self-serving, helped to lessen the demonization of the AIDS victim, with the reminders that a dying son is still a dying son. Murray demonstrates as well that the bodies of AIDS victims have failed to hide secret taboos and present challenges to traditional masculinity. The paradox of the early AIDS epidemic, as social hygiene reformers had discovered when confronting venereal diseases in the early twentieth century, was that the marginalization, or "othering," of the gay population put the larger society at risk. Only through broader acceptance and tolerance—which allowed gay couples to live openly in monogamous relationships, avoid drug use, and access regular health care—could the larger community embrace the marginalized within the public health network.

As the chapters by Ric Caric and Heather Murray demonstrate, the bodies of heterosexual and gay males were discursive objects relating to socio-economic transformations, disease and tabooed states, and even the fundamental nature of gender and sex differentiation. The men in both chapters suffer not only from the diseases of alcoholism and AIDS, respectively, but from lack of control over their bodies. How men experience health is an aspect of masculinity that transcends sexual preference. The acceptance of a lack of control over bodies is a signifier of femininity: the experiences of menstruation, childbirth, fertility, and menopause demonstrate to women, regularly during their adult lives, the reality of the unpredictable nature of the female body.

Whether taking a feminine or masculine perspective, agency is another issue to be considered when reading these chapters. The images, information, attitudes, and conclusions may be transmitted by the writer, vendor, or advertiser, yet the receiver has the choice, or agency, to accept or reject what is offered. Freedom of choice, however, may be within very circumscribed parameters. Here is a contemporary example. Many North American hospitals, as elsewhere, are experiencing outbreaks of infections resistant to antibiotics and leading to illness and deaths. These outbreaks are usually traced to inadequate hospital cleaning and careless hygiene practices of the medical staff. Public health authorities have advised patients to ask their physicians to wash their hands after entering the examination room. Consider the chain of events. As cost-cutting measures, hospitals have privatized cleaning services and awarded the contracts to suppliers who clean the hospitals at the lowest possible cost, which may encourage substandard practices. Busy doctors, nurses, and other hospital staff are careless in maintaining hygienic practices, which encourages the spread of infection. But the nervous and debilitated patient is to begin his or her precious short contact time with the physician, who hopefully has the power to cure, by ordering the physician to wash his or her hands, thereby impugning the doctor's hygienic practices. What is the likelihood that the average patient will do so? And if the patient does not, is he or she to blame for the spread of hospital infection?[11]

Such public health advisories, while seemingly more objective than messages communicated to sell commercial products, are also influenced by considerations of class, gender, ethnicity, and other social differentiations. It is important to note those considerations, particularly when certain groups are targeted—intentionally or not—in such cultural transmissions. The chapters in this collection tease out some of the underlying messages, presuppositions, and intents of a variety of cultural artifacts relating to gender and health, and readers are encouraged to consider all the layers of messages given and messages received.

Notes

1 Some of the books that analyze gender, health, and popular culture are the following: Janine Marchessault and Kim Sawchuk, eds., *Wild Science: Reading Feminism, Medicine, and the Media* (London: Routledge, 2000), which is informed by a history-of-science perspective; Virginia Berridge and Kelly Loughlin, eds., *Medicine, the Market and the Mass Media: Producing Health in the Twentieth Century* (London: Routledge, 2005), which is a British contribution. American scholars have been more active in the field. Important works include Nancy Tomes, *The Gospel of Germs: Men, Women, and the Microbe in American Life* (Cambridge: Harvard University Press, 1998); Leslie Reagan, Nancy Tomes, and Paula Treichler, eds., *Medicine's Moving Pictures: Medicine, Health, and Bodies in American Film and Television* (Rochester: University of Rochester Press, 2007); Naomi Rogers, *Dirt and Disease: Polio before FDR* (New Brunswick, NJ: Rutgers University Press, 1992); Thomas Robertson et al., *Televised Medicine Advertising and Children* (New York: Praeger, 1979); Joan Brumberg, *Fasting Girls: The History of Anorexia Nervosa* (New York: Vintage, 2000); Patricia Fallon and Melanie Katzman, *Feminist Perspectives on Eating Disorders* (New York: Guilford Press, 1994); Allan M. Brandt and Paul Rozin, *Morality and Health* (New York: Routledge, 1997); David Sloane and Beverlie Sloane, *Medicine Moves to the Mall* (Baltimore: Johns Hopkins University Press, 2003); Clive Seale, *Health and the Media* (Oxford: Blackwell, 2004); Vincent Vinikas, *Soft Soap, Hard Sell: American Hygiene in an Age of Advertisement* (Ames, IA: Iowa State University Press, 1992); Kathryn Grover, *Fitness in American Culture: Images of Health, Sport and the Body, 1830–1940* (Baltimore, MD: Johns Hopkins University Press, 1974); Daniel Hill, *Advertising to the American Woman, 1900–1999* (Columbus, OH: Ohio State University Press, 2002); Mary Jacobus and Evelyn Keller, *Body/Politics: Women and the Discourses of Science* (New York: Routledge, 1990); Judith Leavitt, *Typhoid Mary: Captive to the Public's Health* (Boston: Beacon Press, 1996); Julia Grant, *Raising Baby by the Book: The Education of American Mothers* (New Haven, CT: Yale University Press, 1998); and Rima Apple, *Vitamania: Vitamins in American Culture* (New Brunswick, NJ: Rutgers University Press, 1996).

There are few Canadian books relating to the history of health, gender, and popular culture, although the subject is approached in the following texts: Cheryl Krasnick Warsh and Veronica Strong-Boag, eds., *Children's Health Issues in Historical Perspective* (Waterloo, ON: Wilfrid Laurier University Press, 2005); Georgina Feldberg, Molly Ladd-Taylor, Alison Li, and Kathryn McPherson, eds., *Women, Health and Nation: Canada and the United States since 1945* (Montreal and Kingston: McGill-Queen's University Press, 2003); Wendy Mitchinson, *Giving Birth in Canada, 1900–1950* (Toronto: University of Toronto Press, 2002); Veronica Strong-Boag, *The New Day Recalled* (Toronto: Copp Clark Pitman, 1988); and Katherine Arnup, *Education for Motherhood* (Toronto: University of Toronto Press, 1994).

2   Stuart Hall, "The Rediscovery of Ideology: The Return of the Repressed in Media Studies," in John Storey, ed., *Cultural Theory and Popular Culture: An Introduction*, 4th ed. (London: Pearson Education, 2006).

3   Storey, "Introduction," *Cultural Theory*, p. 3.

4   Ernesto Laclau, "Discourse," in R.E. Goodin and P. Pettit, eds., *A Companion to Contemporary Political Philosophy* (London: Blackwell, 1993).

5   Storey, *Cultural Theory*, p. 100.

6   See, for instance, the following works by Michel Foucault: "The Confessions of the Flesh," in Colin Gordon, ed., *Power/Knowledge: Selected Interviews and Other Writings 1972–1977* (New York: Pantheon Books, 1972, 1980), pp. 194–228; "Truth and Power," in James D. Faubion, ed., *Michel Foucault Essential Works: Power* (Harmondsworth: Penguin, 2001); *The Archaeology of Knowledge* (London: Routledge, 1989); *Discipline and Punish: The Birth of the Prison*, trans. Alan Sheridan (New York: Vintage Books, 1977, 1995); and *The History of Sexuality*, vol. 1, *An Introduction* (New York: Vintage Books, 1990).

7   Sarah Stage, *Female Complaints: Lydia Pinkham and the Business of Women's Medicine* (New York: W.W. Norton, 1979).

8   I discuss Fletcher's Castoria in "Vim, Vigour and Vitality: Power Foods for Kids in Canadian Popular Magazines," in Marlene Epp, Franca Iacovetta, and Valerie Korinek, eds., *Edible Histories, Cultural Politics: Towards a Canadian Food History* (Toronto: University of Toronto Press, forthcoming).

9   For more on the body as a contested, or "carceral" space, see Foucault, "Confessions of the Flesh" and *History of Sexuality*.

10   Judith Williamson, *Decoding Advertisements* (London: Marion Boyars, 1978).

11   This is an example of Antonio Gramsci's notion of hegemony, whereby dominant groups seek to obtain the consent of subordinates through a process of "exchange and negotiation." See Storey, *Cultural Theory*, p. 8, for a brief summary.

I: The Transmission of Health Information

Confined: Constructions of Childbirth in Popular and Elite Medical Culture in Late-Nineteenth-Century Australia

Lisa Featherstone

In late-nineteenth-century Australia, a woman had numerous sources for information about pregnancy and childbirth, including her family, friends, and neighbours. Yet by this period, biomedicine and, in particular, gynecology and obstetrics had increasingly replaced women's traditional knowledge as the authority over the birthing process. The disciplines of obstetrics and gynecology functioned to define, order, and treat the reproducing body, and the strict regimen of the hospital informed even the home birth.

This chapter explores the multiple ways in which the medical disciplines attempted to discursively understand and describe childbirth in both elite and popular texts. As historians have suggested, pregnancy and childbirth were pathologized, turned into medical disorders that required the expert intervention of the doctor.[1] Yet this chapter suggests that medical advice differed substantially, depending on the perceived audience. Specifically, the concerns raised in popular self-help guides published by doctors were substantially different from the debates found in medical journals and professional texts; there are notable differences in the medical descriptions of the seemingly static act of birth. This chapter considers the similarities and differences in the constructions of pregnancy and childbirth in popular culture and elite medical discourse. Through this analysis, it suggests that there are multiple ways in which childbirth is socially, rather than biologically, constructed. This has important implications for studies of childbirth, both historically and in the contemporary world, where birth must be understood as culturally specific and as mediated and understood through the wider frameworks of society.

The chapter begins with a brief overview of both popular and elite medical sources, and then considers the general attitude of popular self-help texts toward pregnancy and labour via a consideration of the narrative dichotomies of "natural" and "unnatural." It examines the ways in which the medical profession discursively negotiated the realities of difficult or protracted labour, including the need for instruments or surgical intervention. Medical journals were concerned largely with the abnormal, the interesting, even the bizarre, with little room for consideration of the ordinary. In contrast, self-help guides were preoccupied with domestic preparations and considered only the mundane, offering little guidance if problems did occur. This chapter suggests that concepts of normality and pathology were constantly redefined. Medical discourse was constructed through the perceived reader, whether popular or professional, rather than around the physicalities of childbirth itself.

This is not necessarily unexpected. The literary theorist Mary Poovey has noted the extensive tensions and ambiguities within medical attitudes toward the female body. Medicine, alongside other dominant Victorian discourses, lacked the certainty that its scientific ideologies demanded.[2] This chapter teases out some of these inconsistencies in medicine through a consideration of narrative and audience in popular and elite medical writing.

Medical Narratives in Late-Nineteenth-Century Australia

The second half of the nineteenth century saw a proliferation of medical discourses surrounding pregnancy and childbirth, including the establishment and expansion of medical journals, the professional mouthpieces of doctors.[3] Such journals serve to indicate the public image desired and formed by the medical profession itself. Medical journals offer an unmediated view of how doctors wanted to be perceived. They also offer a view of what doctors were reading: the journals were not necessarily meant for mass consumption, since they were written and produced for their peers. Medical journals did not necessarily represent the views of all doctors—in fact, they were probably rather elitist, indicating a view of medicine that was formed by the doctors in the upper echelons of practice. Yet such records were concerned with building a body of gynecological and obstetric knowledge, educating doctors with the wider view of decreasing maternal mortality and ensuring the centrality of doctors to the process of childbirth.

There was also a wide variety of medical texts written for and consumed by the general public. The market for popular medical texts on domestic medicine expanded enormously in the Victorian era.[4] In Australia, such texts were particularly popular because the vast expanses outside the urban areas meant that pregnant and birthing women did not always access medical care. In a country where only one third of the population lived in cities, women needed to be able to perform basic first aid, as well as deal with more complicated problems if they arose.[5] Even within the cities and towns, domestic texts were popular because of the high cost of medical care. Popular texts then aimed to fill a void. Many were inexpensive, aimed specifically at the working classes.[6] Some of these self-help texts were enormously popular: George Fullerton's domestic guide, for example, ran to eight editions, with the first edition selling five thousand copies alone.[7] This chapter draws extensively on these popular self-help texts, as well as on elite medical journals for comparative purposes.[8]

There are, however, certainly problems with the use of medical texts (whether popular or elite) as evidence. These texts were focused almost solely on white women, as I have argued elsewhere.[9] The experience of indigenous women is lost in these sources, for in this period Aboriginal women were marginalized from medical discourse. In part, this was because Australian doctors only rarely treated Aboriginal women, who were excluded from many hospitals and could not afford private treatment. But there was also a broader conceptual issue. Late-nineteenth-century medicine focused on women's bodies largely in terms of obstetrics and the saving of maternal and infant lives. The generic maternal body was understood in this period as a white body. The Black woman's body or the Black mother's body was therefore rendered both peripheral and invisible in medical texts.

There are other problems, too. Most obviously, medical journals appear to slant case studies toward the positive, reporting the best-case scenarios and the "heroic" breakthroughs rather than the ordinary and the mundane. Medical self-help texts, in contrast, focus on the domestic case and include little advice regarding medical complications. Differences between practice and theory may also have existed—there is nothing to say that local doctors followed the practice of specialists, for example, or that case studies in journals replicated common problems in the home or hospital. Further, doctors who chose to write self-help texts may have stood on the margins of legitimate medicine and may have held opinions considerably different from the medical norm. This is certainly so in the case of the infamous Australian doctor James George Beaney, whose self-help tracts on sex were both popular and controversial. Beaney, the senior surgeon and administrator of operative surgery at the Melbourne Hospital, was widely condemned by the antipodean medical profession. This was partly because of his association with abortions in the 1860s but also because his popular writings on sexology were deemed to belong more in the realm of quackery than of real medicine.[10] Beaney was operating from outside the strictures of the wider profession, and his opinions may therefore have been different from those of his less adventurous colleagues.

There is also the issue of audience. Medical texts, like all texts, were written *to* an audience, yet they were also shaped *by* this audience. Texts written by doctors for doctors reflect their mutual scientific frameworks; together, both author and audience spoke and understood a language of medicine. Popular texts written by doctors but aimed at women still reflected scientific frameworks, including, at a very fundamental level, medical beliefs about women's bodies and pregnancy and childbirth. But an awareness of what readers wanted and/or needed to hear did shape the writing of these popular texts.[11] Further, there is no certainty that a text will be read as the writer intended or that it will be passively received and understood.[12] Women reading self-help texts might have done so in quite a sophisticated, active fashion, translating and creating the text through their own knowledge and experience. As Regina Morantz-Sanchez has shown in her histories of British and American gynecology, inter-relationships between the patient (in this case, the reader) and the practitioner are complex.[13] Patients did have some autonomy in the decision-making process and, on an individual level, were not entirely controlled by the regimes of medicine.

In this chapter, medicine is presented as a discourse of power and authority, but also as a discourse with internal flaws, inconsistencies, and tensions, and subject to negotiation between audience and practitioner. With this in mind, the analysis is largely textual, and popular culture will be narrowly considered through readily available self-help books written by doctors for women's consumption in their own homes. The examination retains its focus on medical texts rather than women's narratives. I am not attempting to examine the ways women constructed or experienced childbirth, and in some ways the women themselves remain rather shadowy within this analysis. Women do, of course, have some agency here. As consumers of popular culture texts, they drove the production and consumption of these books and their numerous republications. Yet women remain largely inarticulate in medical narratives, and I have not sought out their voices in diaries or letters. Instead, the aim is to explore the ways in which medicine constructed childbirth, dependent on the perceived reading audience; the ways in which confinement was created and produced in popular and elite forms of scientific narrative.

Nature and Pathology

One of the clearest markers of difference between self-help texts and elite medical journals was in attitudes toward childbirth as pathology. As Moscucci has noted, doctors, as the dominant commentators on the body, defined womanhood in terms of pathology: within medicine, "woman was, by definition, disease or disorder, a deviation from the standard of health represented by the male."[14] The body of the woman was not only irregular but also pathological.[15] By the late nineteenth century, the impact on childbirth is clear: within medical narratives, confinement was seen as a crisis urgently requiring the expert intervention of a doctor. Most doctors believed that medical management over childbirth was not only preferable but essential. As Sir James Graham, surgeon at the Women's Hospital in Sydney, suggested, "the pregnant woman, from the professional point of view, during her terms of pregnancy, is practically on the sick list ... the border line between the normal and the pathological is very narrow, indeed."[16] All pregnancy and childbirth, whether complicated or not, were linked with sickness and ill health; death in childbed was reflected back on the whole.

Thus, in the elite medical journals, there was a strong and almost unmediated focus on pathology and illness. During the second half of the nineteenth century, the medical management of women's bodies changed significantly. The latter decades saw a proliferation of a range of new, advanced operations, including abdominal surgery. Surgeries for gynecological problems included ovariotomy (the removal of the ovaries) and hysterectomy, vesico-vaginal fistula, and vaginal and uterine prolapse.[17] Other diseases and problems treated surgically included malformations of the ovaries and tubes, particularly ovarian cysts; vesico-vaginal fistula; perineal tears; uterine tumours; fibroids; polyps; and prolapse of the uterus or vagina.[18] In obstetrics, women became subject to all manner of interventions, including forceps and, most dramatically, caesarean section.[19] Surgery became a crucial part of the treatment of childbirth and the broader diseases of women. These surgeries were lovingly detailed in medical journals as examples of medical advancement and ideal medical practice. It was this aspect of childbirth, the extreme and the pathological, that was the focus of elite medical journals.

In contrast to the dominant scientific views, popular self-help texts, even those written by doctors, tended to focus on the naturalness of childbirth. For these doctors, labour was a "natural" function that required little interference. As Arthur Albutt suggested, "A well-formed healthy woman has rarely anything to fear. If the time of pregnancy had been well spent in taking care of the health, labour will present little difficulty."[20] Similarly, Benjamin Fawcett, the author of *Childbirth without Danger and Nearly Painless*, claimed that childbirth was as natural for a woman as it was for a "tree to produce flowers and fruit," for her organs were specifically modified for the reproductive process. He believed that childbirth should not be painful in a healthy system, only in a diseased nervous system.[21] Others noted that labour was not a disease but a natural process.[22]

Doctors who wrote self-help texts appear far less interventionist than doctors writing in elite medical journals. For example, in a letter to the editor of the *Australasian Medical Gazette (AMG)* in 1883, George Read claimed, not disapprovingly, that "the vagina is now made a kind of toy-shop for all kinds of extraordinary instruments."[23] By the 1890s, journals recorded a strong increase in the use of forceps, not only for mothers whose lives were in danger, but for any woman who may face protracted labour.[24] Certainly, many prominent Australian doctors promoted the regular use of forceps. T.W. Corbin of Adelaide used forceps in one in every 3.8 cases, claiming they were a "humane proceeding of modern midwifery."[25] Joseph Beeston, a Newcastle doctor, used forceps once in every three births. Beeston claimed the forceps were useful in a large number of cases, for they lessened both maternal and infant mortality. He felt that forceps decreased the recovery time, as labour was shorter, and therefore they also decreased the incidence of postpartum hemorrage and uterine disease.[26] Certainly some women required intervention in childbirth. Yet forceps were also used and promoted for the convenience of the practitioner: hastening a protracted labour, for example, so the doctor could leave sooner.[27]

If by the 1890s the use of forceps was a common part of obstetric practice, routinely praised in medical journals for both efficacy and convenience, doctors writing popular self-help texts were less enthusiastic. This was based on their belief in labour as a natural process. Doctors writing self-help texts regularly insisted that "meddlesome midwifery" (interfering with the "natural" process) was unnecessary and even harmful. Chavasse suggested, for example, that the doctor was needed only at certain points of the labour, to ensure that the confinement was progressing smoothly. Nature, which was sometimes personified, was to be left alone to manage the process.[28] Authors of self-help texts were sometimes surprisingly detailed in their condemnation of their fellow doctors' interventions in labour. One doctor noted that supporting the perineum was not only useless but harmful: "the natural labour needs no manual local interference."[29] Numerous popularist doctors suggested that instruments were used far more frequently than needed.[30] Others blamed drugs and "instruments of torture" for high death rates of women in confinement.[31]

Doctors who authored self-help texts tended to advise intervention only when absolutely necessary rather than as a routine measure. Yet when forceps or other interventions were needed, the mother was advised to place herself entirely in the professional hands of the doctor: he must "act as he thinks best."[32] Thus, the woman was neither to demand the use of forceps (to hasten labour) or to refuse them; all agency lay with the doctor himself.

This suggests that, despite the strong emphasis on the "naturalness" of childbirth for women, confinement was still constructed as an immediate danger. Even in popular texts, women were always teetering on the edge of pathology. To prevent the plummet into disease and death, childbirth had to be controlled and monitored by the medical professional. There is a fundamental paradox in the ways in which popular medical texts sought to explain pregnancy, childbirth, and maternity. While they were sold quite explicitly to poor women, almost as a substitute for direct medical care, they constructed themselves as merely a supplement. In all difficult cases, the woman reader was advised to consult her doctor. In Albutt's *The Wife's Handbook: How a Woman Should Order Herself during Pregnancy, in the Lying-in Room, and after Delivery*, the very title is suggestive of a definitive guide. Yet this popular text suggested that a doctor should be consulted if there was a problem with diagnosis of pregnancy; if a previous pregnancy had ended in miscarriage; during early pregnancy; and, more generally, during later pregnancy.[33] Certainly the confinement itself was to be a medicalized event. Albutt even claimed that after the labour pains began, the mother should "do nothing" and wait for the arrival of the doctor before commencing labour.[34] The need for medical attention was therefore universalized even within texts sold as self-help tracts. A few home remedies might be given, such as a cocaine solution for toothache and lead lotion for vaginal itching, but for anything more serious, the doctor was to be called.[35]

So even in popular texts, despite their overarching emphasis on the "naturalness" of childbirth, it was but a short step to danger and pathology. Albutt, for example, claimed that the lying-in room could readily become a "chamber of suffering ... painful, lengthy and highly dangerous."[36] Yet if medical advice was followed, this spectre of suffering and death could be readily subverted and childbirth could become "easy, and in most cases entirely free from danger."[37]

Maintaining Medical Control in Popular Culture

To prevent this slippage into pain and suffering, the mother must hand herself over to a strict medical regime. Popular self-help texts maintained medical control through this regime. The woman must "order herself," take care of herself, avoid disease, follow a strict pregnancy diet, and so forth, in order to have a healthy and successful pregnancy and confinement. All of the self-help medical guides of the period had comprehensive lists of problems associated with pregnancy. *Healthy Mothers and Sturdy Children*, for example, listed six pages of problems associated with pregnancy, from morning sickness to excessive salivation and toothache. It also emphasized the psychological impacts of pregnancy, including the possibility of mania, which was seen as a common "side effect."[38] Such problems, it was suggested, could be treated through adherence to the medical model. The list of curtailments was long: pregnant women should avoid "violent exertion," fatigue of any kind, balls and parties, the riding of bicycles, sea-bathing, showers, crowded drawing-rooms, dancing, and all other "feverish pleasures." While not to be regarded as an invalid, she must severely curtail her activities; in the later months, home was seen as the best place for the pregnant woman.[39] In the most radical of these texts, even pain during labour was seen to stem from an unwillingness to follow "rational" medical advice. Pain, therefore, was the fault of the mother herself.[40] Perhaps not surprisingly, then, even in books designed for home care, the subtext prioritized medical influence and management. Above all, women were told to "trust in her doctor, and all will be well."[41]

These medical orders were in general carefully and intensely detailed. Self-help texts placed a particular emphasis on controlling the diet of the mother. As Lisa Forman Cody's chapter (in this volume) shows, medical advice on diet suggested that "the smallest misstep could endanger a future baby's welfare."[42] Although doctors in the United States tended to avoid giving nutritional advice (the kitchen was the place of women, not professional medics),[43] in Australia, doctors were quite prescriptive. With their professional status more clearly defined, Australian doctors were more concerned to subjugate all aspects of pregnancy to medical control.[44] Popular texts suggested that an improper diet would rapidly lead to pathology.[45] The diet during pregnancy was to be plain but nourishing. Most doctors recommended that no alcohol be taken,[46] though some doctors allowed the judicious use of "medicinal" beverages.[47] Water should be filtered, which seems unlikely given the working-class audience of such texts, but no less likely than the diet itself. This was to consist of plentiful vegetables, roasted meat, fish, egg and bacon for breakfast, milk, and ripe fruit (including exotics such as grapes, raspberries, oranges, figs, and raisins).[48] Such a diet must have been a dream for the many poor women subsisting largely on bread and tea. And women who studiously followed the dietary regimes may have been sorely disappointed to find that they did not have a "pain-free birth," as some texts suggested was possible.[49]

Clothing too was to be strictly monitored. Underclothes were to be made of wool to guard against sudden changes in temperature.[50] Stays were to be abandoned, but from five months, an abdominal bandage should be used to "give support to the body, and to prevent the womb from falling too far forward."[51] The regimen for the healthy, natural pregnancy was also to include some exercise. There was no need to neglect general household duties, though heavy lifting should be avoided.[52] Even in a text aimed at the working classes, a daily walk of about an hour was seen as ideal, and pregnant women were advised to take an afternoon rest.[53] Again, the social and economic impossibility of such rest and recreation for the working classes indicates a wide chasm between the women and the medical practitioners, even within popular self-help texts.

Older folkloric advice was more likely to reappear in popular medical texts than in the more scientific elite journals and papers. For example, drawing on age-old ideas of maternal impression, Albutt recommended that the pregnant woman avoid everything of a "disagreeable" nature, every care and worry, in order to have a healthy child.[54] Similarly, the anonymous author of the Melbourne-published text *Healthy Mothers and Sturdy Children* noted that the mother should enjoy "pleasant pictures and books" to "improve herself and her child," while she should avoid "violent exertion, fatigue of any kind, exciting plays, sensational novels, ball and parties."[55] In these popular texts, it was purported that the imagination of the mother-to-be could be easily overexcited (by attending a tragic play, by seeing a "cripple" in the street) and that this could directly impact on the formation of the fetus and later child.[56] This is a notable contrast to medical journals, which were, by the late nineteenth century, attempting to consolidate themselves as vehicles of scientific knowledge and authority.

The Birth in Popular Medical Texts

In both elite medical journals and popular medical texts, instructions for birth generally indicated that a doctor would be present. It is clear, however, that in Australia this was not always the case. Midwives were a practical necessity and not every woman had a doctor present for her confinement. It is impossible to estimate the precise number of Australian women who were confined by midwives, though local history suggests that it was substantial. In Ballarat, over 50 per cent of women were attended by a midwife, while in Townsville in 1890, 73 per cent of children were delivered by a midwife.[57] Women in rural areas generally engaged a midwife as routine and contacted a doctor only if there were complications.[58] In rural Queensland, in particular, there were not enough doctors to cover all confinements.[59] Other women chose not to have a doctor in attendance, for some women did not like the idea of a man examining them.[60] If distance and modesty were of no concern, finances was probably the chief reason that women used a midwife. In 1877 the doctor's fee for a confinement was recommended by the *Australian Medical Journal (AMJ)* at a minimum of three guineas when the wage of a labourer was six or seven shillings per day.[61]

If it is difficult to establish just how many women were confined by a midwife, there are no records of the numbers of women who underwent labour with no professional assistance. Outside the urban centres, conditions were particularly harsh; at times, distances prevented rural women from having the aid of either a doctor or midwife.[62] There is also evidence to suggest that, in Sydney at least, the poorest of urban women sometimes had no assistance at all.[63] Yet self-help texts, while offering themselves as guidebooks for pregnancy and childbirth, offered little in the way of assistance to women enduring a difficult or complicated labour.

Instead, the emphasis in self-help books was on the ordering and preparation of the birthing room. The medical profession developed its own rituals surrounding confinement, many related to the purchase of "necessary" items. Most self-help texts included exhaustive lists of purchases necessary to confinement and the lying-in. Many of these items would have been beyond the reach of a large proportion of women.[64] For example, at a time when most women used and reused homemade towelling for menstrual bleeding, doctors recommended the use of disposable towels. As Vostral suggests, the purchase of commercial products for menstrual (and in this case postpartum) bleeding was constructed as part of what it meant to be a good, clean, "modern" woman.[65] In addition, the doctor required sheeting, towels, binders, oilcloth, and a variety of vessels, including a bedpan, a container for the placenta, washbasins, and a pail. The doctor also required a douche, boiled water, Lysol, and items for the baby.[66] It was also desirable to have a spare rubber sheet, hot water bottles, a sitz bath, a brush, and washcloths.[67] Fullerton specified a "hair mattress" rather than one made of feather and gave a detailed paragraph on the preparation of the bed.[68] Despite his audience of working-class women, Albutt was particularly demanding, including the call for "<u>new</u>" waterproof sheeting.[69] He claimed that it was a "dirty" habit to be confined in ordinary day clothes (suggesting it was probably common), and instead he requested a nightgown and a flannel petticoat.[70] Others described the dress for labour in much detail: A clean nightgown was to be rolled up around the waist. On top of this was to be a short bed-gown, reaching the hips, a flannel petticoat to meet the bed-gown, and a dressing gown on top.[71]

This rigorous sense of order and discipline in popular medical tracts indicates that the medicalization of childbirth was strong even outside the hospital, the traditional site for the medically controlled, regulated birth. Increasingly, the spectacle of the hospital came to influence the home birth, which became increasingly sanitized. In contrast to the earlier birthing scene, when family and neighbours participated, often in a rowdy throng, by the 1890s doctors were recommending a more austere setting. Doctors criticized the noise and cost of the neighbourhood party and called for only the doctor and a nurse to be present.[72] Thus, even before the hospital became the site for general childbirth, confinement was increasingly subject to the strictures of medical authority and hegemony, even within popular advice texts. While medical journals do not offer these detailed and elaborate descriptions of childbirth rituals, the dominant idea of birth remained the same: it was to be legitimated through medical control and monitored through the strictures of medical advice and authority.

Yet a key difference in the approach of elite medical journals and popular texts is found within attitudes toward the complicated or problematic labour. That doctors did not discuss with any specificity the most complicated scenarios in popular medical guides is not surprising. The problematic case was not perceived to be the concern of "unskilled" women (midwife, neighbour, or the mother herself) but the realm of the medical professional. Self-help texts were written as reassuring narratives, determined not to alarm the mother-to-be or harm her unborn child. Just as importantly, the readers themselves may have driven this paternalism. While doctors may have enjoyed (personally or professionally) reading about the thrills of a complicated case and the scientific mastery over the body, women may have sought comfort from the narrative of the normal birth. The frequency and consistency of the constructions of childbirth as "natural" in self-help texts suggests that it must have been gently reassuring to the reader. Thus, the audience may have helped shape and produce these medical texts in crucial, formative ways.

Albutt was rare in discussing the problematic birth in a popular text. Even here, however, the text described birth as a medical event rather than acting as a guide for an inexperienced woman to help herself or another during birth. The forceps, for example, were described as "artificial hands" to guide and assist the child through, shortening a "long, tedious and painful labour."[73] While this advice may have been a comfort during pregnancy, it is unclear how useful it would have been during a difficult labour. Such descriptions, however, inculcated in the mother-to-be notions of docility and obedience. Here, as elsewhere, the mother was instructed to be passive and "do as she is told," with the doctor and his instruments doing the hard "labour" of delivery.[74]

At times, some complications were gently mentioned. Fullerton, for example, recommended that the birthing assistant carefully support the perineum to prevent "the melancholy accident" of a fistula.[75] Yet in self-help texts, it was extremely rare for doctors to even mention the worst-case scenario, the caesarean section. In medical journals in the 1880s and 1890s, the use of caesarean section was under rigorous debate and clinical trial, with the majority of doctors approving of the search for new surgical means of assisting the protracted or undeliverable labour. In the journals, there was a general sense that the operation itself (classic caesarean section or its cousin, Porro's operation, where the uterus was removed along with the baby) was not yet perfected but that further surgical advancement would rapidly render it useful. In practice, of course, death rates from caesarean sections were extremely high in this period, far exceeding maternal mortality for other radical surgeries such as craniotomy.[76]

Of those surveyed, only one popular text mentioned the caesarean section as an option. George Fullerton, in his *Family Medical Guide* (1884) offered a fairly realistic view, far more so than the journals, which tended to stress the positives of scientific advancement and heroism. In contrast, Fullerton wrote that the caesarean section was a perilous operation. He suggested that, because of its clinical difficulties and high death rates, doctors were often unwilling to perform the surgery; he noted also that patients and their families were often afraid to permit it. Fullerton suggested that the operation was so unrefined that as many mothers spontaneously recovered as survived the hazards of the caesarean.[77] No other self-help guide recommended caesarean section for the difficult birth. If the focus was on the natural and normal birth, the potential horrors of the caesarean were to be avoided, in practice and in narrative.

The Case of Puerperal Fever

Puerperal fever was another problem of childbirth that was considered very differently in elite medical culture and popular texts aimed at women. Puerperal fever was a serious condition, much debated in the medical journals of this period. A postpartum (or post-abortive) illness, puerperal fever was caused either by an external infection or by sepsis resulting from putrid matter in the mother's own body. In the nineteenth century, it was most commonly caused by the transmission of bacteria to the mother. This occurred during delivery, obstetric examinations, or surgery; fever passed most readily into a wound caused by the use of instruments. It could also be spread without medical intervention, through contaminated linen or sanitary towels, or even on the clothes or in the nasal passages of the attendant. The infection could then spread from the uterus out through the pelvis and the peritoneal cavity. It was highly contagious: a doctor who treated one patient with the disease was likely to spread it to other women during confinement, as did doctors involved in autopsies.

Death from puerperal fever was both swift and excruciatingly painful, and puerperal fever was a very common cause of mortality: it likely accounted for at least half of all maternal deaths.[78] The only treatment was prevention, and mirroring debates over the illness itself, there was intense debate over the forms that this prevention should take.

Like their European counterparts, Australian doctors were slow to develop vital antisepsis policies. Medical journals of the 1880s and 1890s show no definite consensus on the worth of such precautions.[79] Some doctors realized the importance of rigorous cleanliness, but the adoption of Listerian practice was by no means universal.[80] Further, resistance to antisepsis was fundamental to self-conceptualization of the medical profession itself. Doctors did not like to view themselves as either contaminated or contaminators. Such an idea would cut across the notions of class, gender, and science that the profession had so carefully established. But not all doctors looked outside the profession for the cause of puerperal fever. The eminent Australian gynecologist James Jamieson admitted as early as 1879 that medical men, himself included, were capable of spreading the illness from a septic patient to women in confinement.[81] Yet for the most part, doctors tried to displace fears of fevers onto women, either the patients themselves or the midwives who cared for them.[82]

Debates over puerperal fever (its etiology, prevalence, and prevention) were omnipresent in medical journals during this period. But the complex debates that so absorbed the premier obstetricians in this period were not replicated in self-help tracts. If mentioned at all, puerperal fever was simplified and rendered uncomplicated and manageable. Some practical tips for the avoidance of fever were often given in popular texts. Albutt, for example, recommended that the afterbirth be quickly removed from the birthing room, as it would rapidly become offensive.[83] No context was given, however, to suggest the very real dangers of puerperal fever. The anonymous author of *Healthy Mothers and Sturdy Children* noted that childbed fever was prevalent, and, probably quite legitimately, he believed that most of the cases were preventable. His understanding of puerperal fever was a mix of the medical and the pseudo-scientific. He believed it was caused by inflammation of the system (caused by diet), the use of drugs during and after delivery, and the contusions and bruises from instruments. In the last instance, he was certainly correct, though it is difficult to agree with his statement that "it is within the power of every woman" to avoid puerperal fever.[84]

Of all the self-help texts considered here, only one had a substantial, useful consideration of puerperal fever. Rezin Thompson's *The Medical Adviser: Full and Plain Treatise on the Theory and Practice of Medicine Especially Adapted to Family Use* (1884) was a general guide to family medicine rather than a text aimed specifically at pregnant women, yet it contained a long discussion of common obstetric problems, including miscarriage. Thompson did consider puerperal fever in depth, but this discussion was not found in the midwifery section; rather, it was hidden within the section on fevers. Nor was it indexed, making it less than obvious to the parturient woman or her helpers. Nevertheless, Thompson gave a strong and accurate description of puerperal fever, allowing for good amateur diagnosis.[85] He was, as were many doctors in this period, less confident of the cause. Covering all options (and suggesting a familiarity with contemporary scientific debates), Thompson suggested that puerperal fever could be brought on by inflammation of the uterus or its surrounds, from violence done to the uterus, or from a contagion or epidemic.[86]

Thompson suggested that puerperal fever, like all peritonitis, must be treated aggressively and with skill, lest the "patient be lost." He outlined a rigorous program of care for those who could not seek medical advice. This was quite specific, including precise measurements for pharmaceuticals: "two grains of opium or one of morphine, and then give Dover's powder in doses of two or three grains every hour."[87] The use of opium could be generous to keep the patient "easy."[88] In addition, poultices were to be applied to control the inflammation of the uterus.[89] Thus, despite the fact that puerperal fever was one of the chief dangers of childbed in this period, Thompson was unusual in his detailed examination and explanation of its diagnosis and treatment. Most doctors in self-help texts downplayed its significance and passed treatment back to the consulting physician.

Conclusion

Childbirth was clearly constructed differently in elite medical texts and in popular culture medical guides. All doctors' writing suggests that pregnancy and childbirth were a "normal" part of womanhood, with maternity viewed as women's social and biological destiny.[90] Yet the extent and functioning of this "normality" was constantly under negotiation, shifting and destabilizing all too readily into pathology in various forms. In elite medical journals, the emphasis was on the pregnant and labouring body as constantly under threat. Paradoxically, if it were "normal" to reproduce, it was nevertheless problematic: it was only a short step into pathology, illness, and even death. This meant the labouring woman was always treated clinically as if she was morbid and described narratively as a body in ever-present danger.

Self-help texts conceptualized and negotiated the pregnant and labouring body differently from texts written for doctors. Aimed at a female readership, they conveyed the sense that nature would prevail and that a healthy mother could and would produce a healthy baby through a natural labour. Yet defining "natural" was nonetheless complicated; even in self-help volumes, childbirth was to be a labour monitored and controlled by the doctor. Despite the emphasis on the mother, self-help texts offered little agency to women. The doctor was still the preferred authority on pregnancy and childbirth. Thus, the writers of self-help texts constructed the female body as capable, but capable only with medical assistance. The birthing mother was not fully pathologized, yet the threat of danger was again fundamental.

This chapter has suggested that in late-nineteenth-century Australia, the matters of pregnancy and childbirth were continually under negotiation within medicine. Science was not a coherent discipline. The doctors who chose to publish chapters in major and elite medical journals constructed childbirth and the female body differently from those doctors who chose to write self-help texts for Australian women. Childbirth was thus narrated and packaged differently by various medical men. Birth is clearly a cultural event, not merely biological. Doctors negotiated and wrote about the meanings and practices of birth differently, depending on the perceived audience: for women themselves or for medical peers. The constructions of childbirth itself, therefore, were destabilized and dependent on the audience, either popular or elite.

Notes

1 The literature here is vast. See Carroll Smith-Rosenberg and Charles Rosenberg, "The Female Animal: Medical and Biological Views of Woman and Her Role in Nineteenth-Century America," *Journal of American History* 60 (1973–74): 332–56; Jo Murphy-Lawless, *Reading Birth and Death: A History of Obstetric Thinking* (Cork, Ireland: Cork University Press, 1998); Paula A. Treichler, "Feminism, Medicine, and the Meaning of Childbirth," in Mary Jacobus, Evelyn Fox Keller, and Sally Shuttleworth, eds., *Body/Politics: Women and the Discourses of Science* (New York: Routledge, 1990), pp. 113–38; Barbara Ehrenreich and Deirdre English, *For Her Own Good: 150 Years of the Experts' Advice to Women* (London: Pluto Press, 1979).

2 Mary Poovey, *Uneven Developments: The Ideological Work of Gender in Mid-Victorian England* (Chicago: University of Chicago Press, 1995), p. 12.

3 The most prominent among these were the *Australian Medical Journal (AMJ)* (1856–95 and 1910–14), the *Australasian Medical Gazette (AMG)* (1881–1914), and later, the *Medical Journal of Australia (MJA)* (1914–present).

4 Christopher Gardner-Thorpe, "The Land They Left Behind," in John Pearne, ed., *Pioneer Medicine in Australia* (Brisbane: Amphion Press, 1988), p. 8.

5 See Graeme Davison, "The Exodists: Miles Franklin, Jill Roe and the 'Drift to the Metropolis,'" *History Australia* 2.2 (June 2005): 35–42.

6 H. Arthur Albutt, *The Wife's Handbook: How a Woman Should Order Herself during Pregnancy, in the Lying-in Room, and after Delivery* (Sydney: Modern Medical Publishing Co., 1890s), p. 3; Rezin Thompson, *The Medical Adviser: Full and Plain Treatise on the Theory and Practice of Medicine Especially Adapted to Family Use* (Melbourne: Standard Publishing Co., 1884), p. 526.

7 Edward Ford, *Bibliography of Australian Medicine, 1790–1900* (Sydney: Sydney University Press, 1976), p. 88.

8 To provide an Australian history, the focus has been on Australian medical journals and self-help texts. I have also included overseas authors whose work was published in Australia. The rationale for this was simple: texts published locally were presumably read locally, thus framing and influencing local opinions. Their accessibility is the crucial issue here.

9 Lisa Featherstone, "Imagining the Black Body: Race, Gender and Gynaecology in Late Colonial Australia," *Lilith* 15 (2006): 86–96.

10 C. Craig, "The Egregious Dr. Beaney of the Beaney Scholarships," *MJA* 1 (1950): 593–8; Bryan Gandevia, "Some Aspects of the Life and Work of James George Beaney," *MJA* 1 (1953): 614–9; Bryan Gandevia, "Beaney, James George," *Australian Dictionary of Biography, 1851–1890* (Melbourne: Melbourne University Press, 1966), pp. 124–6.

11 See Robert Crosman, "Do Readers Make Meaning?" in Susan R. Suleiman and Inge Crosman, eds., *The Reader in the Text: Essays on Audience and Interpretation* (Princeton, NJ: Princeton University Press, 1980), pp. 149–64. See also Sharra Vostral's chapter in this volume, "Advice to Adolescents: Menstrual Health and Menstrual Education Films, 1946–1982."

12 For ideas on the reception of popular culture, see Lawrence W. Levine, *The Unpredictable Past: Explorations in American Cultural History* (New York: Oxford University Press, 1993), pp. 304–8.

13 Regina Morantz, "The Lady and Her Physician," in Mary S. Hartman and Lois Banner, eds., *Clio's Consciousness Raised: New Perspectives on the History of Women* (New York: Harper Torchbooks, 1974), pp. 38–53; Regina Morantz-Sanchez, *Sympathy and Science: Women Physicians in American Medicine* (New York: Oxford University Press, 1985);

Regina Morantz-Sanchez, *Conduct Unbecoming a Woman: Medicine on Trial in Turn-of-the-Century Brooklyn* (New York: Oxford University Press, 1999). See also David Armstrong, "The Doctor–Patient Relationship: 1930–80," in Peter Wright and Andrew Treacher, eds., *The Problem of Medical Knowledge: Examining the Social Construction of Medicine* (Edinburgh: Edinburgh University Press, 1982), pp. 109–22.

14 Ornella Moscucci, *The Science of Woman: Gynaecology and Gender in England, 1800–1929* (Cambridge: Cambridge University Press, 1990), p. 102.

15 Moscucci, *Science of Woman*, p. 102.

16 Sir James Graham, "Obstetric Nursing with Special Reference to Savage Races," *Australasian Nurses Journal* 2 (1904): 54.

17 Moscucci, *Science of Woman*, 108. See also Janet McCalman, *Sex and Suffering. Women's Health and a Woman's Hospital: The Royal Women's Hospital, Melbourne 1856–1996* (Melbourne: Melbourne University Press, 1998), pp. 43–7, 117–20, 138–42.

18 Moscucci, *Science of Woman*, p. 131.

19 See Lisa Featherstone, "The Kindest Cut? The Origins of the Caesarean Section in Australia," in Marie Porter, Patricia Short, and Andrea O'Reilly, eds., *Mother Power? Contemporary Feminist Voices* (Toronto: Women's Press, 2005), pp. 25–40.

20 Albutt, *Wife's Handbook*, 15. See also P.H. Chavasse, *Man's Strength and Woman's Beauty: A Treatise on the Physical Life of Both Sexes* (Melbourne: Standard Publishing Co., 1879), pp. 255–9, and Anonymous, *Healthy Mothers and Sturdy Children: A Book for Every Family, Giving the Best Methods of Maintaining Health and Curing Disease, as Taught by Eminent Physicians* (Melbourne: Pater & Knapton, 1893), p. 33.

21 B. Fawcett, *Childbirth without Danger and Nearly Painless* (Sydney: F. Cunningham and Co. Printers, 1882), p. 7. Fawcett himself was a homeopath who practised extensively in western rural New South Wales. He was not medically trained, but his text has been included here as it was very much part of the popular culture of medicine in this period. See Ford, *Bibliography*, p. 83.

22 Chavasse, *Man's Strength*, 281; George Fullerton, *The Family Medical Guide* (Sydney: William Maddock, 1884), p. 5.

23 George Read, "Letter to the Editor," *AMG* (November 1883): 51.

24 David Hardie, "The Forceps in Labour, with Special Reference to a Resistant Cervix," *AMG* (June 1893): 182–3; T.W. Corbin, "Midwifery Experiences," *AMG* (May 1892): 222–4.

25 Corbin, "Midwifery Experiences," pp. 222–4.

26 Joseph L. Beeston, "Obstetrical Statistics—A Record of 800 Cases of Midwifery with Analysis and Observations," *AMG* (September 1891): 355–6.

27 Dr. Little, speaker at the sixteenth General Meeting of the Medical Society of Queensland, *AMG* (May 1893): 148; J.A.G. Hamilton, "Midwifery Experiences," *AMG* (April 1892): 183.

28 Chavasse, *Man's Strength*, pp. 255–7.

29 Anonymous, *Healthy Mothers*, p. 35.

30 Anonymous, *Healthy Mothers*, p. 39; Chavasse, *Man's Strength*, pp. 95, 256.

31 Fawcett, *Childbirth without Danger*, p. 3.

32 Chavasse, *Man's Strength*, p. 259.

33 Albutt, *Wife's Handbook*, pp. 7, 14.

34 Albutt, *Wife's Handbook*, p. 17.

35 Albutt, *Wife's Handbook*, pp. 11–13.

36 Albutt, *Wife's Handbook*, p. 2.

37 Albutt, *Wife's Handbook*, p. 2.

38 Anonymous, *Healthy Mothers*, pp. 10–16.

39 Chavasse, *Man's Strength*, p. 207; George Black, *Everybody's Medical Adviser and Consulting Family Physician* (Sydney: William Dobell and Co., n.d.), p. 743.

40 Albutt, *Wife's Handbook*, p. 15; Anonymous, *Healthy Mothers*, p. 33.

41 Albutt, *Wife's Handbook*, p. 19.

42 See Lisa Forman Cody's chapter in this volume, "Eating for Two: Shaping Mothers' Figures and Babies' Futures in Modern American Culture."

43 Cody, "Eating for Two."

44 The medical status of Australian doctors in this period was generally regarded as relatively high. See Evan Willis, *Medical Dominance: The Division of Labour in Australian Health Care* (Sydney: George Allen and Unwin, 1983), and T.S. Pensabene, *The Rise of the Medical Practitioner in Victoria* (Canberra: Australian National University, 1980).

45 Anonymous, *Healthy Mothers*, p. 18.

46 Anonymous, *Healthy Mothers*, p. 7; Albutt, *Wife's Handbook*, p. 8; Black, *Everybody's Medical Adviser*, p. 743; Fullerton, *Family Medical Guide*, pp. 417–8.

47 Christian U.D. Schrader, *Popular Medical Guide* (Sydney: Direct Supply Co., 1887), p. 115.

48 Albutt, *Wife's Handbook*, p. 8; Anonymous, *Healthy Mothers*, p. 20; Anonymous, *Wife, Maid and Mother* (Sydney, 1883), p. 24.

49 Anonymous, *Healthy Mothers*, p. 18.

50 Albutt, *Wife's Handbook*, p. 9.

51 Albutt, *Wife's Handbook*, p. 9.

52 Albutt, *Wife's Handbook*, p. 10.

53 Albutt, *Wife's Handbook*, p. 10.

54 Albutt, *Wife's Handbook*, p. 14

55   Anonymous, *Healthy Mothers*, p. 8.

56 Anonymous, *Healthy Mothers*, p. 11. See also Cody, "Eating for Two."

57 W.V. Jakins, "Ruptures of the Uterus," *AMJ* (15 November 1881): 491; W.B. Nisbet, "The Education of Midwives," *AMG* (June 1891): 270.

58 Jakins, "Ruptures of the Uterus," p. 491; "Letter to the Editor," *AMG* (June 1888): 227.

59 C.F. Marks, "Address on Medicine as a Department of State—A Suggestion," *AMG* (20 February 1897): 89; Nisbet, "Education of Midwives," p. 270; Kay Saunders and Katie Spearritt, "Is There Life after Birth? Childbirth, Death and Danger for Settler Women in Colonial Queensland," *Journal of Australian Studies* 29 (June 1991): 70–1; M.J. Thearle and Helen Gregory, "Childbirth by Choice: Midwifery in Queensland from Pre-history to the 1930s," Fourth Biennial Conference of the National Midwives Association, Brisbane, 1985, p. 8.

60 See, for example, E.J.A. Haynes, "Abdominal Extra-Uterine Foetation of Eight Months Duration—Operation," *AMG* (October 1892): 370, and Fullerton, *Family Medical Guide*, p. 438.

61 Willis, *Medical Dominance*, p. 101.

62 Philip E. Muskett, *The Illustrated Australian Medical Guide*, 2 vols. (Sydney: William Brooks and Co., 1903), p. 33; Thompson, *Medical Adviser*, p. 526.

63 *Report of the Benevolent Society of New South Wales. For the Year Ending 31st December 1888* (Sydney: Benevolent Society of New South Wales, 1889), p. 12.

64 Muskett, *Illustrated Australian Medical Guide*, pp. 33–5; Alexander Francis, *Pregnancy and Normal Labour: A Practical Guide for the Use of Mothers and Nurses Living in the Bush* (Brisbane: Outridge and Co., 1891), p. 13.

65 Vostral, "Advice to Adolescents."

66 F.C. Richards and S. Edin Eutalia, *Ladies Handbook of Home Treatment* (Melbourne: Signs Publishing Co., 1905), pp. 109–10.

67   Richards and Eutalia, *Ladies Handbook*, p. 110.

68   Fullerton, *Family Medical Guide*, p. 417.

69   Albutt, *Wife's Handbook*, p. 18 (underline in original).

70   Albutt, *Wife's Handbook*, p. 18.

71   Chavasse, *Man's Strength*, p. 265.

72   Anonymous, *Healthy Mothers*, p. 34. See also Francis, *Pregnancy and Normal Labour*, p. 12; Chavasse, *Man's Strength*, p. 265; Albutt, *Wife's Handbook*, p. 16.

73   Albutt, *Wife's Handbook*, p. 20.

74   Albutt, *Wife's Handbook*, p. 20.

75   Fullerton, *Family Medical Guide*, p. 419.

76   Walter Balls-Headley, "Case of Porro's Operation," and Clement Godson, "Porro's Operation," *British Medical Journal* 26 (January 1884): 549, 142–60; Frank A. Nyulasy, "Notes on a Case of Craniotomy—Subsequent Successful Induction of Premature Labour—Child Incubated," *AMG* (1898): 347; W. Edward Warren, "Notes upon Three Successful Craniotomy Operations, All in the Case of the Same Patient," *AMG* (August 1884): 245.

77   Fullerton, *Family Medical Guide*, p. 408.

78   Irvine Loudon, "Deaths in Childbed from the Eighteenth Century to 1935," *Medical History* 30 (1986): 22. Using statistics from Coghlan, the rate was closer to 35 per cent; however, it is likely that many cases were under-reported. T.A. Coghlan, *The Wealth and Progress of New South Wales, 1900–01* (Sydney: William Applegate Gullick, 1902), p. 59.

79   James Jamieson, "The Present State of the Puerperal Fever Question," *AMJ* (June 15, 1884): 247; James Jamieson, "Recent Contributions to the Antiseptic Method," *AMJ* (July 15, 1885): 289–91.

80   Jamieson, "Present State," p. 250; T.N. Fitzgerald, "Presidential Address, Medical Society of Victoria," *AMJ* (January 15, 1880): 26.

81   James Jamieson, "Puerperal Fever: Its Causes, Prevalence, and Prevention," *AMJ* (January 1879): 5. For earlier British conceptualizations of fever, doctors, and midwives, see Alison Bashford, *Purity and Pollution: Gender, Embodiment and Victorian Medicine* (New York: St. Martin's Press, 1998), pp. 73–83.

82   William S. Byrne, "Fevers of the Puerperal State," *AMG* (August 1890): 274. See also Annette Rubinstein, "Subtle Poison: The Puerperal Fever Controversy in Victorian Britain," *Historical Studies* 20 (1983): 420–38.

83   Albutt, *Wife's Handbook*, p. 21.

84   Anonymous, *Healthy Mothers*, p. 55.

85   Thompson, *Medical Adviser*, pp. 321–2.

86   Thompson, *Medical Adviser*, p. 323.

87   Thompson, *Medical Adviser*, p. 325.

88   Thompson, *Medical Adviser*, p. 326.

89   Thompson, *Medical Adviser*, p. 327.

90   M.U. O'Sullivan, *The Proclivity of Civilised Woman to Uterine Displacement: The Antidote. Also Other Contributions to Gynaecological Surgery* (Melbourne: Stillwell and Co. Printers, 1894), p. 8; Dr. Meyer, "President's Address, Vic Branch BMA," *AMG* (January 1895): 26; E.J. Jenkins, "Presidential Address, NSW Branch BMA," *AMG* (April 1896): 131.

Eating for Two: Shaping Mothers' Figures and Babies' Futures in Modern American Culture

Lisa Forman Cody

Since the 1980s, American parenting magazines, pregnancy guidebooks, and advertisements have admonished pregnant women to monitor their food and drink. Pregnant women of the late twentieth century may suspect that compared to the recommendations given to mothers in earlier decades of the twentieth century, they have been expected to follow a peculiarly—but necessarily—strict dietary regime. Women in the 1950s may have smoked and drank while pregnant, but now expectant mothers are expected to forgo caffeine, alcohol, sugar, and junk food, not to mention tobacco and drugs. The advice in recent years has been exacting but sometimes contradictory, suggesting that the smallest misstep could endanger a future baby's welfare. Oysters, for example, might increase the odds of conceiving, but once pregnant, oysters can cause toxoplasmosis leading to miscarriage. Ginger soothes nausea during pregnancy, but too much can cause maternal arrhythmia.[1] Although the tone in 1980s popular parenting materials about prenatal nutrition could certainly be considered anxious, if not alarmist, it would be a mistake to view the concern—and contradictions—about diet and reproduction as belonging only to the late twentieth century.

This chapter explores prenatal nutritional advice given by both medical professionals and popular authors from the late nineteenth century onward. Because both popular and medical works guiding expectant mothers (and fathers) have, until very recently, depicted the typical pregnant woman to be white, middle-class, married, and Protestant, this chapter's sources reflect a normative view in the literature of gender, class, and the culture of food.

There is evidence, of course, that large groups of American women lacked access to the food and practices recommended by mainstream physicians and lay advisors. Anxious mothers in the early twentieth century wrote to the staff at the Federal Children's Bureau, for instance, worrying about their diets and questioning the advice given by their neighbours and friends. These women's letters hint at the variety of America's different culinary customs and the very limited resources available to many families far into the twentieth century. Most pregnancy experts ignored the variety of American diets and the high cost of good nutrition. When they did discuss such issues, they tended to do so in order to chide the mother who rejected a middle-class diet or who foolishly thought good food was too costly.[2]

Authors' dietary advice to pregnant women has been more than simply hewing to a contemporary nutritional ideal. Though they emphasized their expertise as doctors, nurses, learned mothers, or even critical feminists, authors discussing prenatal nutrition did not so much simply report and filter the latest evidence-based research on caloric requirements, specific nutrients' roles in fetal development, substances that pass the placental barrier, or fetal exposure to alcohol, caffeine, and prescribed (or street) drugs, for instance. Experts advising expectant mothers about weight gain and diet reveal as much about recent obstetrical evidence as about broader cultural beliefs about women's bodies. But even more than simply reflecting normative expectations about women's bodies, experts' admonitions about food, drink, and weight gain speak to deep, contradictory, and largely unresolved beliefs about women's fundamental physiological (and moral) obligations to the life of an unborn child.

Over the centuries, midwives and other mothers traditionally offered advice about what to eat and what to avoid in order to become and to stay pregnant. Much of their commentary was aimed at helping a mother with "morning sickness" to make her way through the pregnancy, but very little was said before the late nineteenth century about what a mother *should* consume for the health of her unborn child. When men entered obstetrics after the 1750s, they had relatively little to say about nutrition—most likely because food preparation was so clearly viewed as a feminine and domestic occupation in the eighteenth and nineteenth centuries. In the first decades of the twentieth century, obstetrical and parenting texts began cautiously discussing prenatal nutrition as scientists discovered vitamins and were able to make empirically demonstrable claims about the chemical composition of food. By 1940, however, obstetrical authors were opining extensively about every aspect of a pregnant woman's life, including her dress, diet, and weight gain. In the 1950s and 1960s, mainstream advice books were hard on mothers, typically ordering them not to gain more than 15 pounds.

The popular "natural" childbirth books that emerged in the 1950s and beyond did not, as might be expected, adopt a laissez-faire approach about nutrition and weight gain in contrast to obstetricians' dietary orders. Some works that pitched themselves as opposing male medical control continued to give specific, abstemious orders about food, and, perhaps surprisingly, adopted their own judgmental tone. By the 1980s and 1990s, most popular works on pregnancy, whether written from a medical or feminist point of view, recommended that expectant mothers control their eating and drinking in multiple ways. The trajectory here is thus inversely related to the rise of male, medicalized childbirth: as doctors asserted control over childbirth, prenatal nutrition was of little concern to them, but as women regained some control over their reproductive bodies, both medical professionals and alternative childbirth advocates emphasized diet, with both camps placing great and grave responsibility on expectant mothers for the well-being of their unborn children.

Professionalizing Pregnancy, Dismissing Domesticity

Male medical professionals' quest to gain status in the United States during the nineteenth century drove them to distinguish their enterprise from the domestic, common pursuits of the kitchen and household. American mainstream and elite practitioners successfully emphasized obstetrics as a medical, not domestic, practice, and one that required scientific expertise and the calm, disinterested demeanour that only a well-trained man could offer. By minimizing nutrition and diet, the nineteenth-century M.D. naturally set himself apart from traditional and poorer female midwives. Perhaps nineteenth-century obstetricians and family doctors actually did discuss food or prenatal nausea with their pregnant patients, but their texts suggest otherwise.

Mainstream obstetrical texts barely discussed diet, typically saying nothing more than, as in the case of Calvin Cutter, M.D., that pregnant women should avoid meat during the summer as it was "warming"—and this from the author of one of the most popular physiological textbooks used in American medical schools.[3] Professor John Bate, M.D., offered more specific advice: "The diet [during pregnancy] also requires particular attention, using light and nutritious food, and avoiding all alcoholic drinks, fatty, acidulous, and indigestible foods." He noted in another section of his treatise that dangerous foods included "port wine, syrup of pine-apples, mushrooms roasted and steeped in salad-oil." Yet these evils were mentioned in a long list of *drugs* to be avoided during pregnancy at the end of the book. Ultimately, Dr. Bate was less interested in food than genes. Like many nineteenth-century and early-twentieth-century experts, he opined at length about eugenic factors. "Puny" infants did not result from poor maternal nutrition but from disparity in the age of the mother and father or from the "breeding in-and-in" of the Jews. In other words, the unborn child could be affected by parents being of the same or different races but could not be particularly shaped by what its mother ate, drank, or inhaled during pregnancy.[4]

Alternative medical practitioners, however, distinguished themselves from the mainstream in part by incorporating nutrition into their arguments. John Ellis, one of the founding fathers of American homeopathy, for example, suggested that as far as the best prenatal diet was concerned, it was simply like the best diets in general. Because coffee and tea and especially spices were pernicious for all, and vegetarianism led to the greatest vitality, this was no less true during pregnancy.[5] Or consider Seth Pancoast, M.D., a late Victorian, esoteric practitioner and author who wrote on the cabbala, light therapy, vegetable matter, the miasmatic transmission of cholera, the dangers of masturbation, and women's health concerns. Unlike his more conventional brethren, Dr. Pancoast focused particularly on women's supposed psychosomatic role in shaping their unborn children, emphasizing the importance of a cheerful disposition, exercise, and sound diet. He inveighed against adulterated food, heavy spices, caffeine, and alcohol. The final section in Pancoast's 1899 work offered women advice about practical health matters and was penned by Cornelius Clifford Vanderbeck, M.D., who interwove his recommendations with physiological explanations:

> The pregnant woman should exercise some care of her diet. Meat should be eaten but once a day; rich soups and highly seasoned foods avoided, and all alcoholic and other stimulants strictly shunned. She should eat rather less during early pregnancy than at ordinary times; for while it is true she has two to provide for, yet she has less drain upon her system, from the fact that she no longer is unwell, and the foetus, up to the third month, is not much larger than an egg. An overloaded stomach also may favor the distressing nausea and morning sickness of early pregnancy. During the latter months of pregnancy the diet should be fuller, for if it is too light it is likely to make the mother a poor nurse for her child, both in the quantity and quality of her milk.[6]

The recommendations to avoid coffee, alcohol, and rich food probably resonated with many mothers' own inclinations in the first trimester, a period most liable to nausea, especially when smelling pungent odours. At the same time, Dr. Vanderbeck's advice to "eat rather less" implied that women should control their weight during pregnancy—a point that would become an obsession among later obstetricians and popular health advisors.

Vanderbeck and Pancoast explained to their lay audience that a child absorbed every substance imbibed by a pregnant or lactating mother. Though neither expert offered a detailed list of foods or recipes, they explained why women should monitor what they ate and drank—as well as how they should feel emotionally. "It is to be remembered that during a prolonged period mother and child form together but one living system, and whatever injures the mother's constitution also involves that of her progeny," warned Vanderbeck. He described the potential peril here:

> It should be borne in mind that the period of intrauterine life is one full of danger to the health of the foetus; not only does ill health in the mother react upon the defenceless little creature, but it may be, her thoughts, her mental and moral states, her passions, are reproduced in the child. It is of the utmost importance then that she be surrounded with comfort, cheer, and happiness; that no unkindness be shown her by her husband or family; that she have all advantages of mental ease and comfort to implant in the miniature human being qualities good and noble. How readily mothers believe in birthmarks, and yet how ignorant or negligent are they of prenatal impressions affecting health and morals.[7]

Unlike mainstream nineteenth-century physician-authors, who characterized pregnant women as invalids, Vanderbeck and his colleagues emphasized expectant mothers' responsibility to be and act well. They admonished fathers to be healthy and cheerful at all moments in the reproductive process: "It must be borne in mind that the health of the father, at the time of the impregnation, also influences very much the future child's welfare."[8] Elite physicians established their authority over pregnant women by mystifying knowledge about pregnancy; alternative doctors argued contrarily that pregnancy was knowable and controllable, yet they too failed to give many dietary specifics.

But what did mothers actually eat, or want to eat? Many of the specific recommendations made both by conventional and alternative practitioners about alcohol, "stimulants," spices, meat, and oil-soaked mushrooms might imply that these were foods that pregnant women customarily ate or desired. Information from mothers themselves indicates that pregnancy was popularly considered to be fraught with danger. The Federal Children's Bureau received a letter from a Nebraska woman in 1922 asking, "What foods should a expectant mother eat. Is it so that if she eats certain foods it will kill the baby. I have been told that no vinegar or pep[p]er should be used especially red pep[p]er please explain those matters to me."[9] A 1919 text described a "prejudice ... against onions, asparagus, and celery" (which in fact were explained to be "harmless" by the medical author),[10] again suggesting the prevalence of beliefs about the dangers of specific foods. It is difficult to gauge how much women followed popular lore (or professional advice) in practice because turn-of-the-century sources recording women's own experiences during pregnancy said little about diet except to note prenatal nausea. For instance, when Stanford researcher and physician Clelia Duel Mosher interviewed nearly fifty educated women at the turn of the twentieth century, several of her questions opened potential discussion about diet and experience during pregnancy. Aside from recalling experiences with prenatal nausea, these women said next to nothing about what they ingested during pregnancy. Instead, the few who responded to Moser's prompts about "prenatal influence" discussed the after-effects of their emotional feelings during pregnancy. One respondent noted that her daughter was "very sensitive; feelings easily hurt," and she attributed this to her emotional state during pregnancy, "hav[ing] always laid it to prenatal influence, as I was unnaturally and morbidly sensitive during the 9 mos. preceding her birth."[11]

These claims that the feelings during a mother's pregnancy had the power to shape the disposition (or even the physiology) of an unborn child were centuries old. Despite elite physician-authors' attempts to eradicate such beliefs, women across classes often subscribed to such views, as did many alternative practitioners. Dr. Seth Pancoast included a lengthy chapter lifted almost verbatim from a sixteenth-century French treatise on how women's fears and desires could turn their fetuses into "monsters," presenting it as *modern* evidence of the dangers of the maternal fears and bad moods.[12] These beliefs in the physiological force of mothers' ideas failed to dissipate in the twentieth century—one woman from Florida who wrote the Federal Children's Bureau in 1922 for advice about her pregnancy asked whether her fears had the power to shape her child: "I am expecting the Stork the latter part of August and have had some very harrowing frights that keep me more or less alarmed—I have one perfect son 3½ yrs old and can't bear the idea of a deformed child.... lend me what help you can; am 14 miles from nearest doctor and have constant dread of what might happen. Yours in distress."[13]

This sort of evidence suggests that mothers (and even some practitioners) believed that maternal emotions had greater impact on the future welfare of unborn children than maternal nutrition during pregnancy. In this regard, popular beliefs about prenatal development and maternal emotions were little shaped by the medicalized, "rational" stance of elite physicians who rejected such mind-body connections. It was not simply the poor, but also the well educated, as in the case of Dr. Mosher's informants, who strongly maintained faith in their feelings having the power to shape their offspring.

The Science of Motherhood

Since the American Medical Association excluded female physicians (and any other "irregular" practitioner) after 1900, women doctors and nurses were forced to carve out special areas of expertise that wed their "traditional" or "natural" knowledge about babies, women, and domesticity with the latest advances in scientific medicine.[14] Female physicians and nurses practising among poorer patients witnessed the debilitating effects of poverty and inadequate diet on the health of mothers and babies, and these health advocates in the trenches lobbied for over a decade before Congress created a Federal Children's Bureau in 1912. The Children's Bureau was designed to gather data about maternal, infant, and pediatric health, plus offer advice to women and communities about scientific motherhood. Ultimately, advocates of the Children's Bureau were able to win congressional passage of the *Maternity and Infant Act* of 1921, popularly known as the *Sheppard-Towner Act*, which offered grants-in-aid to states to alleviate conditions of poor maternal and child health. Beginning in 1913, the Bureau distributed millions of its pamphlet *Prenatal Care* and was roundly applauded for having reduced the infant mortality rate and improved the health of infants through its advice, including its recommendation that pregnant women consult obstetricians early and often in their pregnancies.[15]

For all their work in creating a role for female medical expertise and their focus on real mothers' needs, the Children's Bureau nonetheless ultimately shared the position with mainstream doctors that obstetricians—presumably male—knew best. Twentieth-century physicians advised expectant mothers to "go to your doctor as soon as you know or suspect that you are pregnant."[16] They thus extended the length of the doctor–patient relationship from typically about twenty weeks to at least forty weeks, which became standard in the twentieth century, and they consequently helped to reinforce the position that a doctor, not a woman herself, determined her fitness for motherhood. Herbert Guttmacher, M.D., explained his view on this in 1973: "A prize cow or thoroughbred mare is not mated until it is determined the animal is in optimal condition. In theory and in fact, a woman should consult her doctor and not attempt pregnancy until he gives her the green light."[17] Female medical providers who established the Children's Bureau and worked in the field certainly witnessed the experiences of varied populations and the prenatal importance of nutrition, but they, perhaps paradoxically, urged expectant mothers to defer to medical doctors—who actually received very little training, if any, in nutrition before the late twentieth century.

As "professional" or "scientific" motherhood gained stature among the public in the 1910s and 1920s, male physicians emphasized recent advances in bacteriology, chemistry, and research medicine. Whereas nineteenth-century texts spoke more about the qualities of recommended and prohibited food, such as "rich" soups, "warming" meats, and "light" diets, twentieth-century medical texts began naming specific foods, sorted into food groups of vegetables, fruits, grains, dairies, and meats. Doctors' shift toward making these more concrete recommendations surely reflected new research into nutrition from the 1880s forward. Though the chemical composition of certain foods was not entirely worked out, researchers recognized that certain grains, fruits, vegetables, and dairy products had a positive effect on nutritional deficiencies; doctors thus tended to echo this general advice that mothers eat a varied, rich diet based on the different food groups, including dairy.[18] In other words, as soon as research medicine could lay claim to a scientific understanding of nutrition, the world of kitchen and diet reappeared in popular obstetrical and family care texts. As Yale biochemical research physician J. Morris Slemons explained in 1919, "Pregnancy is essentially a problem in nutrition."[19]

Rima Apple has shown that the popular press, drug companies, and retailers immediately latched onto the wonders of vitamins, extolling their virtues to the public. By the 1920s, works on "scientific motherhood"— many written by female physicians and nurses—and the popular press, such as *Good Housekeeping,* ordered mothers to learn about vitamins and to secure them for themselves and their children through cod-liver oil and supplements.[20] Vitamins may have been wildly popular among the early-twentieth-century public, but they were not among physicians, especially when it came to recommendations about prenatal nutrition. The American Medical Association (AMA) opposed the use of vitamin supplements in general, arguing that their effects were "'worthless'" and, as late as 1961, "pure superstition."[21] This stance resulted in large part from the organization's concern that the public's use of vitamins amounted to self-diagnosis and self-medication and thus competed with mainstream physicians' authority. With AMA physicians on board, the advice given by *Good Housekeeping* and other popular women's magazines was simply for women to consult their doctors on the matter of prenatal nutrition.[22] Even the softer, gentler medical guide from 1950, *Understanding Natural Childbirth*, dismissed the idea of women determining for themselves what supplements they should take: "[I]f vitamins or any other special foods should be added, or if any particular foods should be avoided, the doctor will direct the expectant mother. He is her guide."[23]

Despite advances in twentieth-century nutritional research, physicians disagreed about certain foods. Nineteenth-century texts about pregnancy had encouraged women to avoid meats almost altogether (and did not make up the deficit with legumes or other appropriate meat substitutes). Into the 1940s, many doctors recommended drastically limiting meat intake during pregnancy. As one woman reported to the Federal Children's Bureau in 1926, "'According to one doctor, I am allowed to eat everything 'on earth' while another doctor tells me to eat nothing but milk, potatoes, butter; no eggs, vegetables or meats. I am in a great predicament as which is which.'"[24] In 1942 author and nurse Lona L. Trott explained to the expectant mother in her scientific *Red Cross Home Nursing*, "Most doctors will say the mother may have all the fruits, vegetables, cereals, and milk that she wants. But there is some difference of opinion about the amount of meat and eggs allowed under certain conditions."[25]

The 1940s marked a turning point. A training text for obstetricians and nurses told its readers that "there is no reason why a normal pregnant woman should not eat meat in moderation, notwithstanding an old superstition to the contrary" because "modern investigation" showed that "abundant salt for seasoning and … eating highly spiced foods" was far more dangerous than eating meat.[26] Like many female medical authors working under the aegis of the established male medical professional, Nurse Trott ultimately deferred the specifics of prenatal nutrition to each mother's obstetrician: "A doctor's guidance about which foods should be increased will spare the mother a great deal of anxiety."[27] Obstetricians themselves agreed, recommending to their colleagues and nurses that "the physician should not assume that the patient eats sensibly just because she appears strong. He should give his patient a definite diet."[28]

Women's Shapes and Women's Movements

In keeping with a century focused on physical beauty, clothing, cosmetics, and slenderness, twentieth-century obstetrical texts from the 1920s also began focusing on weight gain, with an underlying assumption that (middle-class) female readers had easy access to food and drink—which they should limit in the primary interest of staying thin. Eating too much would not improve fetal health, according to the experts, but only fatten the mother: AMA vice-president William J. Carrington warned that "excessive calories do not go into the baby's sinews but are stored as fat in odd and embarrassing places about the body of the mother." What those odd, embarrassing places might be was not explicitly identified, but like nearly every other obstetrical advocate of slight weight gain, Dr. Carrington suggested that a dangerous contingent existed somewhere in women's worlds that advocated obesity during pregnancy: "It is a mistake to overeat, although many bridge table experts give the gratuitous advice that 'a mother expecting must eat for two.'"[29]

Dr. Carrington located the hazardous advice to fatten up in the self-important opining of non-experts: the bridge-playing gossip. Others emphasized how "Grandma knew, or thought she knew" the facts but she had nothing more than "her collection of misinformation, lack of information and old wives' tales."[30] Old superstitions about such things as the power of an expectant mother's cravings to mark a fetus with a birthmark apparently did continue to circulate,[31] but it is much harder to locate anybody writing on pregnancy who advocated the "old wives' tale" of "eating for two" either before or after the 1940s, when obstetricians began chiding pregnant women about weight gain. Even when Nurse Louise Zabriskie in 1946 described how "the pregnant mother is eating for two people," she qualified the situation: "the second person is so very tiny in the beginning that no extra quantity of food is needed." Only after the fifth month should the mother consider "a slight increase in quantity" of food, and in the end, the typical mother should gain twenty-five pounds.[32]

I have yet to find any text explicitly advocating "eating for two" in a literal sense; instead, I have found that both nineteenth- and twentieth-century pregnancy guides mostly advocated some type of *reduction* in diet or drink of some sort, such as cutting out meat, sugar, or butter, or even cutting total caloric intake. Nonetheless, the rhetorical design of the postwar obstetrical expert was clear: by distinguishing the scientifically learned author from the laywoman gossip or old-fashioned advisor of the past, the modern authority underscored his (or her) expertise as rational, scientific, and managerial. After all, the recommended diets to gain only ten pounds or so in a pregnancy required precise measurements and proscriptions. (Carrington's emphasis on not overeating seems, however, peculiarly contradicted by his suggestion that "cream, butter, cheese, oils and fat meats … should be included liberally in the diet unless there is nausea or obesity" and that "[s]ugars are the quickest 'pick-ups' available with which to combat fatigue.")[33]

By the late 1940s, a svelte pregnancy dominated American expectations, despite the fact that research on vitamins, minerals, and the sad effects of starvation during World War II on the caloric needs of the unborn baby proved the need for maternal weight gain. Experts' emphasis on gaining only fifteen, or even as little as seven, pounds might seem contradictory to this scientific research, but the admonition to gain so little weight simply reflected the widespread idea that the fetus absorbed what it needed from its mother. Dr. Carrington put it baldly: "Babies, like tapeworms and other parasites, help themselves to what they want, mother getting along as best she can on leftovers."[34] Comparing infants to tapeworms is hardly sentimental, yet the point in the baby boom era was made blatantly transparent here: baby

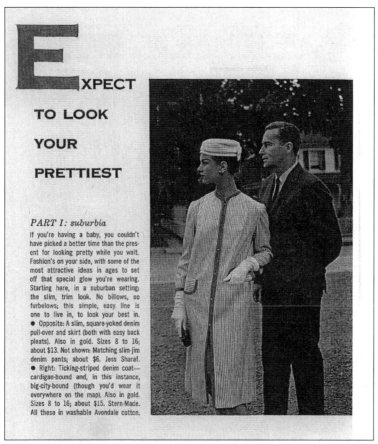

EXPECT TO LOOK YOUR PRETTIEST

PART I: suburbia

If you're having a baby, you couldn't have picked a better time than the present for looking pretty while you wait. Fashion's on your side, with some of the most attractive ideas in ages to set off that special glow you're wearing. Starting here, in a suburban setting: the slim, trim look. No billows, no furbelows; this simple, easy line is one to live in, to look your best in.
● Opposite: A slim, square-yoked denim pull-over and skirt (both with easy back pleats). Also in gold. Sizes 8 to 16; about $13. Not shown: Matching slim-jim denim pants; about $6. Jess Sharaf.
● Right: Ticking-striped denim coat—cardigan-bound and, in this instance, big-city-bound (though you'd wear it everywhere on the map). Also in gold. Sizes 8 to 16; about $15. Stern-Made. All these in washable Avondale cotton.

Figure 1   Fashion for expectant mothers. Under the heading "Expect to Look Your Prettiest," the text states, in part: "Starting here, in a suburban setting, the slim, trim look. No billows, no furbelows ..." *Good Housekeeping* 150 (1960), p. 67.

came first, biologically and physiologically, while the mother was simply a vessel, a caretaker, a second stringer, stuck with the "leftovers." Thus, if babies were parasites, they could get what they needed easily enough from seven or fifteen pounds weight gain, and the debased status of mother as gleaning the leftovers was mitigated by the fact that gaining so few pounds would make her pregnancy barely noticeable: the parasite was almost invisible.

Popular literature reinforced the ideal that pregnant women and new mothers should focus on limiting their weight gain, apparently mostly for fashion. Keeping baby—whether a parasite or not—invisible was echoed in clothing patterns from 1945 (fig. 1). Popular women's magazines pushed "the

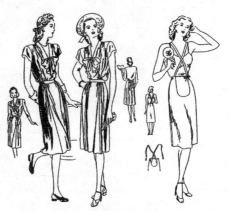

2. MOTHER'S CLOTHES

DURING pregnancy clothes should be comfortable, attractive, light in weight, and suited to the weather. They should prevent fatigue through support given the breasts, abdomen, and back. All tight bands should be avoided because they interfere with the circulation and may cause swelling, make a difference in a person's mental outlook, which is very important in this period. Clothes also afford an added opportunity for diversion.

DRESSES AND SLIPS

Dresses made in surplice, wrap-around, or two-piece styles in attrac-

FIG. 19. (*Left*) Vogue maternity dress pattern, No. 5312. (*Right*) Vogue maternity skirt pattern, No. 7609. (Copyright, 1945, The Condé Nast Publications, Inc.)

cramps, or general discomfort. Clothes that allow for change in form save expense and much bother. If clothes are made so as to fit well and are kept fresh and clean, the pregnant mother will always feel well dressed. Clothes tive materials are the most satisfactory. Various accessories do much to freshen a dress and detract attention from the changes in the figure (Fig. 19). Slips of wrap-around or adjustable styles are excellent (Fig. 20).

Figure 2 Vogue maternity-dress patterns, highlighting a svelte pregnancy. Condé Nast Publications, Inc., 1945, reprinted in Louise Zabriskie, *Mother and Baby Care in Pictures* (Philadelphia: J.B. Lippincott Co., 1946), p. 31.

slim, trim look" with "no billows, no furbelows" in 1960 (fig. 2).[35] One nurse's manual described how women typically considered "pregnancy and lactation" as "unbecoming, because they leave them with flabby breasts and protruding abdomen."[36] Food advertisements reassured women in 1960: "If you're one of the many young mothers who has to weight-watch, both before and after a new baby comes, you'll be glad to know that Velveeta's extra goodness comes from the **non-fat** part of the milk," which helped confirm the ad's rhetorical question: "Having babies and keeping slim is a job, isn't it?"[37] Though Velveeta's ad campaign, which offered different monthly episodes of "The Big Job of Being a Mother" in *Good Housekeeping* and other homemaking

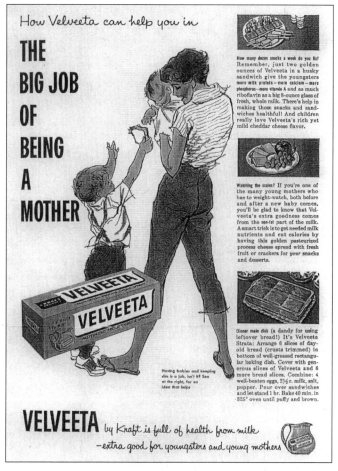

Figure 3   The ideal young mother within months of giving birth. "The Big Job of Being a Mother," advertisement for Velveeta, *Good Housekeeping*, January 1960, p. 15.

magazines of the period, highlighted the delights of raising toddlers, the copy here and elsewhere played into two underlying dynamics of the age that help us better understand the cult of thin in relation to pregnancy (fig. 3).

Demographically, the youngest wives in American history were those who wed in the postwar period—the average age of marriage for women in the 1950s was twenty compared to twenty-five at the turn of the twenty-first century. Mothers of the baby boomers were themselves barely adults, so it's not surprising that Velveeta's ad campaign—as well as the popular glorification of the young, nymph-like pregnant figure in popular texts—depicted the "young mother" as a big sister. While "children really love Velveeta's rich yet mild cheddar cheese flavor," the young mom should remember that "a smart trick is to get needed milk nutrients and cut calories by having this golden pasteurized process cheese spread with fresh fruit or crackers for *your* snacks and desserts."[38] After all, a young mother's tastes were not much different from those of her children. Though Velveeta and a host of popular sources reflected the demographic reality that the typical pregnant consumer was young and likely had more adolescent than urbane tastes, the ad campaign also captured the reality for the tens of thousands of very young postwar mothers who found themselves raising children, and lots of them: this was "a job," but one that was hardly glamorous. Asserting that mothering was a "big job" both acknowledged the challenge of staying at home with children and suggested that what these mothers did counted, in the same way that having a remunerative occupation or profession did.

Given that the ideal for women's figures from the 1920s onward was thin and even childlike, it is unsurprising that mainstream obstetrical texts reinforced slimness in expectant mothers, but doctors also claimed that scientific evidence showed weight gain during pregnancy to be unsafe. Because some studies during World War I in Germany showed that rates of eclampsia *declined* as food supplies were depleted, many obstetricians recommended that pregnant women gain little weight. As Dr. Danforth happily noted of hungry German women in the First World War, "provided their own nutrition was not impaired, the inability to overeat was a blessing in disguise." Unlike nineteenth-century doctors and midwives who did not specify how much a pregnant woman should gain, twentieth-century doctors specified quite precisely a mother's weight increase. In the 1940s, Danforth recommend "20 pounds, or at most 25."[39] After World War II, when the sorry effects of the Dutch famine on low birth weights, stillbirths, and heightened infant mortality were recognized, obstetricians no longer explicitly cited the positive effects of reduced calories during World War I as Danforth had done in his 1941 volume. Yet until the 1970s, authors kept telling women to gain no more than twenty pounds and to do this by eating no more than 1,800 calories a day throughout the entire pregnancy.[40] This amount is in marked contrast to pre–World War texts that, although they never advocated "eating for two," did describe typical weight gains to be around thirty pounds during pregnancy, and to texts written after the 1980s, which describe weight gains of thirty-five pounds as healthy.[41]

There were critics of this postwar emphasis on keeping the pregnant woman as trim as possible. President Eisenhower's Secretary of Agriculture, Ezra Taft Benson, reported in a 1960 issue of the AMA's popular magazine, *Today's Health*, that the National Research Council had amassed numerous studies showing that "the housewife ... tends to skimp on her own diet." One study out of Iowa "showed that the diets of at least one-half of the housewives provided less than 80% of the recommended levels for calcium, ... Vitamin C, and Vitamin A," while another study on "mothers-to-be" in Massachusetts "linked complications of pregnancy in part with low nutrition."[42] Perhaps doctors should have been encouraging pregnant women, if not to eat for two, at least to eat for one. But even in a special issue of *Today's Health* devoted entirely to family nutrition in October 1965, nothing was said about prenatal nutrition requirements.

Perhaps the most surprising aspect of the mid-twentieth-century emphasis on thin pregnancy was how female authors, including those ultimately advocating natural childbirth methods, were just as concerned about plump mothers as mainstream obstetrician authors; in fact, they recommended gaining even less. Dodi Schultz's 1970 *Have Your Baby—and Your Figure Too!* recommended a fifteen- to twenty-pound weight gain, which is not surprising given the book's title.[43] But Erna Wright, a Lamaze educator and natural childbirth advocate, recommended gaining even less: "The total weight gain for an average-sized woman should be 20 pounds throughout the whole pregnancy. People who are shorter than 5 feet 3 inches shouldn't put on more than 10 pounds maximum." And just in case the expectant mother read this as encouragement to eat "sugar and pastries" like "the majority of pregnant women," they should not: "This does not mean that you *must* put on that amount of weight. There are some people who put on 7 pounds during the whole pregnancy; they're fine, and so is the baby. Don't try to push it up. Try rather to keep it down."[44]

For Wright, Schultz, and other authors of the 1950s to 1970s, carbohydrates were the bug-bear of pregnancy and weight gain. Erna Wright offered a classic bait-and-switch: "You can eat anything and everything, and as much as you like," she began, but then warned, "*except* for the foods called *carbohydrates*. These include bread, potatoes, sugar, pastries, cake, chocolates, sweets and alcohol." She ordered women not to eat cornflakes for breakfast "because you eat sugar with them." Bacon and eggs were preferable. Milk—a sugar— also was not so necessary: "if you hate milk, you needn't feel any longer that you are sinning against yourself and your child if you don't drink it." Wright admitted the importance of calcium but encouraged women to eat cheese or yogurt instead. "But go easy on the sugar." Such abstemious advice might naturally lead to a warning about alcohol consumption during pregnancy as well, but Wright, like so many of her contemporaries in the 1960s, was far more forgiving about alcohol than pastries. "The odd drink, the odd glass of sherry, a glass of wine with your dinner—these are fine." Too much alcohol was dangerous, she admitted: "if you're accustomed to drinking three cocktails before every meal and then a bottle of wine as well, look out!" Not only was "[a]lcohol, remember, ... converted sugar," it also might "render ... you somewhat incapable" and "you might fall and hurt yourself. This, however, is a secondary consideration. Alcohol, like starch and sugar, is fattening, and therefore an enemy."[45]

These mainstream texts and the popular press in the twentieth century targeted the particular market of middle-class, white women. These American mothers were more likely than the nation's poor and working classes to be able to afford obstetrical care and a varied diet, including dairy and such fresh and out-of-season fruits as citrus every day (not to mention books on pregnancy and childcare).[46] Occasionally, mainstream texts scolded readers, presumably those who were less affluent, that obstetrical care was not as expensive as they might fear and that they should eschew female midwives because "they lack scientific knowledge."[47] Yet, for the most part, mainstream medical professionals played upon popular anxieties about beauty and fitness. Even works aimed at poorer urban populations, such as the training materials put out by the Visiting Nurse Association of Brooklyn, reminded the reader that "a good diet does not necessarily mean a high cost diet."[48] And it was only these works designed for specific neighbourhoods and populations like multi-ethnic Brooklyn that acknowledged dietary differences among religious groups and the importance of "racial customs."[49] The popular press and mainstream works presumed that pregnant women mixed milk and meat and could access fresh citrus, and said nothing positive about spicy food or "certain nationality dishes."[50]

By the late 1950s, some women and prominent medical researchers in the United States, Europe, and the Soviet Union began resisting medicalized aspects of birth, including the use of sedatives and episiotomies. Ferdinand Lamaze's *Painless Childbirth* (1956), Grantley Dick-Read's *Childbirth without Fear* (1944), and Helen Heardman's *A Way to Natural Childbirth* (1948) inspired mothers to learn more about their parturient bodies and about ways to reduce pain during delivery without the use of drugs. American texts popularizing natural childbirth methods did not always address diet, but many did. Though the tone of such works as Frederick Goodrich's *Natural Childbirth* (1950) was less hectoring when it came to diet (as well as other matters) than typical mainstream texts of the 1940s and 1950s, the author noted the difficulties of "excessive" weight gain. Like his contemporaries, Goodrich argued that gaining more than twenty pounds caused complications, especially in natural births.[51]

The women's movement led expectant mothers to discuss their concerns more freely in "rap" sessions and in such works as *Our Bodies, Ourselves* (1971). As women became more educated health care consumers, they pressured the medical profession and hospitals to let women stay awake during delivery and to eschew anesthesia. The first printings of *Our Bodies, Ourselves* offered unusually specific advice about what exactly to eat during pregnancy, telling the female reader: "We are very ignorant. We are taught very little about nutrition." But women were not alone in having little understanding the importance of diet. Doctors also knew little about nutrition as it related to pregnancy, the book reminded readers.

> It's important for us to know that our doctors don't agree with one another about the role of nutrition in pregnancy…. While all doctors would agree that we all should eat milk, eggs, green leafy vegetables, and fruit, they will disagree about our intake of salt, our weight gain, the number of calories we need, the value or harmfulness of diet pills. Up till now we have accepted our doctors' words as truth. For example, many of us who had children recently were advised not to gain much weight and were put on low-salt, low-calorie diets. We accepted these restr[i]ctions. We didn't intelligently question our doctors…. Now we're learning about a large and growing body of research which criticizes those "traditional" pregnancy diets we had.[52]

This work, like others critical of mainstream medicine, offers elliptical evidence that modern obstetrical practice commonly imposed difficult, even unhealthy diets on many pregnant American women and that diet pills may have been much more commonly prescribed in practice than obstetrical texts themselves would reveal.[53]

Our Bodies, Ourselves, like other "consciousness-raising" works of the period, asserted that proper nutrition was more than a matter of simply eating what was wholesome and healthy. More importantly, the hungry mother needed to grasp intellectually the physiological requirements of pregnancy while exploring her emotional, personal feelings about food: "[I]t's clear that food means different things to different people. Custom, religion, and the region we live in determine what we eat." Here the reflective exercise was designed to learn not so much about nutrition per se, but about one's emotional history in order to liberate oneself from the past: "It will be helpful for you to explore the meaning foods have for you. They might mean warmth and care. They might mean a restrictive home.... (For instance, milk might symbolize home and mother, so this very necessary food will be ignored to the detriment of pregnant mother's and fetus's health)."[54] Although *Our Bodies* came from the opposite political vantage point than most popular pregnancy texts written by male authors, both sources depicted what a woman learned from "Grandma," "the bridge-playing gossip," or even one's own "restrictive" parental household as somehow detrimental and potentially damaging. Mainstream texts placed authority in the rational, scientific knowledge of the male doctor, while the early feminist alternative used doctors' condescending advice as a consciousness-raising exercise of feminist liberation.

Our Bodies and other volumes in this genre of modern self-help books encouraged these personal meditations on food's private meanings for each individual, but by the early 1980s, most editions of these works asserted quite specific advice about the food women should eat and why, and if women found certain foods unpalatable or exotic, they suggested recipes to infuse a diet with large doses of vitamins and calcium. The "Best Odds Diet" of the *What to Expect When You're Expecting* series included suggestions for the "Double-the-Milk Shake," with one-third cup of powdered skim milk added to a cup of liquid skim milk, a frozen banana, cinnamon, and vanilla to "pacify your sweet and snacking tooth."[55] Unlike works written by doctors, texts written by women, including *Our Bodies,* encouraged mothers to eat liver and other organ meats at least once a week, and to eat eggs, lean protein, and as much as a quart of milk a day. The modern women's movement endorsed natural childbirth and self-knowledge about prenatal nutrition as means to challenge institutional and male medicine. Yet the alternative pregnant path did not necessarily give women complete freedom, as Erna Wright's chastising tone about carbohydrates suggests, or the repeated warnings about fat, sugar, alcohol, processed food, caffeine, and more in the *What to Expect* series.

As in earlier works with a bait-and-switch tone to the mother about substances, feminist and popular health books downplayed the effect of alcohol, caffeine, and illegal drugs when calming women's worries about what they imbibed "before they knew they were pregnant." But then these authors usually doubled back, warning that no amount of any of these substances was recommended once a woman realized she was expecting. "There's no evidence that a few drinks on a couple occasions early in pregnancy will prove harmful to your baby," reassured *What to Expect*, an advice book whose origins lay in one of the author's anxiety about "the wine I'd sipped nightly with dinner, and the gin and tonic I'd downed more than a few times before dinner in my first six weeks of pregnancy ... the coffee I'd drunk, and the milk I *hadn't*; the sugar I'd eaten, and the protein I hadn't." Yet, although the authors laid out paragraphs of pros and cons, in the end, they turned against alcohol, coffee, and especially sugar. For instance, they warned, "[T]here is no assurance that [a glass of wine nightly] is a wise practice. The safe daily alcohol dose in pregnancy, if any, is not known."[56]

The efforts of natural birth advocates, a feminist and post-feminist popular health movement, and the profit-making needs of hospitals have combined forces since the 1970s and 1980s to give women seemingly greater control over their pregnancies. Hospitals have banished the routine use of restraints and general anesthesia and encouraged mothers' partners to take part in the delivery of their babies. They have incorporated prenatal education classes and made hospital labour rooms look more like "home." These innovations have altered the experience of childbirth in the late twentieth century, but not without mixed results. Prenatal education classes do not necessarily give expectant mothers an open forum but instead can serve to acculturate women in the expectations of hospital protocol.[57] Late-twentieth-century popular literature that emphasizes the latest scientific rationale behind dietary recommendations demystifies prenatal nutrition, but the high expectations for mothers to eat fresh fish, more expensive organic fruits and vegetables, and labour-intensive unprocessed foods, plus to renounce alcohol, caffeine, sugar, tobacco, and even such medication as antidepressants from conception onward places responsibility for a child's well-being on the mother almost entirely. The nature of the challenges facing mothers has changed across the decades in the United States, to be sure, from mothers being ordered to be of good cheer in the late nineteenth century, to staying svelte in the 1950s, to regulating every aspect of diet in the 1980s and beyond, but one thing has remained consistent. Though the many twentieth-century advocates for women's control over their reproductive bodies and pregnancies have succeeded in giving mothers more of a say in the management of their births, they paradoxically have conveyed a message similar to that long promoted by male doctors: mothers either do not know what is good for them nutritionally or they crave what is indulgent and damaging. Either way, mothers are implied to be inherently and naturally likely to endanger themselves and their babies, so they need to be trained otherwise.

Few authors in the twentieth century suggested that eating (or dieting) properly during pregnancy was easy. As Velveeta's 1960 ad campaign put it, "Having babies ... is a job, isn't it?" It implied that, like all aspects of motherhood, feeding the fetus properly was demanding and likely required sacrificing one's alimentary desires. The twentieth-century expectation that mothers must renounce aspects of their regular diet—whether alcohol, coffee, sugar, fat, sushi, or excessive calories—can be interpreted as representing something more than knowledge about nutrition or even cultural beliefs about women's bodies and desires. When doctors and lay authors opine about whether a pregnant woman should drink a martini or a milkshake, their discussions stand in for larger ethical and legal questions about what responsibility women do (or do not) have for their unborn children.

Authors writing for pregnant American women have, in the twentieth century, uniformly suggested that good mothers do and should make sacrifices for their fetuses, but some of their comments about this state of affairs betray ambivalence and apparent contradictions. At mid-century, when advisers fretted far more about maternal weight gain than fetal inebriation, few facts were known about what the fetus absorbed and at what physiological benefit or cost. Dr. Carrington's 1944 description of an unborn child as a "tapeworm or parasite" that absorbed what it needed while the mother got the "leftovers" revealed more than contemporary and limited knowledge about prenatal nutrition. It also symbolized women's secondary status to the fetus in an age before the pill and legal access to abortion. By the 1970s, as experts learned more about the physiological relationship between mother and child, they worried less about women gaining weight than about what they—and their unborn children—consumed. But even here, authors' pronouncements may seem contradictory. Consider the *What to Expect* series' reassurance that drinking alcohol before becoming aware of being pregnant is probably fine, but even a sip after knowing one is pregnant is harmful and unacceptable. Though *What to Expect*, like every other guide to pregnancy, avoids discussing abortion, *Roe v. Wade*, and so on (even in chapters on prenatal screening for fetal abnormalities), this paradoxical passage about the toxic effects of alcohol consumption can be read as standing in for a quietly pro-choice stance about a mother's moral obligations to the unborn: once she knows of her pregnancy—a polite proxy for *choosing* motherhood—a woman is fully responsible for the health of her unborn child, even if that means sacrificing her own desires and needs.

The modern American mother, as so many guides have advised across the decades, should not "eat for two," but for one. Though mid-century authors intended to emphasize the miniscule caloric needs of the fetus here, the advice can also be read ironically: the one person out of two being fed first is not the mother but the child. Since the late 1960s and 1970s—the age of the sexual revolution, the artificial control of reproductive cycles through hormonal birth control, and the legalization of abortion with *Roe v. Wade*—pregnant women may have gained their reproductive rights, but they continue to eat for baby first. They have been reminded by all the experts (not to mention restaurant staff who refuse to serve them alcohol) that they are morally obligated to renounce their habits and desires for an unborn child—even when they simultaneously have the legal right to terminate that pregnancy. This is, at the very least, a cultural paradox. And it is one unlikely to be resolved any time soon as science uncovers more information about prenatal nutrition and fetal development while Americans debate, in court and out, what the balance of rights is between a woman, her unborn child, and the interests of others.

Notes

1. Peter Nathanielsz and Christopher Vaughan, *The Prenatal Prescription* (New York: HarperCollins, 2001); Jeremy Groll and Lorie Groll, *Fertility Foods: Optimize Ovulation and Conception through Food Choices* (New York: Simon & Schuster, 2006). The history of fetal alcohol syndrome, "crack babies," and so on is vast but beyond the scope of this chapter. See, for example, Elizabeth M. Armstrong, *Conceiving Risk, Bearing Responsibility: Fetal Alcohol Syndrome and the Diagnosis of Moral Disorder* (Baltimore: Johns Hopkins University Press, 2003); Karen D. Zivi, "Who Is the Guilty Party? Rights, Motherhood, and the Problem of Prenatal Drug Exposure," *Law and Society Review* 34.1 (2000): 237–58.

2. The first popular work to acknowledge racial and ethnic difference was the Boston Women's Health Course Collective's *Our Bodies, Ourselves* (Boston: New England Free Press, 1971), and from the 1980s onward, numerous pregnancy guides have marketed themselves to particular ethnic and religious communities.

3. Calvin Cutter, *First Book of Anatomy* (Philadelphia, 1854), p. 58.

4. J.W. Bate, *The Book of Secrets and Private Medical Adviser* (Chicago, 1895), p. 193 on diet, p. 302 on bad foods, pp. 67–8 on May–December couples and Jewish degeneration.

5. John Ellis, *The Avoidable Causes of Disease, Insanity and Deformity* (New York, 1860).

6. C.C. Vanderbeck, in S. Pancoast, *The Ladies' New Medical Guide*, rev. ed. (Philadelphia: John E. Potter, 1890), pp. 584–5.

7. C.C. Vanderbeck, in Pancoast, *Ladies' New Medical Guide*, p. 585.

8   C.C. Vanderbeck, in Pancoast, *Ladies' New Medical Guide*, p. 585.
9   Kristin Barker, "Birthing and Bureaucratic Women: Needs Talk and the Definitional Legacy of the Sheppard-Towner Act," *Feminist Studies* 29.2 (Summer 2003): 344.
10 J. Morris Slemons, *The Prospective Mother: A Handbook for Women during Pregnancy* (New York: D. Appleton & Co., 1919), p. 93.
11 "Blank No. 11," 17 (d), in Clelia Duel Mosher, *The Mosher Survey: Sexual Attitudes of 45 Victorian Women*, eds. James MaHood and Kristine Wenburg, intro. Carl N. Degler (New York: Arno Press, 1980), p. 124.
12 Pancoast, *Ladies' New Medical Guide*, pp. 202–8. Pancoast draws upon Ambroise Paré, *On Monsters and Marvels*, trans. Janis L. Pallister (1571; Chicago: University of Chicago Press, 1995).
13 Barker, "Birthing," p. 343.
14 Barbara Ehrenreich and Deirdre English, *For Her Own Good: 150 Years of the Experts' Advice to Women* (London: Pluto Press, 1979), p. 73.
15 Richard W. Wertz and Dorothy C. Wertz, *Lying-In: A History of Childbirth in America* (New Haven, CT: Yale University Press, 1989), pp. 203–11; Rima Apple, *Perfect Motherhood: Science and Childrearing in America* (New Brunswick, NJ: Rutgers University Press, 2006), pp. 34–55; E.R. Schlesinger, "The Sheppard-Towner Era: A Prototype Case Study in Federal–State Relationships," *American Journal of Public Health* 57.6 (1967): 1034–40.
16 William C. Danforth, *A Woman's Health* (New York: Farrar & Rinehart, 1941), p. 144.
17 Herbert Guttmacher, *Pregnancy, Birth, and Family Planning: A Guide for Expectant Parents in the 1970s* (New York: Viking Press, 1973), p. 76. This was the "modernize[d]" edition of Guttmacher's *Into This Universe: The Story of Human Birth* (New York: Viking Press, 1937); the earlier edition encouraged seeing the physician as soon as the mother missed her period (p. 117).
18 Danforth, *Woman's Health*, pp. 162–4.
19 J. Morris Slemons, *The Nutrition of the Fetus* (New Haven, CT: Yale University Press, 1919), p. 7.
20 Rima Apple, *Vitamania: Vitamins in American Culture* (New Brunswick, NJ: Rutgers University Press, 1996).
21 Apple, *Vitamania*, pp. 82, 77.
22 Kim Chuppa-Cornell, "Filling a Vacuum: Women's Health Information in *Good Housekeeping*'s Articles and Advertisements, 1920–1965," *The Historian* 67.3 (2005): 454–73.
23 Herbert Thoms, with Laurence G. Roth, *Understanding Natural Childbirth: A Book for the Expectant Mother* (New York: McGraw-Hill, 1950), pp. 40–1.
24 Barker, "Birthing," p. 345.
25 Lona L. Trott, *American Red Cross Home Nursing* (Philadelphia: Blakiston Co., 1942), p. 201.
26 F.L. Adair, ed., *Maternal Care: The Principles of Antepartum, Intrapartum, and Postpartum Care for the Practitioner of Obstetrics*, 2nd ed. (Chicago: University of Chicago Press, 1941), pp. 14–15; Anne E. Stevens, *Maternity Handbook for Pregnant Mothers and Expectant Fathers by the Maternity Center Association, New York City* (New York: G.P. Putnam's Sons, 1932). Stevens recommended that a pregnant woman "should *never* eat more than one serving of meat or fish a day" (defined as two ounces; p. 48).
27 Trott, *American Red Cross Home Nursing*, p. 201.
28 Adair, *Maternal Care*, pp. 13–14.
29 William J. Carrington, *Safe Convoy: The Expectant Mother's Handbook* (Philadelphia: J.B. Lippincott, 1944), p. 64. Others who described the eat-for-two rule as commonplace

(and wrong) include Slemons, *Prospective Mother*, p. 85; Slemons, *Nutrition of the Fetus*, p. 46; Guttmacher, *Into This Universe* (1937), p. 131; Mario Castallo and Audrey Walz, *Expectantly Yours: A Book for Expectant Mothers and Prospective Fathers* (New York: Macmillan, 1943), pp. 32–3; Frederick W. Goodrich, Jr., *Natural Childbirth: A Manual for Expectant Parents* (Englewood Cliffs, NJ: Prentice-Hall, 1950), p. 83; William H. Genné, *Husbands and Pregnancy: The Handbook for Expectant Fathers* (New York: Association Press, 1956), p. 32.

30 D.A. Dukelow, "School for Expectant Families," *Today's Health* (March 1950): 31, 53.

31 Nathan Fasten, "The Myth of Prenatal Influence," *Today's Health* (October 1950): 27, 42; "What You Can Do about Birthmarks," *Good Housekeeping* (September 1960): 131.

32 Louise Zabriskie, *Mother and Baby Care in Pictures*, 3rd ed. (Philadelphia: J.P. Lippincott, 1946), pp. 10, 14.

33 Carrington, *Safe Convoy*, p. 65.

34 Carrington, *Safe Convoy*, p. 66.

35 "Expect to Look Your Best," *Good Housekeeping* (January 1960): 66–73.

36 *Suggested Material for Teaching Mothers' Classes* (Brooklyn: Maternity Center Division of the Visiting Nurse Association of Brooklyn, 1941), [p. 4].

37 Velveeta Advertisement, *Good Housekeeping* (January 1960): 15.

38 Velveeta Advertisement, *Good Housekeeping* (January 1960): 15.

39 Danforth, *Woman's Health*, p. 161. For another positive view of the World War I German famine's effect on pregnant women, see Guttmacher, *Into This Universe*, p. 90; for a post-World War II vague reference to "Observations made in Germany during the war," see Sol T. De Lee, *Safeguarding Motherhood* (Philadelphia: J.B. Lippincott, 1949), p. 46.

40 Guttmacher, *Into This Universe*, p. 132; for 1,800 calories a day, see De Lee, *Safeguarding Motherhood*, p. 55.

41 Slemons, *Nutrition of the Fetus*, p. 7.

42 Ezra Taft Benson, with Theodore Irwin, "American Nutrition Paradox: Want Amidst Plenty," *Today's Health* (May 1960): 23–5, 66–7, quotations from p. 24. By 1970 the National Research Council was recommending at least 2,200 calories a day for pregnant women. The Committee on Maternal Nutrition, The National Research Council, *Maternal Nutrition and the Course of Pregnancy* (Washington, DC: National Academy of Sciences, 1970), p. 196.

43 Dodi Schultz, *Have Your Baby—and Your Figure, Too!* (New York: Pyramid Books, 1970), p. 2.

44 Erna Wright, *The New Childbirth* (New York: Hart Publishing, 1966), pp. 49–51.

45 Wright, *New Childbirth*, p. 51.

46 Lee A. Craig, Barry Goodwin, and Thomas Grennes, "The Effect of Mechanical Refrigeration on Nutrition in the United States," *Social Science History* 28.2 (2004): 325–36.

47 Trott, *American Red Cross Home Nursing*, p. 199.

48 *Suggested Material*, [p. 11].

49 *Suggested Material*, [p. 9].

50 Genné, *Husbands and Pregnancy*, p. 33.

51 Goodrich, *Natural Childbirth*, pp. 4–5.

52 Boston Women's Health Course Collective, *Our Bodies, Ourselves*, n.p.

53 "Diet pills" could have been diuretics or even methamphetamines. For the use of diuretics, see J. L. Walker, "Methyclothiazide in Excessive Weight Gain and Edema of Pregnancy," *Obstetrics and Gynecology* 27.2 (1966): 247–51. For the use of stimulants, see B.I. Coopersmith, M.D., who concluded that because adjusting thyroid hormones was "toxic in many cases," Dexedrine sulfate was preferable as "a safe and effective

drug to use in controlling weight gain during pregnancy." The Smith Kline & French Inter-American Corporation, Dexedrine's manufacturer, incorporated this ringing endorsement for speed in its professional advertisements. B.I. Coopersmith, "Dexedrine and Weight Control in Pregnancy," *American Journal of Obstetrics and Gynecology* 58.4 (1949): 664–72; untitled advertisement placed by Smith Kline, *Canadian Medical Association Journal* 65 (August 1951): 153. By the late 1960s, medical and science journals published research demonstrating the toxic effects of stimulants and other "weight loss" substances on the fetus. Whether American general practitioners and obstetricians commonly continued to prescribe drugs like Dexedrine, and for how many years into the 1970s and beyond, are far more difficult questions to answer beyond reporting anecdotal evidence, including this quote from *Our Bodies.*

54   Boston Women's Health Course Collective, *Our Bodies, Ourselves*, n.p.

55   Arlene Eisenberg, Heidi Eisenberg Markoff, and Sandee Eisenberg Hathaway, *What to Expect When You're Expecting* (New York: Workman, 1984), pp. 87, 85.

56   Eisenberg, Markoff, and Hathaway, *What to Expect*, pp. 15, 55. See also Caterine Milinaire, *Birth: Facts and Legends* (New York: Harmony Books, 1974). Milinaire explained that "grass," narcotics, barbiturates, and LSD were "relaxing" but ultimately dangerous for the fetus. Milinaire's book also warned that vitamins were probably unnecessary.

57   Elizabeth M. Armstrong, "Lessons in Control: Prenatal Education in the Hospital," *Social Problems* 47.4 (2000): 583–605; Wertz and Wertz, *Lying-In*, pp. 234–305.

Advice to Adolescents: Menstrual Health and Menstrual Education Films, 1946–1982

Sharra L. Vostral

M any women born after 1940 in the United States hold vivid memories of menstrual education during their teenage years. Some had mothers or sisters to explain menstruation; others learned from their physical education instructors. Most, though, were part of a nation-wide audience subjected to menstrual education films shown at school. These films came in two basic varieties: those produced by organizations that promoted public health and wellness, and those sponsored by corporations that manufactured menstrual hygiene technologies and crafted a role in public health education.[1] These two sponsor types had different goals that were apparent in the films' narration, production, and acting. Health and wellness films stressed caring for the body, eating right, and bathing. Corporate films stressed these same points, as well as the importance of managing menstruation with multiple changes of a sanitary napkin, which, not coincidentally, happened to be manufactured by the companies sponsoring the films.

To better understand the relationship of menstrual movies to menstrual technologies, I utilize the framework of scripting, which has multiple meanings in this context. In a very obvious sense, actors perform scenes for the films based upon a scripted text. The narrative of the film provides a literal and visual script instructing girls about menstrual health and how to use menstrual hygiene technologies. In historical terms, this type of source material is often referred to as prescriptive literature, in part because it emanates from an authoritative body to provide very specific instructions about how to act or think.[2] It prescribes behaviour, but whether or not recipients follow the advice is altogether another question. Both Lisa Forman Cody and Lisa Featherstone discuss medical advice literature about pregnancy and childbirth in this volume. Featherstone makes the important point that this literature did not necessarily predict actions: patients maintained a degree of autonomy concerning decision making about their own medical care. In addition, this prescriptive literature is useful to assess idealized outcomes and to consider which stakeholders would benefit from certain belief systems or behaviours, and how women in turn shaped larger discussions with their own actions. Thus, examining the film script is one component for understanding the menstrual education genre.

I also employ the framework of scripting in terms of analyzing technologies, and ultimately the portrayal of menstrual hygiene technologies, in these films. Though scripting is most often associated with text, it can be usefully applied to objects. Madeline Akrich, who works within the field of sociology of technology, argues that designers inscribe a kind of scenario, or technical conceptual map, into a technology or object concerning the ways it should be used and how it will evolve once out in the world.[3] She calls this a "script" or "scenario" for the technology. Designers hold a "projected user" in mind, but a "real user" must eventually encounter the object. Akrich defines this relationship between object, meaning, designer, and real and imagined user as "de-scription."[4] Thus, built into the menstrual hygiene technologies are assumptions of how they should be used and subsequently how they must be "read" or even decoded by users. Because the knowledge of using menstrual hygiene technology is not innate, how to extract information from the technology—figuring out what the technology scripts to a user—must be learned. Menstrual hygiene print advertising and educational films spent a great deal of energy scripting information to young, potential users. Therefore, this chapter assumes a dual scripting of both language and object concerning menstrual hygiene technologies.

This scripting was necessary for the domestication of menstrual hygiene technologies into American households, and in particular into teenagers' hands, during the twentieth century.[5] The concept of domestication helps to explain how a seemingly outrageous technology becomes normalized, and even rendered invisible, with daily use. Because of the potential for tampons to be understood in a negative light due to their phallic-like shape and their potential to break a virginal hymen, manufacturers worked to neutralize, tame, and domesticate them for adolescents' use. Thus, advertising scripts, film scripts, and technological scripts denatured the potentially dangerous implications of young, sexualized women using menstrual hygiene by rendering the technologies inert. Analyzing the menstrual education film within the context of popular culture offers a means to unfurl the relationships of adolescence, gender, menstrual health, and popular culture in the United States during the mid- to late twentieth century through ubiquitous, yet veiled, menstrual hygiene technologies.

Throughout this chapter, I rely on the menstrual hygiene film collection compiled by A/V Geeks, a video distributor devoted to the preservation and dissemination of "ephemeral film"—that is, films produced by a sponsor for a particular purpose, including training or social guidance.[6] Housed under the name *It's Wonderful Being a Girl*, the collection presents a variety of menstrual education films. I look at two categories of film: those produced by the makers of menstrual hygiene products and those sponsored by non-profit organizations for public health dissemination. The public health films include *Growing Girls* (The Film Producers Guild, National Committee for Visual Aids in Education, 1949), *Personal Health for Girls* (Coronet Instructional Films, 1972), and *Girl Stuff* (Churchill Films, 1982). Films produced by corporations include *The Story of Menstruation* (Kimberly-Clark, 1946), *It's Wonderful Being a Girl* (Johnson & Johnson, 1968), and *Naturally a Girl* (Johnson & Johnson, 1973). Overall the films are indicative of the mid- to late twentieth century and, in general, were targeted at white, middle-class girls and teenagers.

Through this genre of the menstrual education film, I analyze three significant themes that will be developed in this chapter. First, the films scripted ideal behaviour in terms of femininity and expectations of motherhood. Both corporate and non-profit films consistently stressed that menstruation was about completing the circle of life so that girls could be mothers.[7] They also scripted clear paths to follow to attain an ideal femininity as a teenager. How to become attractive emerged as a worthy, tangible goal for girls. Second, how to decode the enscripted use of menstrual hygiene technologies and what kind of technologies girls should use for their first periods constituted a good portion of many of the films. Third, the films scripted what amounted to a vital skill that every girl should learn, a circumscribed and feminized version of rugged individualism. The films reinforced the notion that girls could display their true grit by overcoming the limitations of menstruation and their own uncooperative bodies through the use of menstrual hygiene technologies, and in essence "pass" as normal and act as if they were not menstruating.[8] Gone were the days of enforced withdrawal from social engagements during one's period, afforded to privileged white women up through the 1920s. Now, whether or not girls felt cramps, fatigue, or bloating, they were expected to "buck up" and forge ahead. In total, the films reflected societal anxieties about teenagers and their menstrual health, but they scripted ideal behaviour to inform teenaged girls' gender identity and development.

Education Films

Movies have provided entertainment for audiences since the early twentieth century. Using film to send an educational message capitalized on people's love for motion pictures, while simultaneously acknowledging their disinclinations to learn about syphilis or drunk driving through more traditional venues of the doctor's office, school lecture, or community meeting hall. Films proved to be very powerful in distributing information about government programs during World War II. For example, moviegoers were shown, through the antics of Donald Duck in the Disney production *The Spirit of '43* (1943), that citizens should save money and exercise frugality. The omniscient narrator warned the audience, "Every dollar you sock away for taxes is another dollar to sock the Axis."[9] Health practitioners and physicians also discovered that films reached patients and created medical literacy more successfully than could otherwise have been achieved.[10] Organized medicine took a strong lead in collaborating with filmmakers and producers to ensure accuracy of content.[11] Audiences viewed films on the subjects of tuberculosis, venereal disease, and breast cancer in theatres as well as doctors' offices. One-minute shorts, such as the public health reminder *Don't Spread Germs* (1948), demonstrated that even a common sneeze deserved proper hygienic intervention to reduce the dissemination of disease-causing bacteria.[12] The themes of these films were broad and represented a concerted public health effort to change individuals' behaviours.

Children were a special audience for the films, however, because of the assumed pliability of their young minds and the belief that if children were trained properly, bad or unwanted behaviours might be nipped in the bud. The messages directed at girls and young teens seemed to have a particular urgency because they represented the future of American democracy.[13] If girls could be trained in their formative years, the common thought went, then American society as a whole might produce ideal adult women and mothers in the future. These women would uphold citizenship and help support the status quo. In this way, male (and white) patriarchy would be maintained and renewed.

According to Ilana Nash, a scholar of teen film, movies accomplished this educational task by tapping into long-held beliefs and concerns about teenagers in two particular ways. First, films presented what she calls "the chrysalis moment," defined as "the carefully manipulated scenario in which an adolescent female is shown crossing a threshold of sexual maturity, like a caterpillar's transition to butterfly."[14] The chrysalis moment evokes desire and anxiety, for the teenager is alluring yet innocent. I contend that it is because of this anxiety over the teen's liminality between the worlds of woman and child that education films emerged to channel and police burgeoning sexuality. Thus, the menstrual education film was calculated to reach pre-menarchal girls before their emergence from the metaphorical cocoon. Second, Nash identifies an assumption about the "emptiness" of teenagers' minds and a desire—sexual and otherwise—to fill that void as key to the teen film genre.[15] This emptiness is significant because it refers to a girl's lack of sexual consciousness, of intellect, and of self-knowledge. Indeed, when girls are so constructed as "clueless," it becomes paramount to fill these lacks with a socially acceptable and scripted model of femininity. Bearing the burden of sexual and civic inexperience, yet crucial to the stability of propagating future generations, young women were shaped by the menstrual hygiene film for the necessity of motherhood, the proper traits of femininity, and the appropriate use of technologies.

Menstrual Education

Addressing girls about their periods emerged in the late 1920s and early 1930s, when it became apparent to corporations that to attend only to adult users was shortsighted. Corporations believed that teenaged girls needed to be reached at an early age in order to become lifelong consumers of menstrual hygiene technologies. Becoming a modern teenager meant consuming products of all sorts, systematically maintaining a good-smelling and hygienic body, and emerging as a consumer-citizen.[16] By the 1930s, marketers increasingly came to think of teenagers as a distinct group, having their own set of aesthetic tastes and purchasing patterns.[17] The acts of consumption, as well as the use of body-management technologies such as manufactured sanitary napkins, created a set of generational practices that were often very different from those of their mothers, and contributed to a collective identity for the group.[18]

Kimberly-Clark Corporation, which first successfully sold Kotex sanitary napkins in 1921, recognized this adolescent market early on and published booklets intended to educate girls about their periods. Unlike a trip to visit the doctor, where a girl might receive a lecture about menstruation, the 1928 booklet "Marjorie May's 12th Birthday" relayed advice in the form of a story, which seemed more palatable than heavy-handed warnings from a physician. Of course, distribution of these booklets was not just a public service. Corporations carefully crafted booklets, filmstrips, and then films to be used in tandem with health and hygiene classes, or sex education courses. The new genre of the menstrual education film emerged with *The Story of Menstruation*.[19] Sponsored by Kimberly-Clark Corporation and produced by Walt Disney Productions in 1946, the film ushered in a new era of educational media. It skilfully manipulated colour animation to present a forbidden topic as unsensational, wholesome entertainment, thus cleverly domesticating it. One reviewer felt that *The Story of Menstruation* succeeded in presenting menstruation with "an air of good cheer."[20] It differed significantly from sensational sex hygiene films and drug films, which often sought to scare children and teens out of their wits and thereby push them onto the straight and narrow path of abstinence. The same reviewer, writing for the *Journal of the American Medical Association*, noted that there was a desperate need to present "material related to the reproductive processes without creating an atmosphere of tension, not to say fear and disgust."[21] The film offered parents, teachers, and concerned school board members a way to teach human reproduction without falling into the trap of prurience. One school board member lamented, "I wish it were possible to present sex to girls in such a way that they would not thereafter associate the whole subject with old bewhiskered doctors threatening venereal disease."[22] The *Journal of the American Medical Association* reviewer claimed, "This film is the answer to the problem." Many others agreed. The film received the "Good Housekeeping Seal of Approval," and Kimberly-Clark claimed that more than 105 million girls viewed it over thirty-five years.[23] The film became the gold standard of the menstrual hygiene educational film genre. The film was also unique for Disney in terms of business collaboration, since it was one of the few films that Disney did not possess in full ownership.[24]

What marked this film as artistically sophisticated was its animation. The film did not rely on simple stick figures or overwrought acting. It was a remarkably pleasant artistic endeavour, featuring soft colours, floating flowers, and soothing music. The female protagonists were characteristic of Disney, with creamy white complexions, pleasing curves, and perky rear ends that prefigured Peter Pan's Tinkerbell.[25] Kimberly-Clark published "Very Personally Yours" to correspond with the film, and the characters in this booklet possessed large heads, peg legs, and no feet. These cute, stylized storybook characters helped to lull, domesticate, and constrain sexuality through a tale about health, reproduction, and hygiene, reducing menstruation to mere entertainment. Most importantly, the story helped to define femininity as a system, one that needed to be learned and practised daily, and that could be maintained through technology.

Motherhood and Femininity

The Story of Menstruation began with the multiple notions of motherhood. The female narrator first asked, "Why is nature always called Mother Nature?" "Perhaps," she continued, "it's because like any mother she quietly manages so much of our living, without our even realizing there is a woman at work."[26] The film employed the traditional depiction of nature as a maternal woman devoted to providing food and shelter to her dependants. This personification naturalized woman's nurturing role in the family, while ignoring the effort involved.[27] A woman's nature thus sets her on an inevitable course to become a selfless mother. The film often referred to nature to explain that menstruation was part of the cycle of life, a cycle that, not surprisingly, was dictated by Mother Nature. The reference also segued into a more physiological explanation that later films did not always follow. "Mother Nature controls many of our routine body processes through automatic control centers called glands." Mother Nature provided the rhetorical link to the relatively new concepts of hormones, the function of the pituitary gland, and physiology.[28] "As a girl moves from blocks to dolls to books," the film explained, "her body is obeying the orders issued by the pituitary gland."[29] Since Mother Nature designed the pituitary gland, a girl had no choice but to "obey" orders. This skilfully articulated representation of menstruation affirmed maternal determinism: the biology of the body dictated a teenager's maternal destiny.

This destiny was further established through a none-too-clear discussion of human reproduction. Following the talk about pituitary glands and "maturing hormones," the schematic presented a two-dimensional image of the uterus, ovaries, fallopian tubes, and a pipe-like vaginal opening. Although the film was in colour, the reproductive organs were conspicuously in dark and light grey tones. After discussion about the production of eggs, the narrator states, "If the egg is impregnated, which happens when a woman is going to have a child, the egg will stay within the uterus; the thickened lining will provide nourishment for the budding human being in the early days of its development."[30] In this scenario, it is as if the woman gets herself fertilized and somehow makes herself pregnant. The conspicuous absence of the sperm made impregnation seem either automatic or self-induced. "Most eggs pass through without being fertilized," the narrator assures, yet "when this happens there is no use for potential nourishment and it passes from the body." This nourishment was identified as menstruation, depicted as a grey fluid-like substance pouring out of the vagina. A teenaged viewer would be hard-pressed to locate this "external opening" without a few more clues. Utterly unlike the grey liquid flowing out of the body in a matter of seconds, menstrual fluid remained unidentifiable. This crass representation dismissed sexual feelings but celebrated fertility, perpetuating the empty-vessel stereotype of teen students. Solely focusing on the end result of motherhood, it bypassed the process by which one might arrive there while reinforcing its inevitability. The laws of nature were now presumed to be abundantly clear. Menstruation was "one small part of nature's eternal plan for passing on the gift of life." This gift of life was repeated in the conclusion through life cycle tropes, moving from a toddler playing with a doll, to a girl at school studying a book, to a young woman in a formal wedding dress, to an adult woman cooing over a baby. In clear and accessible terms, the film scripted the path for the ideal white, maternal, hetero-normative woman of post–World War II America.

Just as motherhood was portrayed as a natural part of life, so too was femininity. Although learning to be feminine takes a lot of work, the film reduced the practices of femininity to mere "common sense." Though presented as an intuitive operation, femininity was shown to be a learned exercise in need of vigilant study and rehearsal. A good presentation of feminine demeanour meant attending to hygiene in all its forms. *The Story of Menstruation* suggested that girls "just use common sense" when bathing or doing exercise. Warned to avoid extremes, like picking up a large chair with one hand in order to vacuum underneath it, girls were nonetheless assured that "you can do practically everything you normally do." The image correlating with this assurance was a teenaged girl dancing with a boy. Wearing a lovely dress while he sported a suit, jacket, and tie, the girl danced a slow waltz. But when the two suddenly burst into swing, their clothes changed too. She morphed to wear a more casual skirt and sweater, while he sported a T-shirt, cardigan, and pants. The narrator chided, "Oh come now, we said [you can do] *practically* everything." Energetic movement pushed the limits, and the two quickly morphed back to the tame and measured waltz. Restraint and physical containment were shown to be hallmarks of feminine decorum.

As this last scene suggests, menstruation sparked transitions within relationships. As a whole, the educational film genre applauded female friends and encouraged supportive friendships while warning against those who constituted a bad influence. The girl smoker prompted the chastising comment: "Smoking, alcohol and drugs can damage the body and mind," raising fears of delinquency and sexual immorality. The girl smoker was no friend of femininity.[31] Alternatively, mothers might become friends rather than dictators. Films portrayed a companionate parenting model that must have been more fantasy than reality. Advice columns in popular magazines such as *Parents* warned of the danger that mothers represented for their impressionable daughters. Elizabeth Woodward reprimanded mothers' inadequacies and announced: "Maybe you're the one who has filled her with fear and superstition! You passed on to her what information you had. You dug into your own experience … and shared with her some of the bogey ideas you picked up when you were a teen-ager."[32] Blaming mothers for these superstitions, "the curse," and not bathing, along with failing to take up the mantle of femininity reflected a backlash against gender equity on the World War II homefront. Woodward lamented, "No wonder your daughter may be afraid to talk things over with you." No daughter, she implied, would wish to learn of the negative aspects of becoming a woman.[33] Woodward begged mothers, "[I]f *you* can't tell her what she wants to know adequately, sanely, unemotionally, scientifically … why not choose the source of her information?" Not surprisingly, this source was *The Story of Menstruation.*[34] The experts insinuated that mothers and daughters might experience improved relationships through the translational narrative of the menstrual education film.

The Story of Menstruation was recycled many times, so that women coming of age well into the 1960s still viewed it. In 1973, women's liberation levelled an influence on menstrual education films. The film *Naturally a Girl*— produced for Johnson & Johnson, makers of Modess, Stayfree, and Carefree brands of menstrual hygiene products—ended on a rather upbeat note: "Being a woman is one of the things I like best about myself." The feminist and the women's health movements inspired the narrative's content and tone. The film ended optimistically, telling young girls, "If you can dream, you can do it." Images of a teacher, secretary, flight attendant, and even telephone line repair person flashed on the screen to confirm the opportunities available to women, with the implication that after beginning menstruation, one would be able to participate in the new abundance afforded to liberated women.

Yet the film made a strong statement about the norms of femininity. *Naturally a Girl* opened with an off-camera interviewer asking, "What is menstruation?" to on-camera teens. Many girls smiled, nervous and too embarrassed to say much. Some said it was when a woman can have a baby. Others talked about a monthly cycle. The person who provided a perfect, textbook definition of menstruation was a white, teenaged boy. Even though a young man, he emerged as the expert, already vested with male authority. A few frames later, an African American teenaged boy shyly smiled and said, "Oh, I know what that is." The juxtaposition of the knowledgeable white boy with the befuddled girls and embarrassed black boy reinforced a disparity in the ability to access knowledge, power, and privilege.

The film stressed that being a woman means taking care of the body. Ideally, a girl would take care of her body for her own feelings of self-worth. The film also communicated the message that good grooming habits are performed for others, however, not just for oneself. "It's smart to keep looking smart," the film asserted, and pointed to the necessities of bathing and washing one's hair. *The Story of Menstruation* also promoted bathing, telling girls to take a warm bath and not overtax or shock the system with a cold or hot shower. This challenged the commonly held notion that bathing, regardless of temperature, might stop the menstrual flow.[35] *Naturally a Girl* stressed that the body sweats and produces more oil during menstruation so bathing is essential. In *Personal Health for Girls* (1972), a public health film, the setting of a department store provided ample opportunity to find products to maintain feminine standards of cleanliness. Not only invoking the skills a woman needed as a shopper, the film urged the use of deodorant, brush and comb, toothpaste, and acne treatment, if necessary. Young women were being trained to be highly self-conscious of natural body odours and their physical appearances. They were learning to objectify themselves by decorating themselves and masking their smells with the consumption of objects and purchase of technologies. In addition, *Personal Health for Girls* emphasized that the body is made more pleasing through exercise, which keeps the body "firm and attractive." This advice was juxtaposed against the image of a menopausal woman. Two girlfriends shopped for hats, scarves, and perfumes, and bumped into a heavy-set woman, who clearly had body odour. The girls scrunched up their faces in disgust at the smell; this woman was the antithesis of femininity. She appeared no longer to be fertile and seemed not to have cared for her body like an ideal woman should.

Decoding Technologies

The films worked hard to naturalize their scripting of femininity to make it seem that the learned performance was part of innate womanhood. In a like manner, technologies were presented as simply part of being a woman. Yet technologies—encompassing artifacts, knowledge, and practice—are not necessarily intuitive and must be learned.[36] The artifacts of menstrual hygiene also require a special skill set and an understanding of what their use means. Users must decode the artifacts to determine the directions and use set forth in the inscription created by designers. Specifically, the elastic belt, a daunting contraption, comes to mind. The dominant fastener of sanitary napkin technology from the 1920s until the early 1970s, the elastic belt with clasps held a pad between a woman's legs and near her crotch. Securing a sanitary pad with long tabs and discerning the subtle difference between the front and back of the pad were not intuitive acts, nor was the method to customize the pads to fit more comfortably between the legs. Lacing one's body through the belt, looping the sanitary pad through the tabs, then smoothing out undergarments and clothing took practice and flexibility. The gauze also had a tendency to chafe the inner thighs. The films sponsored by menstrual hygiene manufacturers explained and promoted menstrual hygiene in a broader attempt to domesticate the technologies and make them safe for adolescents to use regularly. The corporations skilfully merged product placement into the classroom, further legitimating menstrual hygiene as domesticated technologies, safe for teenagers.

The Story of Menstruation did not show sanitary pads outright, but Kimberly-Clark Corporation was identified as the sponsor. Following the film, a school nurse, teacher, or public health practitioner would talk about the film and hand out supplies of sanitary napkins. *It's Wonderful Being a Girl* (1968) depicted girls watching a similar film, creating the sense that girls going through puberty were all spectators of menstrual hygiene education films. Johnson & Johnson used "soft sell" in this film to alert viewers to stock up on feminine napkins and sanitary panties, made evident by the protagonist's mother, who kept her chest of drawers filled to the brim with the requisite supplies. *Naturally a Girl* (1973) encouraged girls to wear sanitary pads with a belt or the new technologies of sanitary and mini-pads with adhesives in order to "be prepared." It was hardly practical to wear a pad at all times, but the film implied that a girl nonetheless was irresponsible if she did not use available technology to manage her body at every moment. Technological management was the practice necessary to achieve the goal of menstrual health.

Naturally a Girl adopted a non-committal tone toward tampons, which were "small but absorbent" with "no worry of odour," thus neutralizing what had been a contested technology. With this technology, girls could swim during their periods instead of succumbing to constructs of menstrual inabilities. Condoning tampons, even ever so briefly in the film, departed from earlier films, which had ignored them. Tampons raised sensitive issues of sexuality, which the films were so adept at skirting. From their origin in 1936, tampons were deemed threats to a girl's virginity and vilified as sexual stimulants. Health practitioners debated the danger of tampons to the hymen, the anatomical proof of virginity. Many physicians advised against them. Mary Barton, a medical practitioner, confirmed the problem of a falsely lost virginity in "Review of the Sanitary Appliance with a Discussion on Intra Vaginal Packs." "It is difficult," she explained, "for virgins to use any internal pad without causing partial or total rupture of the hymen with regular use." She indicated that the "rupture has only forensic significance" but that "it is worth considering from the individual standpoint."[37] The prevailing wisdom held that virginal girls were just too young, too sexually inexperienced, for tampons. *Naturally a Girl* challenged this wisdom, however, in effect decoding and rewriting the tampon technology. Manufacturers pressed for a tame and innocuous inscription of tampons instead of the more titillating and phallic reading.

By the 1980s, health concerns for teens had shifted to becoming critical not of tampons but of all feminine hygiene practices. *Girl Stuff* (1982), sensitive to the concerns of public health, took the unusual step of discouraging teens from using vaginal sprays and douches. The film explained that the hymen, vaginal lining, and clitoris were very sensitive and that these chemicals did more harm than good. Despite a more anatomically correct discussion of the reproductive organs and this rather anti-corporate message, the link between purchasing menstrual hygiene technologies and femininity proved to be already fully ingrained in viewers. One teenager interviewed for the film said, "It makes me feel more feminine to have a nice fresh-smelling pad."[38] Fresh-smelling pads were generally heavily perfumed, and perfumes were identified as the culprit in many uncomfortable vaginal rashes. Perfumes were part of the technological arsenal to mask one's period and to "pass" as normal—as a non-bleeder, at least temporarily—so as to carry on with one's life as a happy-go-lucky teenager.[39]

Rising to the Challenge of Menstruation

To a certain degree, each film espoused a critical element of the menstrual script: the "buck-up camper" approach to menstrual management. First, the films assumed in girls a degree of trepidation, grumpiness, and poor attitude about menstruation. They also presumed that this disgruntlement would have an effect upon others. It was therefore presented as a girl's individual responsibility to have a proper attitude and mindset. Girls could test their mettle by suppressing any sign or sense of distress about their periods, thus enacting the feminine version of "pulling herself up by her bootstraps."[40] Suppressing the physical signs was assumed to ease presumed psychological discomfort, which made "toughing it out" more achievable through technological intervention. This circumscribed behaviour would not only benefit others, who would no longer have to endure her teenaged drama, but the teenager might find strength and even joy in overcoming the throes of her period and in sacrificing her personal feelings for the greater good. It reinforced the traits of being a selfless nurturer, which she was naturally supposed to be. I suggest that in suppressing her discomfort, the menstruating teenager could "pass" as her "normal" self, as if menstruation were not occurring and regardless of the fact that menstruation is normal and healthy for most teenagers and women. The films balanced carefully this dual argument that menstruation is natural and normal but nonetheless must be masked and made invisible.

The films encouraged girls to keep a personal calendar and mark off the days during which they menstruated in order to be prepared for the next round of bodily and emotional turmoil set in motion by their hormones. *The Story of Menstruation* explained that "it not only is a useful record of past performance but it comes in handy when you have to plan ahead." Describing menstruation as a performance was telling because it cast it as a willed behaviour. It presumed that a girl could evaluate it as if it were a mental or physical test such as a biology exam or the hundred-metre dash. The recommendation of planning also implied that she had control over her period. The film imposed on her the responsibility for managing her period with the corollary obligation of using a menstrual technology to do so. It also hinted that planning would enable her to hide menstruation from others, and that this was desirable and even a duty. Giving in to menstruation was an ironic lapse in femininity. Warning girls to plan ahead prepared them for using a menstrual hygiene technology, as well as for their fertile times of the month. The underlining notion of fertile times suggested knowledge that young girls supposedly should not possess yet was nearly unavoidable in discussing how and when to use the technology. The result of this early training could help them to track ovulation and become pregnant, under presumably appropriate circumstances, and, just as easily, to avoid pregnancy. By tracking performance, a girl could carry a pad around so that when the periodic event did occur, she could preserve the appearance of a fluid-free body.

The films were quite stern about the importance of overcoming menstrual malaise. *The Story of Menstruation* warned, "Do something about that slouch." By practising what the narrator termed "good living," girls might experience "new poise," which in turn would "lift morale." Succumbing to the throes of menstrual instability was, in essence, just downright rude.

"After all, no matter how you feel," the movie chided, "you have to live with people. You have to live with yourself, too," as if being pleasing to others was necessarily a tenet of one's self-esteem.[41] The movie painted a rather glum picture of girls sobbing in front of their vanity mirrors, lost and out of control of their emotions due to their periods. "And once you stop feeling sorry for yourself and take 'those days' in your stride, you'll find it easier to keep smiling and even tempered."[42] Girls might feel bloated, crampy, and miserably uncomfortable, but they were repeatedly instructed to act as if this were not a problem. Playing the role of the temporarily ill girl undermined the duties of an obedient, cheerful, feminine teenager and her smooth transition into nurturing, uncomplaining motherhood.

The recommendation to look on the sunny side remained a recurrent theme in many of the films. The 1949 public health film *Growing Girls* sympathized, "It's not unusual to have some discomfort the first few days of your period," but suggested glibly, "Try to ignore it."[43] The message was repeated in *It's Wonderful Being a Girl* (1968). "There's no need to mope around just because you're menstruating—but don't overdo it."[44] Gone were the days when women and girls might take time to rest during their periods, although by so doing, they risked this condition being used against them as evidence of their delicate constitutions. In many ways, a significant cultural moment was marked by describing menstruation as a healthy condition rather than as "the sicktime." It hardly seemed right, however, to disregard entirely real bodily signals of pain for the sake of "bucking up." In the film, the protagonist's friend, Jean, disabused protagonist Libby of the notion that she could just sit on the sidelines at the skating rink because she was not feeling so well. "That's no reason not to go," Jean retorted. And in fact, Libby did not successfully "pass" by sitting on the sidelines but rather was made more noticeable by missing out on the fun.

The theme continued with *Naturally a Girl* (1973): "No need to miss out on the fun just because you are menstruating. With a little planning ahead you can be ready and confident for anything."[45] This planning ahead meant packing menstrual hygiene technologies in a girl's purse or bag. By the early 1970s, this menstrual cover-up had become more feasible with the lavender plastic Tampax tampon case and the plastic menstrual wallet. The need to hide these menstrual cover-ups necessitated the use of a purse, a sure sign of a transition from girl to woman and a marker of adult femininity. Finally, the film asked: "Does everyone know when you're menstruating?" Reassuringly, the narrator responded, "No. If you don't tell, there's no way anyone can know."[46] The film reassured, while at the same time confirming that there was something to hide. "Normality" became the suppression of natural biological processes, and "natural" femininity was a learned performance successful only through technology. Women passed as normal by denying nature.

Conclusion

Menstrual hygiene education films were successful in naturalizing menstrual hygiene technology and technologizing menstruation. *The Story of Menstruation* insisted that "there is nothing strange or mysterious about menstruation" while making it something that must be hidden. The 1968 film *It's Wonderful Being a Girl*, sponsored by Johnson & Johnson, did the same. When Libby told her mother "I don't think I'll like it," her mother explained that menstruation was completely natural and "it's part of being a girl." The mother associated menstruation with a fairly pleasant natural process, sewing the seeds of proper behaviour in an appropriate response. Later in the film, when Libby was with her friend Jean at the pool, a third friend said she could not swim because she had "the curse" and was therefore "unwell." Libby and Jean understood menstrual slang but felt sorry for their friend because no one ever taught her proper menstrual demeanour.

The menstrual hygiene education film has become a staple of health and hygiene classes in schools across the United States. Historically for many girls, the rudimentary information about puberty, bodily change, and menstruation conveyed by the films provided the extent of their knowledge on this subject. To laud the films for this public service, however, is to overlook the other messages delivered by them. The legacy of anxious concealment and the mandate for technological intercession still persists. The scripting of femininity and motherhood into the storylines of the films and the artifacts reinforced traditional gender roles. The films also naturalized the concept of technological management of the body with the objects of tampons and sanitary napkins. Simultaneously, the films denaturalized normal bodily functions by requiring technological intervention to manage them. The corporate ties to education and public health, and the consumerism it bolstered, cannot be severed from the films' health claims. The domestication of menstrual hygiene technologies for teenagers' safe use, and the scripting of their meaning for adolescent audiences, sheds light on the intersections of gender, health, and popular culture and the political stakes of managing women's behaviour.

Notes

Thanks to the History of Medicine Reading Group at the University of Illinois, including Leslie Reagan, Paula Treichler, and in particular Matt Gambino, for reading early versions of this paper. Thanks also to Pat Gill for her revision suggestions.

1 There is a growing body of work on sex education, but it does not include menstrual hygiene education. See Robert Eberwein, *Sex Ed: Film, Video and the Framework of Desire* (New Brunswick, NJ: Rutgers University Press, 2000); Jeffrey Moran, *Teaching Sex: The Shaping of Adolescence in the 20th Century* (Cambridge: Harvard University Press, 2000). There is also a literature on menstrual education films, but it does not engage the artifacts of menstrual hygiene as technological. Margot Kennard discusses the politics, messages, and meanings of corporate-sponsored menstrual education films in "The Corporation in the Classroom: The Struggles over Meanings of Menstrual Education in Sponsored Films, 1947–1983," unpublished PhD dissertation, University of Wisconsin (1989), and also in "Producing Sponsored Films on Menstruation: The Struggle Over Meaning," in Elizabeth Ann Ellsworth and Marianne Whatley, eds., *Ideology of Images in Educational Media: Hidden Curriculums in the Classroom* (New York: Teachers College Press, 1990), pp. 57–73. For images of menstruation in film, television, and media, see Janice Delaney, Mary Jane Lupton, and Emily Toth, *The Curse: A Cultural History of Menstruation*, 2nd ed. (Champaign: University of Illinois Press, 1988); Elizabeth Arveda Kissling, "On the Rag on Screen: Menarche in Film and Television," *Sex Roles* 46.12 (2002): 5–12; Michelle H. Martin, "Postmodern Periods: Menstruation Media in the 1990s," *The Lion and the Unicorn* 23.3 (September 1999): 395–414.

2 "Glory of Woman: An Introduction to Prescriptive Literature," Rare Book, Manuscript, and Special Collections Library, Duke University, http://library.duke.edu/specialcollections/bingham/guides/glory/index.html (accessed 2 June 2010).

3 Madeline Akrich, "The De-Scription of Technical Objects," in Wiebe E. Bijker and John Law, eds., *Shaping Technology/Building Society: Studies in Sociotechnical Change* (Cambridge: MIT Press, 1992), pp. 205–24.

4 Akrich, "De-Scription of Technical Objects," p. 208.

5 Roger Silverstone, *Consuming Technologies: Media and Information in Domestic Spaces* (London: Routledge, 1992); Maren Hartmann, Thomas Berker, Yves Punie, and Katie Ward, *Domestication of Media and Technology* (Berkshire, UK: Open University Press, 2005).

6 *It's Wonderful Being a Girl*, film collection, A/V Geeks, n.d. See also the Prelinger Collection and Prelinger Archives, http://www.archive.org/details/prelinger (accessed 27 August 2007).

7 I use the term "girl" in the spirit of Modern Girl around the World Research Group, who argue, "'Girl' signifies the contested status of women who lie outside childhood and outside contemporary social codes and conventions relating to marriage, sexuality and motherhood and is a preferable theoretical alternative to the overdetermined category 'woman,'" in Tani Barlow et al., "The Modern Girl around the World: A Research Agenda and Preliminary Findings," *Gender and History* 17.2 (August 2005): 291.

8 Sharra Vostral, *Under Wraps: A History of Menstrual Hygiene and Technologies of Passing* (Lanham, MD: Rowman & Littlefield, 2008), ch. 2.

9 *The Spirit of '43*, A Walt Disney Donald Duck Technicolor Film (1943), YouTube, http://www.youtube.com/watch?v=WaVTc-Ur89Q (accessed 28 August 2007).

10 Leslie Reagan, Nancy Tomes, and Paula Treichler, eds., *Medicine's Moving Pictures: Medicine, Health and Bodies in American Film and Television* (Rochester: University of Rochester Press, 2007).

11 "Introduction," in Reagan, Tomes, and Treichler, eds., *Medicine's Moving Pictures*.

12 *Don't Spread Germs*, directed by John Krish (UK: Central Office of Information for Ministry of Health, 1948), http://www.archive.org/details/dont_spread_germs_TNA (accessed 1 August 2007).

13 "Introduction," in Moran, *Teaching Sex*; Janet Golden, Richard Alan Meckel, and Heather Munro Prescott, *Children and Youth in Sickness and Health: A Handbook and Guide* (New York: Greenwood, 2004), pp. 85–106.

14 Ilana Nash, *American Sweethearts: Teenage Girls in Twentieth-Century Popular Culture* (Bloomington: Indiana University Press, 2006), p. 23.

15 On teenage consumerism, see Nash, *American Sweethearts*, pp. 25–6. On menstrual advertising, see Debra Merskin, "Adolescence, Advertising and the Ideology of Menstruation," *Sex Roles* 40.1 (June 1999): 941–57; Michelle H. Martin, "'No One Will Ever Know Your Secret!' Commercial Puberty Pamphlets for Girls from the 1940s to the 1990s," in Claudia Nelson and Michelle H. Martin, eds., *Sexual Pedagogies: Sex Education in Britain, Australia, and America, 1879–2000* (New York: Palgrave, 2003); Lara Friedenfelds, "Materializing the Modern, Middle-Class Body: Menstruation in the Twentieth-Century United States," unpublished PhD dissertation, Harvard University (2003).

16 Joan Jacobs Brumberg, "'Something Happens to Girls': Menarche and the Emergence of the Modern American Hygienic Imperative," *Journal of the History of Sexuality* 4.1 (July 1993): 99–127; Joan Brumberg, *The Body Project: An Intimate History of American Girls* (New York: Random House, 1997).

17 Kelly Schrum, *Some Wore Bobby Sox: The Emergence of Teenage Girls' Culture, 1920–1945* (New York: Palgrave, 2004), p. 3.

18 Vostral, *Under Wraps*, ch. 3.

19 *The Story of Menstruation*, Walt Disney Productions, with Kimberly-Clark Corporation (1946).

20 Eric Schaefer, *Bold! Daring! Shocking! True!: A History of Exploitation Films, 1919–1959* (Durham: Duke University Press, 1999).

21 "Review of *The Story of Menstruation*," *Journal of the American Medical Association* 133 (5 April 1947): 1033.

22 "Review of *The Story of Menstruation*."

23 Kennard, "Corporation in the Classroom," p. 35.

24 Stefan Kanfer, *Serious Business: The Art and Commerce of Animation in America from Betty Boop to Toy Story* (New York: Da Capo, 2000), p. 179.

25 Nicholas Sammand, *Babes in Tomorrowland: Walt Disney and the Making of the American Child, 1930–1960* (Durham: Duke University Press, 2005); Steven Watts, *The Magic Kingdom: Walt Disney and the American Way of Life* (Boston: Houghton Mifflin, 1997).

26 *Story of Menstruation*.

27 Catherine M. Roach, *Mother/Nature: Popular Culture and Environmental Ethics* (Bloomington: Indiana University Press, 2003).

28 Nelly Oudshoorn, *Beyond the Natural Body: Archaeology of Sex Hormones* (New York: Routledge, 1994).

29 *Story of Menstruation*.

30 *Story of Menstruation*.

31 *Personal Health for Girls*, Coronet Instructional Films (1972).

32 Elizabeth Woodward, "Do You Scare Her to Death?" *Parents* 24 (1949): 52.

33 "Growing Up and Liking It" (Milltown, NJ: Personal Products Corporation, 1944), p. 5, located at Museum of Menstruation, Menarche Education Booklets, http://www158.pair.com/hfinley/guli44a.htm (accessed 6 November 2000).

34   Woodward, "Do You Scare Her to Death?" p. 52.

35   "How to Tell Your Daughter," *Parents Magazine* 22 (December 1947): 138.

36   Ronald Kline, "Construing 'Technology' as 'Applied Science': Public Rhetoric of Scientists and Engineers in the United States, 1880–1945," *Isis* 86.2 (1995): 194–221.

37   Mary Barton, "Review of the Sanitary Appliance with a Discussion on Intra-Vaginal Packs," *British Medical Journal* 1 (25 April 1942): 524–5.

38   *Girl Stuff*, Churchill Films (1982).

39   Vostral, *Under Wraps*, ch. 6.

40   Daryl Costos, Ruthie Ackerman, and Lisa Paradis refer to this as the "grin-and-bear-it" model in "Recollections of Menarche: Communication between Mothers and Daughters Regarding Menstruation," *Sex Roles* 46.1–2 (January 2002): 49–59. I employ the colloquial "buck-up camper" because it connotes activity and participation rather than "grin-and-bear-it," which implies endurance and suffering.

41   *Story of Menstruation*.

42   *Story of Menstruation*.

43   *Growing Girls*, Film Producers Guild, National Committee for Visual Aids in Education (1949).

44   *It's Wonderful Being a Girl*, Johnson & Johnson (1968).

45   *Naturally a Girl*, Johnson & Johnson (1973).

46   *Naturally a Girl*.

Controlling Conception: Images of Women, Safety, Sexuality, and the Pill in the Sixties

Heather Molyneaux

The history of the birth control pill has become intertwined in North American popular culture and imagination with the so-called sexual revolution of the sixties.[1] Forms of birth control existed prior to the sixties, but the pill is usually depicted by historians as the ultimate material representation of the sexual revolution.[2] Images of the pill in pharmaceutical advertisements in the sixties presented the pill not as a tool for sexual revolution but as a "natural" means of family planning. These advertisements articulated the fears in popular culture of two potential consequences of the pill: negative side effects and immorality.

In the wake of the thalidomide tragedy, where hundreds of children were born with deformities as the result of a sleeping aid, pharmaceutical companies attempted to advertise what was to become a billion dollar industry—the birth control pill. Striving to portray this new form of birth control as "natural," companies depicted women alongside flowers in advertisements for the pill; this visual imagery, published in medical journals, was meant not only to calm public fears about sexual promiscuity but also to alleviate concern about the potential health hazards of the pill.

Images in birth control advertisements not only presented the pill as natural and therefore healthy, but also depicted the consumer of the pill as moral. By presenting the consumer of the pill as a white, middle-class, married woman (sometimes already a mother), birth control pill advertising drew on popular symbols of morality in order to quell fears that the pill would lead to promiscuity.

While there were changes in the depiction of women in pharmaceutical advertisements from the fifties to the sixties, these differences were far from revolutionary. In the sixties, the image of the ideal and healthy Canadian woman remained white, middle-class, and heterosexual. By examining the history of the birth control pill in Canada—more specifically, by analyzing the representation of women in birth control pill advertisements in the *Canadian Medical Association Journal (CMAJ)*[3]—I argue that while the pill was a revolutionary new birth control method, birth control pill advertisements do not present clear evidence of a "sexual revolution" in the sixties.

Sexual Revolution?

The mythical images of suburbs and family values of the post–World War II era and the association of the pill with the sexual revolution of the sixties are stereotypes that reduce the diverse experiences of men and women in postwar North America.[4] Activities associated with the sexual revolution— such as premarital sex, the spacing of births, and the limiting of family size— were already occurring in the fifties, well before the arrival of the pill.[5] That is not to say that changes were not taking place in the sixties, but historians and feminist scholars are now questioning the extent of these changes.[6] Sheila Jeffreys, author of *Anti-Climax: A Feminist Perspective on the Sexual Revolution,* notes that while there was an increased stress on female sexuality, this message was tempered with the notion that women should only be enjoying sex within the confines of marriage.[7]

The case of the so-called sexual revolution demonstrates how greater discourse related to sexuality did not translate into greater sexual freedom. Instead, increased discourse normalized sexuality and created limits. As Michel Foucault argues, increases in the discourse on sexuality did not eradicate taboos surrounding sexuality because discourses on sexuality "never ceased to hide the thing it was speaking about."[8] In the sixties, discourses written by advertisers, journalists, physicians, and scientists attempted to defuse the potential threat that women posed to male power by placing greater emphasis on the institution of marriage as well as on the importance of physician control.

Regulating Menstruation

Early advertisements for the pill were marketed under the name Enovid as a menstrual regulator and not a contraceptive, similar to late-nineteenth- and early-twentieth-century advertisements for purported abortifacients.[9] At first glance, these advertisements appear to be more sexually and socially liberating than later marketing campaigns because they do not focus on women's marital status. However, even early Enovid ads presented both biological and social limitations for women. The first advertisement in the *CMAJ* for the new birth control pill did not explicitly present the medication as a method of contraception (fig. 1). Enovid, first approved by the Food and Drug Administration (FDA) for sale in the United States as a regulator

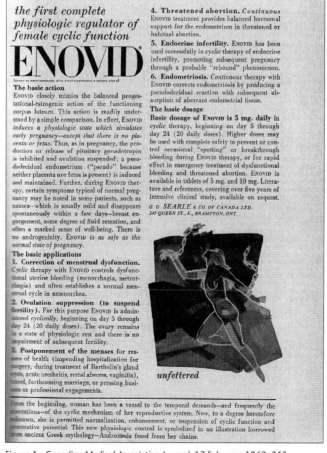

Figure 1   *Canadian Medical Association Journal*, 17 February 1962: 353.

for menstrual dysfunction in 1957, was available in Canada from 1961, though not approved for use as a birth control pill until 1963. Until 1963 advertisements for Enovid in the *CMAJ* did not list "contraception" or "birth control" as an application for the drug. Instead, phrases like "ovulation suppression to suspend fertility" were employed, implying its contraceptive function. By 1959, 1.5 million women in the United States had prescriptions for Enovid. It is doubtful that these women suddenly discovered they had a menstrual disorder; it is quite likely that many of them used Enovid as a contraceptive.[10]

The image on the bottom right-hand corner of the advertisement (fig. 1) represents the Greek mythological figure Andromeda, with her wrists bound by chains. The text explains that the drug Enovid normalizes, enhances, or suspends procreative potential, thus freeing women from the aberration and demands of their cycles. The chains that bind Andromeda represent the reproductive cycle that ties her down and acts as punishment. The imagery and related text in the advertisement present menstruation as negative. The woman is trapped by her menses and is presumably waiting to be rescued by a male hero, perhaps the physician who is needed to prescribe the medication.

The advertisement did not necessarily give physicians an entirely negative representation of women. Application number three in this ad lists not only health as a reason for postponement of the menses but "travel, forthcoming marriage, or pressing business or professional engagements," which suggests that women can engage in travel and business, but not while they are menstruating. While the Enovid imagery and text may seem to be liberating for women, it ultimately has negative connotations. Menstruation is depicted as an oppressive biological function that figuratively (as depicted in the image) chains women and literally (as mentioned in the text) acts as a barrier for women's success in the business world.

Advertisements in which Enovid was marketed as a birth control pill were not published in the *CMAJ* until 1961. Neither were articles on the birth control pill, even though the pill was developed in the fifties. There may have been some hesitation on the part of Canadian physicians to discuss issues of contraception—after all, a section of the 1892 Criminal Code restricted writing on contraception. This section reads: "Everyone is guilty of an indictable offense and liable to two years' imprisonment who knowingly, without lawful excuse or justification, offers to sell, advertises, publishes an advertisement of or has for sale or disposal any medicine, drug or article intended or represented as a means of preventing conception or causing abortion."[11] However, this section of the Criminal Code was not repealed until 1969, long after birth control pills were advertised and written about in the *CMAJ*.

While birth control remained illegal in the twentieth century, this did not mean that birth control information was not circulated. In 1930 factory owner A.R. Kaufman established the Parent's Information Bureau (PIB), and nurses working for the PIB distributed birth control pamphlets to the working class. In 1936 PIB nurse Dorothea Palmer was charged under the Criminal Code with distributing birth control information. She was not convicted during the 1937 trial because she claimed that she was working "for the public good" by giving birth control information only to married women.[12]

Few people were ever tried under this section of the Criminal Code, and only one person was convicted: in 1962 Harold Fine was found guilty of advertising condoms as contraceptives and was subsequently imprisoned.[13] To circumvent the Criminal Code, pharmacists usually advertised condoms as a form of disease prevention. Many Canadian physicians fitted and dispensed diaphragms and spermicidal jelly before the invention of the pill; however, according to a 1962 *CMAJ* article, no physicians were ever convicted. In a *CMAJ* article on the "Legal Implications of the Non-therapeutic Practices of Doctors," Manitoba lawyer G.P.R. Tallin argued that physicians prescribing birth control pills could claim that this practice was "for the public good," and therefore they would not be convicted of misconduct.[14]

Physicians may have avoided dispensing birth control advice because of the Criminal Code, but another, more likely, theory is that physicians did not consider conception and contraception a "scientific" topic until the legalization of the birth control pill. This new contraceptive, in pill form, was seen as a scientific product, a prescribed "preventative medicine."[15] Arguably, the birth control pill was novel and differed from other experimental drugs because it was the first prescription medication in the modern era produced and prescribed for a healthy consumer.[16] FDA officer Dr. Pasquale DeFelice reviewed the Searle application for Enovid and noted that "everything else up to that time was a drug to treat a diseased condition. Here suddenly was a pill to be used to treat a healthy person and for long term use."[17] Some physicians argued that the pill was in fact a preventative medicine. Historian Carole McCann notes that obstetricians in the early twentieth century stated that while pregnancy and childbirth were natural processes, the potential for pathology was ever present.[18] If pregnancy could be viewed as potential pathology, then the birth control pill could be seen as a preventative medicine.

Medical Concerns

While the general public did not express grave reservations about the potential side effects of the pill until the late sixties, physicians expressed some hesitancy about the new contraception in the early half of the decade, partly because of the occurrence of limb malformations associated with the use of thalidomide during pregnancy. Thalidomide was marketed as a sedative or tranquilizer, and was also used as a sleep aid. Assumed to be non-toxic, with no side effects, thalidomide was considered safe for pregnant women.[19] Shortly after its release onto the Canadian market in April 1961,[20] the negative effects of thalidomide became known to physicians. In December 1961 companies began sending letters to Canadian physicians warning against prescribing the drug to pregnant and premenopausal women because of the occurrence of congenital defects—the most severe involving deformation of the limbs, ears, forehead, and lips—as well as "gastrointestinal, cardiac and renal lesions."[21] On 2 March 1962, the drug was pulled from the Canadian market.[22] While Canada did not license thalidomide until four years after its release in Germany, the drug was not removed from Canadian markets until three months after it was banned in Germany, England, and Australia.[23] In less than one year on the market, thalidomide affected between ninety and 125 Canadian children born to mothers who had taken even the smallest amount of thalidomide during pregnancy.[24]

A 1963 *CMAJ* article warned that a similar situation could occur—and that physicians needed to be aware of and diligently report malformations—as a consequence of birth control pill usage.[25] As a result, possible links between the pill and headaches, premature menopause, arterial emboli, asthmogenic effects, and thromboebolic disease were reported in *CMAJ* editorials and letters to the journal from 1966 to 1968.[26] Although some *CMAJ* readers challenged these links,[27] many Canadian physicians prescribed the birth control pill with reservations.

Birth control pill manufacturing in the early sixties was a million-dollar industry for pharmaceutical companies, which needed to alleviate reservations the medical profession held about potential hazards of the pill. By the mid-sixties, birth control pill advertisements revolved around the crucial idea that the pill, while chemically engineered, was "natural" because it was safe and simulated a woman's natural menstrual cycle. The 1966 "In Harmony with Nature" Norlestrin birth control pill advertisement may not seem to symbolically represent a woman (fig. 2). A birth control pill dial dispenser is shown nestled on daisy leaves. The light in the photograph is diffused, resulting in soft pastel colours and amorphous lines. The light pink of the

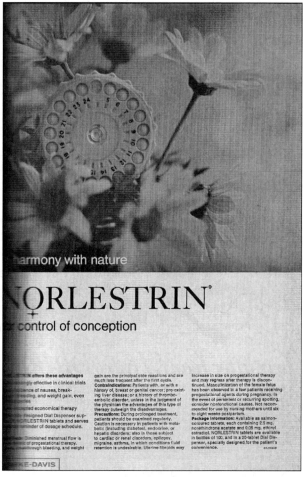

Figure 2   *Canadian Medical Association Journal,* 12 March 1966: 15.

pills and the baby blue hue of the dispenser contrast with the muted green, yellow, and white of the daisies and stems.

The package is emphasized because before 1962 women were expected to take twenty pills, count five days, and start again. This method was difficult at times because the day women started again would change from month to month. In 1962 the first package specially designed for the pill was created by David Wagner, neither a doctor nor a scientist, but a concerned husband. His prototype, the Dialpack, a round plastic pill dispenser, was later copied by the drug companies Searle and Ortho Pharmaceutical.[28]

While the packaging of the medication is featured, this advertisement also associates the pill with flowers. By showing the pill resting on the leaves of daisies, the pill is depicted as an extension of nature. The image is infused with soft pastel tones synonymous with femininity and ultimately with women. The connection between the pill, nature, and women was not coincidental. The same theme emerged in an Oracon contraception advertisement in 1966 (fig. 3). The ad, which includes the text "So close to nature that it simulates the natural menstrual pattern," does not depict the pill and dispenser. An image of a large white flower in full bloom is superimposed onto the hair, right cheek, neck, and shoulder of a young woman. She has short hair that is curled and styled, and her long eyelashes and full lips convey a serene expression and a subtle smile. Her bare neck and shoulder indicate that she might possibly be naked. Here nature and woman visually and quite literally become one.

The association of the birth control pill Oracon with nature in the imagery of the advertisement not only indicated its safety but also reassured the reader that the so-called natural menstrual pattern would remain. The text on the second page of the advertisement states that Oracon's hormone sequence of estrogen alone for sixteen days followed by estrogen and progestogen for the last five "simulates the natural female cycle, the endometrial response is more normal than with combination products and menstrual bleeding is regular

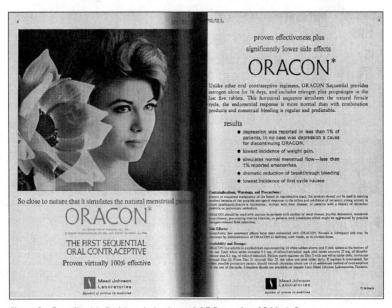

Figure 3   *Canadian Medical Association Journal*, 17 December 1966: 4–5.

and predictable." The birth control pill is described as natural because it does not disturb the menstrual cycle but in fact mimics the "natural" state of menstruation.

Consumers of the Pill

While the advertisements in the *CMAJ* focused on connecting the pill with women and nature, the articles emphasized the scientific importance of the product to humankind. Rather than stating the pill's benefit to women, articles in both popular magazines and medical journals cited the biggest benefit of the pill as population control. *Chatelaine* magazine, and not the *CMAJ*, published the first Canadian article that connected the birth control pill to the issue of population control. This is not surprising, for, as historian Bernard Asbell notes, medical journals were reluctant to publish papers on contraception. Gregory Pincus, one of the scientists responsible for creating the birth control pill, announced at a Canadian conference on hormones in the mid-fifties that he had published the first medical findings on the pill in the *Ladies Home Journal,* a popular women's magazine in the United States.[29]

In her quantitative study of articles on birth control in five major American women's magazines, media arts scholar Dolores Flamiano notes that articles on the pill were published in the fifties. Once birth control became a matter of public policy and the scientific problem of population control emerged, the issue of birth control in the fifties became a "masculine discourse unsuitable for discussion in women's magazines."[30] While coverage on the issue of birth control disappeared from the pages of women's magazines in the United States, such coverage increased in scientific journals.[31]

This was not the case in Canada. During the fifties, the *CMAJ* was silent on issues of birth control, whereas *Chatelaine* published an article on the subject. Medical researchers looked to women's magazines to gauge public reaction to medical technologies. A 1962 article from the women's magazine *Good Housekeeping* was footnoted in a *CMAJ* study on the pill, along with references from the leading medical journals.[32] Historian Valerie J. Korinek's observation that the editors of *Chatelaine* in the fifties and sixties "combined commercial success with a feminist agenda" may account for this difference in the content of American and Canadian women's magazines: *Chatelaine's* editors may have been willing to publish articles on the pill because of their feminist beliefs.[33]

In the 1953 article "The Pill that Could Shake the World," *Chatelaine* author Gerald Anglin discussed the pros and cons of a potential new birth control method in pill form. While Anglin noted that the pill had the potential either to create happier Canadian families or to increase promiscuity and lower morals, the article focused mainly on saving the world from overpopulation.[34] This theme continued in articles in both popular and medical journals. Two of the three articles in the *CMAJ* opened the subject of clinical trials of the pill with an introduction to the necessity of population control.[35] The subject was deemed so pressing to physicians that an article devoted to the topic was published in the journal in 1964 by Vancouver biologist L.S. Anderson. Anderson's article, "The Mushroom Crowd: Social and Political Aspects of Population Pressure," stated that physicians need to be concerned with population pressure because of the influence of overpopulation on standards of living, and, ultimately, on human health.[36] The author praised Japan's efforts at population control while noting that India was in urgent need of birth control.[37]

The birth control pill was hailed by manufacturers as a social policy instrument and a solution to the problem of overpopulation. John G. Searle, chairman of the G.D. Searle Company, stated that the company's greatest "contribution to mankind" was Enovid, not because it in any way liberated women but because "it is a positive answer to a world threatened by overpopulation, and the resulting poor subsistence, poor shelter, and poor education that surplus peoples are forced to endure."[38] Authors in popular and medical journals, as well as scientists and pharmaceutical company representatives, stressed the pill's role in controlling population growth and poverty rather than its role in providing women with control over reproductive health and sexual freedom.

While the early articles focused on population control overseas, the reality is that the pill was destined for North American households, where pharmaceutical companies and physicians could realize lucrative profits. Advertisements for the pill did not emphasize population control or a revolution in women's sex lives. Instead, these advertisements focused on the importance of the pill to white middle-class women in committed (married) relationships.

The emphasis on the pill as a medication for married women is evident in the imagery of birth control pill ads in the *CMAJ*; it can be seen even in the simplest advertising designs. One example is the 1963 birth control pill ad for Ortho-Novum (fig. 4). Like the advertisement for Norlestrin, where the pill dispenser rests on daisy leaves (fig. 2), the packaging of the pill is emphasized. However, so is the hand. It's obvious that the string tied around the finger as a reminder to take the pill is no longer needed, since the pills are nicely sorted out into days of the week. Also, the elegant hand, with smooth white skin

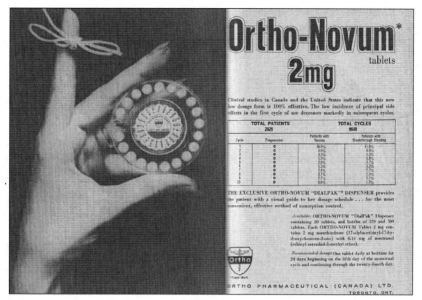

Figure 4   *Canadian Medical Association Journal,* 2 February 1963: 341–2.

and long fingers sporting well manicured and polished nails, indicates that the woman attached to the hand is young, attractive, and wealthy enough to avoid manual labour. In the centre of the page, a gold wedding band shines on the hand's ring finger.

In birth control pill advertisements in the mid-sixties, the image of the married woman took centre stage. A 1966 Lyndiol advertisement presented the pill as an important part of newlywed life (fig. 5). In this advertisement, we are transported to the doctor's office; he is poised and alert, with pencil in hand and paper within reach. From our vantage point, we can clearly see the woman seated in front of him. She is smiling, her head tilted, and is nervously playing with one of the many strands of pearls around her neck. This action gives us an unobstructed view of her left hand and the gold wedding band around her ring finger. Underlined on the second page of the advertisement is the phrase "For your newlywed patients." Further text urges physicians to contact the Canadian office of the Organon pharmaceutical company for sample kits to distribute to patients as a "Special family planning guide."

The image of the birth control pill user in the early to mid-sixties was almost exclusively restricted to married women, but not necessarily to the newlywed. In this 1966 Secrovin ad, a mother and a daughter are seen standing in a wind-blown field (fig. 6). The little girl gleefully skips along

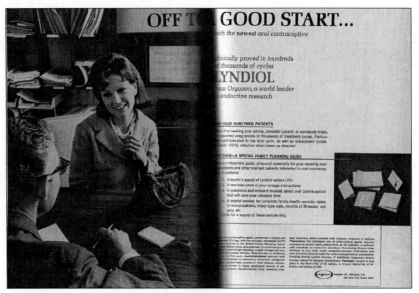

Figure 5   *Canadian Medical Association Journal*, 11 June 1966: 10–11.

while holding her mother's hand. The figures are presented as silhouettes, so it is unclear if the mother is holding her hand up to control her hair or if she is using her hand to protect her eyes from the sun while she gazes across the field of grass. At any rate, the scene is idyllic and implies that this mother, with the aid of the birth control pill Secrovin, is free to lavish individual attention on her daughter and to frolic uninhibited in a field without the fear of an unplanned pregnancy.

The image of the birth control pill user as wife and mother is not a surprising one, since the pill in North America was viewed as a means of family planning. A 1961 editorial in the *CMAJ* on the pill noted that "the fundamental aim of birth control [as opposed to population control, is not] a preventative medicine against pregnancy but as a method to limit the number of pregnancies."[39] Other advertisements and articles presented the married woman as the ideal consumer of the pill. The only explicit mention of an unmarried consumer in the *CMAJ* appeared in a letter to the journal concerning potential side effects, and here the pill was prescribed to control a menstrual dysfunction.[40] The results of the only *CMAJ* survey on birth control pill consumers were published in 1965 and included only the responses of married women. One of the survey questions asked for the husband's opinion of oral contraceptives.[41] Author C.A. Douglas Ringrose did not reveal

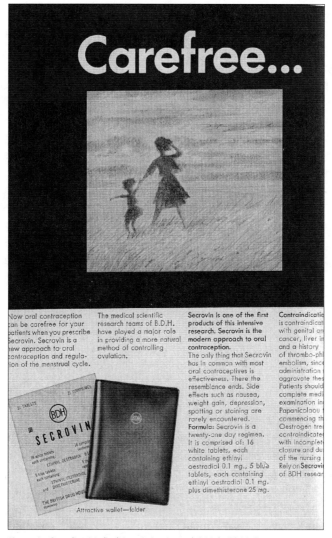

Figure 6   *Canadian Medical Association Journal,* 16 July 1966: 1.

what these husbands' opinions were but notes that 22 per cent of the married women surveyed believed sexual morals would decline because of the pill's ability to abolish the fear of pregnancy and its potential availability to single women or teenagers.[42]

Accessibility

Due to rising awareness about birth control and easier access to the pill, prescriptions for the birth control pill had increased by the mid-sixties. However, accessibility was still an issue.[43] Single women found it difficult to get prescriptions for the pill, and working-class married women found the pill's cost prohibitive. In sixties America, only middle-class women with money could afford the pill. In 1960 the annual retail price for the pill was $100; by 1965 the price had dropped to $25, but even this was too expensive for working-class women. Some American women obtained the pill at a cheaper price in clinics, but it remained unaffordable for many women until the late sixties.[44]

In Canada, the birth control pill was more affordable. A 1961 *CMAJ* editorial listed the physician's cost to be $24 to $36 if the medication was obtained "with discreet purchasing," but the patient's cost would have been higher.[45] A 1962 *Chatelaine* letter to the editor stated the cost to be four dollars a month, beyond some women's means.[46] Canadian women who did not have access to a family doctor or hospital had the most difficulty procuring prescriptions for the pill.

Planned Parenthood clinics offered the pill at a reduced rate, but access was severely limited. In 1937 birth control clinics operated in Toronto, Windsor, and Hamilton.[47] By 1960 the only official Planned Parenthood clinic was in Hamilton, Ontario, while there were 340 Planned Parenthood clinics in Great Britain.[48]

Also, as noted in the *CMAJ*, Canadian medical students received an inadequate education in fertility control.[49] A survey in 1964 concluded that, unlike American medical schools, "routine inclusion of information on birth control in premarital counseling and in postpartum examinations was provided in a minority of schools," and only two out of the seven Canadian medical schools surveyed "taught that instruction in birth control should be given at the request of any patient," not just married women or women with menstrual difficulties.[50] Some Canadian physicians felt that the birth control pill could cause "abortion of a fertilized ovum" and therefore were morally opposed to prescribing the pill.[51] Even if some women did have access to a physician, that physician might not be well informed on the topic and could potentially deny prescriptions.

Changing Imagery?

Attitudes surrounding the pill and its users changed in the late sixties. American historian Lara Marks comments that while the ideal pill consumer was "older women with children, the oral contraceptive was rapidly to become the contraceptive of choice among young women with no children."[52] These young women ideally were married, like the women depicted in many of the *CMAJ* birth control pill advertisements. The mainstream press continued to condemn sexually active unmarried women.[53]

Advertisements in the late sixties, such as the 1969 advertisement for Serial 28 (fig. 7), began to present the birth control pill consumer's marital status as ambiguous. Like the ad for Norlestrin (fig. 2), the text of the Serial 28 ad emphasizes the packaging, no longer a system of twenty pills, but

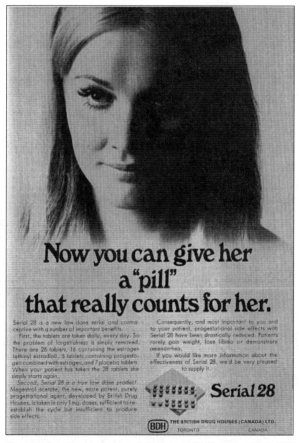

Figure 7   *Canadian Medical Association Journal*, 13 December 1969: 117.

twenty-eight, making it easier for women to determine when to take the pill. The imagery is quite striking. The advertisement presents a head shot of a beautiful young woman. The emphasis here is on her eyes, her long eyelashes, and not her hands. She looks directly into the camera. Her gaze suggests sexual freedom and perhaps even hints at potential promiscuity. Unlike in early advertisements, this pill consumer could be either single or married, yet still under a doctor's supervision.

Even though the married woman was no longer the only type of woman represented, by the seventies, the image of the ideal birth control user remained, for the most part, unchanged. Married women were still represented as ideal users of the birth control pill, even as advertisement images expanded to include more "types of women," such as the 21-Pak Norlestrin advertisement (fig. 8). The first page of the advertisement displays the different faces of seven women, arranged in a circular pattern around a packet of birth control pills. At the centre of the ad, in the middle of the pills, is a floral motif, indicating once again that the pill is natural and therefore safe.

On the second page of the ad, text proclaims that the pill is "now for all of them" and the same images of the women are labelled according to their reasons for needing the medication. Of the seven women depicted, three are labelled as mothers or wives, and a fourth, labelled "primipara," displays a wedding band. The marital status of three of the women, however, remains ambiguous, as their reasons are listed as "irregular," "side-effect prone," and "easily confused." A woman labelled as "irregular" is not necessarily taking the pill for the prevention of pregnancy but for medical reasons. The image

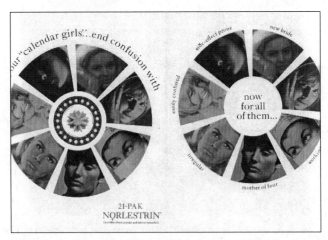

Figure 8   *Canadian Medical Association Journal*, 17 June 1967: 13–14.

associated with "side-effect prone" is a young woman whose face is partially obstructed as a result of the lighting. Both "irregular" and "side-effect prone" are frowning. Perhaps the most interesting image of these three is "easily confused," represented by an attractive young blond woman, the only one of the seven "Calendar" girls who exhibits a toothy grin.

While the image of the pill user changed in the late sixties, the stereotypes about this female-controlled contraception prevailed. This 1970 ad for Orifer, a prenatal supplement, was a direct reflection of the belief that women are irresponsible, liable to forget, and are to blame for the pill's failure (fig. 9). The ad reads, "The other pill: Don't let her forget this one." In smaller text below this image, the ad proclaims that "Orifer is the other pill. The one most women take after discovering they have one of the pills left over." A young woman is depicted as ruefully holding up an Orifer tablet with her left hand, which bears a wedding band. The bottle of prenatal vitamins rests upon her growing stomach. This ad served to reaffirm medical control by indicating that women are unable to control their own minds and bodies, and therefore need medical monitoring.

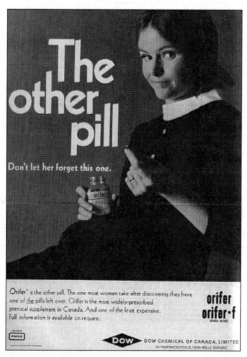

Figure 9   *Canadian Medical Association Journal*, 31 January 1970: 136.

Public Concerns

The pill, declared 100 per cent effective, was not the end of the physician-centred process of reproduction. In the early sixties, physicians speculated on the pill's efficacy. A 1963 *CMAJ* editorial noted that while the pill was effective, "unintelligent use or carelessness can leave the way open for pregnancy."[54] As an alternative explanation, Ron Kenyon, in a 1961 *Chatelaine* article, wrote that women naturally rebel against contraception due to a deep subconscious need to bear children.[55] Lawrence Galton, in his monthly column "What's New in Health," cited a University of Washington study concluding that women who forget to take the pill daily are either immature or do so as revenge against their husbands.[56] In response, Mrs. D. Harrison from Glenbush, Saskatchewan, wrote that the notion of women getting pregnant to spite their husbands was just part of the warped thinking on the part of doctors "who pass themselves off as intelligent men."[57] The Orifer ad argues that where the patient has failed, the doctor will prevail. As the Orifer ad and the *CMAJ* and *Chatelaine* articles indicate, women were blamed for the failure of the birth control pill.[58]

Women were also blamed for some of the pill's side effects. John Rock, one of the pill's creators, noted that "the pill merely provided a natural means of fertility control such as nature uses after ovulation and during pregnancy."[59] Side effects such as weight gain were easily dismissed as results of a state of false pregnancy or a woman's poor dietary habits, not the pill.[60] A 1970 *CMAJ* editorial questioned the links between contraception, depression, and migraine by claiming that these "side effects" were sometimes manifestations of the patient's own neurosis and "related to the previous personality of the individual rather than to the pill."[61] But many Canadian women, Mrs. Harrison included, challenged the notion that women were to blame for the pill's inadequacy.

In the late sixties, just as distribution was legalized,[62] the general public began to question the pill's safety. In 1968 the first Canadian court case involving thalidomide poisoning began.[63] Babies disabled by thalidomide poisoning were growing into visibly deformed children. The timing of these court cases coincided with early-seventies publications on the thalidomide children's plight and a public questioning of the safety of the birth control pill.

Based on a British report on drug safety, a 1970 *CMAJ* article stated that Ottawa authorities were searching for a better pill, one containing a lower dosage of estrogen, to decrease the incidence of clotting.[64] The decision to lower estrogen content, and the appointment of a Special Advisory Committee on oral contraceptives to the Food and Drug Directorate by

Canadian Minister of Health Dr. John Munro, came on the heels of public and professional concern voiced in 1969 and 1970 in American Senate subcommittee hearings and in the British Dunlop Committee.[65] However, the Canadian Medical Association (CMA) insisted that the oral contraceptive was safe for the average healthy female and that, while the pill posed "slight risks," they were far less than the "potential hazards of pregnancy."[66] The CMA disagreed with the Food and Drug Committee Report recommendation to include an explanatory pamphlet in the patient packaging on the grounds that it "will create additional unnecessary patient concern, self-diagnosis, and may in fact detract from already inadequate patient education."[67]

By the late sixties, most Canadian women were aware of the pill's risks but decided that they were outweighed by the benefits. The 1969 McGill *Birth Control Handbook* stated that tobacco and alcohol use were more dangerous and noted that there would be less risk to women's health if the campus promoted coin-operated dispensers of the pill rather than cigarettes.[68] In a 1969 issue of *Chatelaine*, Jack Batten noted that even though it was considered safer than having a baby, many Canadian women were pressured to give up the pill as a result of reported side effects.[69]

Conclusion

Sale of the birth control pill, however, remained strong, and the imagery employed in advertisements continued to emphasize both the "naturalness" and safe nature of the pill, and the role of the pill in the lives of white, middle-class, married women. To mark the end of the sixties, the pharmaceutical company C-Quens published a *CMAJ* advertisement depicting the woman of the seventies (fig. 10). Structured as a photographic collage, the advertisement declares a new era for the birth control industry; however, the images included in the advertisement are reminiscent of sixties imagery.

C-Quens 100 was to be "the oral contraceptive for the woman of the seventies." But who exactly was this new woman of the seventies? The imagery of the advertisement, a photographic collage reminiscent of a family photo album and featuring black-and-white photos of various women accented by a red-and-grey floral motif, strives to answer this question. In every photograph in the advertisement, the new woman of the seventies is shown as young, pretty, white, and middle class. The floral graphic highlighting the brand name reveals not only the feminine nature of the product but suggests that the drug, like flowers, is a natural product. The first woman of the seventies depicted in the advertisement is a young woman with long straight hair who smiles at the reader out of the zero in the "seventies" of the text. She also

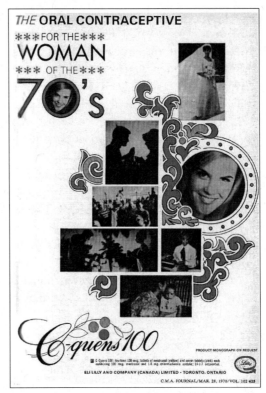

Figure 10   *Canadian Medical Association Journal,* 28 March
1970: 625.

appears in the photographic collage, on the right-hand side near the centre of
the advertisement. She is young and pretty, her marital status is ambiguous,
and she looks directly into the camera.

However, the marital status of some of the other women is clearly
indicated. Prominently featured is a photograph of a young woman in a
wedding dress. The photograph below depicts just the silhouette of a man and
a woman, perhaps a romantic honeymoon snapshot. Underneath is a group
photograph of a family watching acrobats at a circus. The next snapshot is of
a young couple outdoors at a party. The young man is lighting up a cigarette
while the woman holds a drink in her left hand. Underneath the party scene
is a photograph of another young woman at work, wearing a white dress shirt
and scarf, and looking down at her hands while typing. The bottom image
features yet another young woman who is embracing an infant.

The images imply that the woman of the seventies is not one but many
different women. The marital status of most of these women is ambiguous.

However, the images narrate the ideal cycle of a woman's life, which includes marriage, romance, work, and motherhood. The importance of marriage and family is indicated by the prominent placement of the woman in the wedding dress at the top of the ad and the young woman holding a baby at the bottom of the collage. These images emphasize the importance of the pill in a life cycle that includes motherhood. The pill becomes a means for family planning rather than an instrument of sexual revolution. As the McGill *Birth Control Handbook* indicated, the pill had the potential to liberate women; however, this liberation could not happen without broader changes in society.[70] The science behind the pill's creation was justified in the sixties not because it liberated women but because it was a tool for population control and family planning.

Birth control advertisements featuring women were part of the broader discourse in which norms of female sexuality were determined. Physicians were presented with a vision of the ideal patient who, in the early sixties, was white, middle class, and married. In 1969 the imagery was expanded to include other women, but this new image was still narrowly constructed. By the end of the sixties, the depiction of the pill as safe and respectable converges. The C-Quens advertisement (fig. 10) presents the pill as a natural part of a woman's life, which includes marriage and children. While the pill was a revolutionary new birth control method, it alone did not create a sexual revolution. The images of women represented in the advertisements articulated boundaries about appropriate female sexuality, expressed the need for physician intervention, and contributed to the creation of norms and limits of sexual behaviour.

Notes

1 Both Watkins and Allyn note the widely held assumption that the pill created a sexual revolution, although Watkins dismisses this claim. Elizabeth Siegel Watkins, *On the Pill: A Social History of Oral Contraceptives 1950–1970* (Baltimore: Johns Hopkins University Press, 1998), p. 2; David Allyn, *Make Love Not War: The Sexual Revolution: An Unfettered History* (New York: Little, Brown, 2000), 294.

2 Watkins, *On the Pill*, p. 55.

3 While the *Canadian Medical Association Journal (CMAJ)* is not a journal that was read by the masses, the pharmaceutical advertisements within the journal were influenced by popular beliefs.

4 Joanne Meyerowitz, "Introduction: Women and Gender in the Postwar United States," in Joanne Meyerowitz, ed., *Not June Cleaver: Women and Gender in Postwar America, 1945–1960* (Philadelphia: Temple University Press, 1994), p. 1.

5 Lara V. Marks, *Sexual Chemistry: A History of the Contraceptive Pill* (New Haven, CT: Yale University Press, 2003), p. 203; Angus McLaren and Arlene Tigar McLaren, *The Bedroom and the State: The Changing Practices and Politics of Contraception and Abortion in Canada, 1880–1997*, 2nd ed. (Toronto: Oxford University Press, 1997), p. 134.

6 Tom Smith, "The Polls—A Report: Sexual Revolution?" *Public Opinion Quarterly* 54.3 (1990): 419.

7 Sheila Jeffreys, *Anti-Climax: A Feminist Perspective on the Sexual Revolution* (London: Woman's Press, 1990), p. 93.

8 Michel Foucault, *The History of* Sexuality, vol. 1, *An Introduction.* Trans. Robert Hurley (New York: Vintage Books, 1990 [1978]), p. 53.

9 Sarah Stage, *Female Complaints: Lynda Pinkham and the Business of Women's Medicine* (New York: W.W. Norton, 1979), pp. 90–1.

10 Bernard Asbell, *The Pill: A Biography of the Drug That Changed the World* (New York: Random House, 1995), pp. 163–4.

11 McLaren and McLaren, *Bedroom and the State*, p. 19.

12 Linda Revie, "More Than Just Boots! The Eugenic and Commercial Concerns behind A.R. Kaufman's Birth Controlling Activities," *Canadian Bulletin of Medical History* 23.1 (2006): 120, 132.

13 G.P.R. Tallin. "Legal Implications of the Non-Therapeutic Practices of Doctors," *CMAJ* (4 August 1962): 210. Cited in McLaren and McLaren's *Bedroom and the State*; Harold Fine was convicted in 1961 (p. 132).

14 Tallin, "Legal Implications," p. 210.

15 Angus McLaren, "Sexual Revolution? The Pill, Permissiveness and Politics," in *Twentieth-Century Sexuality: A History* (Oxford: Blackwell Publishers, 1999), p. 168.

16 Andrea Tone, *Devices and Desires: A History of Contraceptives in America* (New York: Hill & Wang, 2001), p. 220.

17 Carole R. McCann, *Birth Control Politics in the United States, 1916–1945* (Ithaca: Cornell University Press, 1994), p. 304.

18 McCann, *Birth Control Politics*, p. 66.

19 Insight Team of the Sunday Times of London, *Suffer the Children: The Story of Thalidomide* (New York: Viking Press, 1979), p. 2.

20 Under brand names Kevadan and later Talimol in October 1961.

21 Jean F. Webb, "Special Article: Canadian Thalidomide Experience," *CMAJ* (9 November 1963): 987.

22 Webb, "Special Article," p. 988.

23 Thalidomide Task Force, *Report of the Thalidomide Task Force*, vol. 1 (Ottawa: War Amputations of Canada, 1989), p. 11.

24 The *CMAJ* article is based on the observation of 115 thalidomide babies (1987), 74 of whom were alive at the time the article was published. Vol. 1 of the *Report of the Thalidomide Task Force*, published in 1989, puts the number at 125 (p. 1), while *Suffer the Children* estimates the number to be closer to 90 (p. 134). The two later sources most likely only include those thalidomide children who survived. Symptoms of thalidomide poisoning also varied from physical deformity to internal problems, and it was difficult to diagnose.

25 Webb, "Special Article," p. 992.

26 George X. Trimble, "To the Editor: Vascular Headaches and Oral Contraceptives," *CMAJ* (4 June 1966): 1241; W.F. Baldwin, "To the Editor: True Ovarian Failure?" *CMAJ* (18 March 1967): 681; J.E. Musgrove and M.J. Tushig, "To the Editor: The Contraceptive Pill and Major Arterial Emboli in a Teen-aged Girl," *CMAJ* (12 October 1968): 724–5; Leon Ruben and Arnold Rogers, "To the Editor: Neurological Symptoms and Oral Contraceptives," *CMAJ* (23 March 1968): 609; Editorial, "Thromboembolic Disease and Oral Contraceptives," *CMAJ* (5 August 1967): 302.

27 J.D. Horan and J.J. Lederman, "To the Editor: Possible Asthmongenic Effect of Oral Contraceptives," *CMAJ* (20 July 1968): 130–1; J.C. Whyte, "To the Editor: Oral Contraception and Thromboembolic Disease," *CMAJ* (20 July 1968): 131.

28 Marks, *Sexual Chemistry*, p. 246.

29 Asbell, *The Pill*, p. 136.

30 Dolores Flamiano, "Covering Contraception: Discourses of Gender, Motherhood and Sexuality in Women's Magazines, 1938–1969," *American Journalism* (Summer 2000): 73.

31 Flamiano, "Covering Contraception."

32 J.H. Dickinson and G.C. Smith, "A New and Practical Oral Contraceptive Agent: Norethindrone with Mestranol," *CMAJ* (10 August 1963): 245.

33 Valerie J. Korinek. *Roughing It in the Suburbs: Reading* Chatelaine Magazine *in the Fifties and Sixties* (Toronto: University of Toronto Press, 2000), p. 4.

34 Gerald Anglin, "The Pill That Could Shake the World," *Chatelaine* (October 1953): 17.

35 Dickinson and Smith, "New and Practical"; C.A. Douglas Ringrose, "Current Concepts in Conception Control," *CMAJ* (10 August 1963): 246; Morris P. Wearing, "The Use of Norethindrone (2 Mg.) with Mestranol (0.1 Mg) in Fertility Control: A Preliminary Report," *CMAJ* (10 August 1963): 239.

36 L.S. Anderson, "The Mushroom Crowd: Social and Political Aspects of Population Pressure," *CMAJ* (5 December 1964): 1213, 1222.

37 Anderson, "Mushroom Crowd," p. 1220.

38 Marks, *Sexual Chemistry*, p. 38.

39 "Pills for Birth Control," *CMAJ* (28 January 1961): 227.

40 Musgrove and Tushig, "To the Editor," p. 724.

41 Ringrose, "Emotional Response," p. 1207.

42 Ringrose, "Emotional Response," p. 1208.

43 Marks, *Sexual Chemistry*, p. 205.

44 Tone, *Devices and Desires*, p. 257.

45 "Pills for Birth Control," p. 227.

46 Mrs. E.M. Higgans, Letter to the Editor, *Chatelaine* (February 1962): 92.

47 McLaren and McLaren, *Bedroom and the State*, p. 92.

48 "Physicians and Contraception," *CMAJ* (10 October 1964): 820.

49 "Physicians and Contraception," p. 820.

50 Christopher Tietze et al., "Teaching of Fertility Regulation in Medical Schools: A Survey in the United States and Canada, 1964," *CMAJ* (2 April 1966): 719.

51 A.J. Cunningham, "Letters to the Journal: Physicians and Contraception," *CMAJ* (9 January 1965): 87; countered by "The Editor Replies," *CMAJ* (9 January 1965): 88, and by the Associate Medical Director of Planned Parenthood in New York, Gordon W. Perkins, "To the Editor: Physicians and Contraception," *CMAJ* (29 March 1965): 631–2.

52 Marks, *Sexual Chemistry*, p. 200.

53 Watkins, *On the Pill*, p. 67.

54 "Oral Contraceptives," *CMAJ* (10 August 1963): 270.

55 Ron Kenyon, "The Pill Nobody Talks About," *Chatelaine* (November 1961): 64.

56 Lawrence Galton, "What's New in Health: Who Forgets the Pill?" *Chatelaine* (May 1965): 16.

57 Mrs. D. Harrison, "Letter to the Editor: 'Who Forgets the Pill?'" *Chatelaine* (August 1965): 68.

58 Nicole J. Grant also comes to this conclusion in *The Selling of Contraception: The Dalkon Shield Case, Sexuality, and Women's Autonomy* (Columbus: Ohio State University Press, 1992), p. 19.

59   Marks, *Sexual Chemistry*, p. 130.

60   Beryl A. Chernick, "Blood Pressure and Body Weight Changes during Oral Contraceptive Treatment," *CMAJ* (28 September 1968): 599.

61   Editorial, "Psychopathology of the Pill," *CMAJ* (31 January 1970): 217.

62   Contraceptives were finally decriminalized on 27 June 1969. See Brenda Margaret Appleby, *Responsible Parenthood: Decriminalizing Contraception in Canada* (Toronto: University of Toronto Press, 1999), p. 216.

63   Insight Team of the Sunday Times of London, *Suffer the Children*, p. 134.

64   "Ottawa Drug Authorities Look for Better 'Pill,'" *CMAJ* (31 January 1970): 219.

65   "Hazards of the Oral Contraceptive," Medical News: Special Supplement, *CMAJ* (30 May 1970): 1193.

66   "The Pill: Thousands of Canadian Women have been Needlessly Upset," The Association Speaks, *CMAJ* (14 February 1970): 227; "Hazards of the Oral Contraceptive," p. 1193.

67   "The CMA Comments on the Food and Drug Committee Report 'Hazards of the Oral Contraceptive,'" Association News: Special Supplement, *CMAJ* (19 December 1970): 1417.

68   *Birth Control Handbook* (Montreal: Student's Society of McGill University, 1969), p. 15. McGill's *Birth Control Handbook* was widely read and sold millions of copies in Canada and beyond between 1968 and 1975. For a complete history of the handbook, see Christabelle Sethna, "The Evolution of the *Birth Control Handbook*: From Student Peer-Education Manual to Feminist Self-Empowerment Text, 1968–1975," *Canadian Bulletin of Medical History/Bulletin canadien d'histoire de la médicine* 31.1 (2006): 89–118.

69   Jack Batten, "Is There a Male Conspiracy against the Pill?" *Chatelaine* (July 1969): 17, 40.

70   *Birth Control Handbook*, p. 2.

All Aboard? Canadian Women's Abortion Tourism, 1960–1980

Christabelle Sethna

hanging Places (1975), David Lodge's witty satire of Anglo-American academic life in the 1960s, begins with the startling discovery that Morris Zapp, an esteemed American professor, is the sole male passenger on a packed flight to London. When Zapp learns that all the women on board are heading to the English capital for abortions, his pregnant seatmate, a young, single university student, casually informs him of the package deal she has negotiated: "round trip, surgeon's fee, five days' nursing with private room and excursion to Stratford-upon-Avon."[1]

In this work of fiction, the punchline sends up what has come to be known as "abortion tourism." Arguably an insensitive term that has anti-abortion connotations,[2] abortion tourism is the generic catchphrase for the very real travel women undertake to access abortion services. Travel is one of the central barriers to abortion access: the further a woman has to travel for an abortion, the less likely she is to obtain one and the more likely she is to be young and underprivileged.[3] Yet abortion tourism persists. It is most familiar to Ireland, where abortion is predominantly illegal. Every year, thousands of Irish women leave to seek legal abortion services in England.[4] Often conducted over a long range and across domestic and international borders, abortion tourism remains such a commonplace transnational occurrence that it is documented in academic literature as well as in popular culture productions such as novels, short stories, poems, songs, and cartoons.[5]

Canada has its own little-known history of abortion tourism. Canadian scholars studying abortion have concentrated on analyzing the changes to the status of abortion in the country's Criminal Code.[6] Although compelling evidence indicates that many Canadian women coped with these changes by travelling to access abortion services before *and* after abortion was legalized in 1969, the topic of abortion tourism remains seriously under-investigated in Canada.[7] This chapter focuses on contemporaneous real-life accounts of Canadian women who travelled domestically and internationally for illegal and legal abortions between 1960 and 1980. These accounts appeared in the university student press, mainstream publications, women's magazines, and government-commissioned reports. Cultural productions of abortion tourism were often infused with humour, irony, sadness, or regret. Real-life accounts, which dramatized the Byzantine lengths women journeyed to procure an abortion, were laced with indignation. Bringing women's forced flights to public light provided different constituencies of readers with valuable information on circumventing abortion laws; detailed the consequent financial, emotional, and physical risks involved; and troubled the concept of abortion tourism itself. Indeed, real-life accounts of Canadian women's abortion tourism constructed abortion laws as a "carceral space" within which pregnant women seeking abortion were monitored, disciplined, and punished jurisdictionally but from which only the privileged few could escape geographically.[8]

Abortion and Contraception in Canadian History

The criminalization of birth control in Canada stretches back to the late nineteenth century, when eugenic thought was prevalent. Canadian legislators fearing the prospect of "race suicide" sought to increase the number of offspring born to Anglo-Saxon Christian women.[9] They looked to the example of restrictive British and American birth control laws to prohibit, through the Criminal Code, the sale, advertisement, and distribution of contraceptives and abortifacients. A woman who procured her own abortion could be sentenced to up to seven years incarceration. Abortion providers, who were trained medical or non-medical personnel, were liable to the maximum penalty of life imprisonment.[10] Although suspected abortion providers were rarely tried, guilty verdicts were reached in nearly half the cases before the courts.[11] There was a "good faith" provision that allowed for an abortion to save the life of the mother. This provision eventually led some non-Catholic hospitals in the 1960s to establish therapeutic abortion committees (TACs) composed of physicians who determined whether an abortion was necessary on a case-by-case basis. Still, the possibility of prosecution meant that many doctors refused to perform abortions at all.[12]

Despite its illegality, Canadian women, whether married or single, continued to turn to abortion. Some tried to self-abort by injuring themselves, by ingesting traditional remedies such as pennyroyal, or by introducing slippery elm bark, needles, or hooks into their uteri. Others consumed quack potions or pills advertised for sale as menstrual regulators. Finally, many women depended on abortion providers who had to perform abortions surreptitiously, sometimes under unhygienic conditions. While most women survived their abortions, others died from subsequent septic infections.[13]

Around the World

Sharra Vostral's chapter in this volume discussing postwar advice to adolescent American girls regarding menstruation reveals that the ideal white, hetero-normative woman was believed to be programmed by "Mother Nature" to be a mother. The wilful termination of a pregnancy seriously disrupted this essentially feminine script. However, it was not until the 1960s that illegal abortion came to be recognized as a serious public health problem in Canada. Because illegal abortion was an underground practice, it was difficult to quantify; some conservative estimates set the number at a hundred thousand annually.[14] In this same decade, international organized tourism exploded exponentially. Global pleasure travel, undertaken by upper-class Europeans who benefited from colonial expansion into distant lands, has a long history.[15] Tourism characterized by organized holidays began in the 1840s, when Englishman Thomas Cook standardized package tours within Britain for the working classes. Cook's expeditions to European sites attracted a primarily single female clientele keen on unchaperoned travel.[16] By the 1960s, the expansion of airline companies, transatlantic travel routes, and middle-class disposable incomes made international organized tourism affordable for those living in the West. The World Tourism Organization recorded seventy million annual international arrivals in 1960. The United Nations (UN) declared 1967 International Tourism Year. International bodies even recommended that developing states newly liberated from colonial rule could acquire some financial capital by attracting tourists. Ironically, the imbalance of power between tourist and host countries meant that tourism exacerbated the dependence of developing nations on Western currencies.[17]

As various nations began to liberalize their abortion laws, Western women seeking abortions rode the boom in international organized tourism by travelling to abortion services far from home. In mapping the global itinerary of abortion tourism, one sees, for example, that French women turned to Switzerland for abortions.[18] American women went to Mexico so frequently that one travel agency received an award for selling the most three-day weekends to that country.[19] It was even speculated that American and Canadian women took abortion vacations in Europe.[20] Although abortion was still illegal in Canada, no person at that time could be convicted of an offence committed outside the country.[21] Not surprisingly, many Canadian women seeking abortion services flocked to locales that had also become premier tourist destinations.

Britain (excepting Ireland) proved to be an abortion hot spot. After it was first promulgated in 1861, the British abortion law remained virtually unchanged for many decades, decreeing that it was unlawful to procure a miscarriage. A loophole appeared in 1939 when Dr. Aleck Bourne was charged with performing an abortion. The court acquitted him, accepting that the abortion was lawful because it was intended to preserve the physical and mental health of his patient, a fourteen-year-old girl pregnant as the result of a gang rape. Whereas eugenic fears over race suicide in the late nineteenth century led to the promulgation of Britain's restrictive birth control laws, eugenic revulsion over the birth of disabled children galvanized the loosening of such legislation in the late twentieth century. In the 1950s and 1960s, thousands of British women—along with their European and Canadian counterparts—gave birth to children with malformed or missing limbs after they had consumed thalidomide, a drug marketed as a sleeping and morning sickness aid. Consequently, the 1967 British *Abortion Act* permitted abortions if two doctors agreed there was a risk of fetal anomalies. Moreover, the act allowed for an abortion if the continuation of the pregnancy threatened the woman's life, her physical or mental health, or any of her existing children. As the act did not discriminate against non-residents, European, Canadian, and American women bolted to Britain for abortions. In the year 1973, the number of abortions performed on non-residents peaked at 56,581.[22]

Accounts of Canadian Women's Abortion Tourism

Some scholars distinguish travellers from tourists and denounce the tourist as a status-seeking consumer who has displaced the traveller searching for authentic experiences of place. Other academics reject the validity of this distinction, asserting that both travellers and tourists are marked by their privileged position in relation to the local populace.[23] A tourist, according to Julia Harrison, makes a choice to travel and to return home.[24] Nevertheless, as tourist travel has become so overdetermined by what Raminder Kaur and John Hutnyk call "the articulation of privilege,"[25] it is perhaps more appropriate to categorize abortion tourists with trans-status subjects, refugees, or even exiles. For this group of individuals, journeys from home can be liberating. More often than not, they can also be transgressive and fraught with peril.[26] Although the abortion tourist suffers because of a punitive patriarchy determined to keep her penitent, a complex articulation of privilege embedded in the practice of abortion tourism showcases the socio-economic disparities among women.

The Canadian university student press disseminated some of the earliest real-life accounts of women travelling for illegal abortions. The jump in female student enrolment in universities, the lack of sex education in schools, and the illegality of contraception contributed to a rise in out-of-wedlock pregnancies on campus.[27] Although the birth control pill was available (on a doctor's prescription), I have found that it was clearly intended for married Canadian women, a situation that posed numerous difficulties for both students and doctors at university health services.[28] As Heather Molyneaux shows in her chapter in this volume, advertisements for oral contraceptives that appeared in the *Canadian Medical Association Journal (CMAJ)* routinely featured married women, their wedding rings prominently displayed, as the most appropriate consumers of oral contraception. Young, unmarried couples facing the dilemma of an unwanted pregnancy were increasingly likely to reject a "shotgun" marriage. Aside from adoption, the other option for a young single woman was an abortion. Procuring an abortion was an onerous task because the illegality of the procedure was compounded by the sense of sexual impropriety associated with an out-of-wedlock pregnancy. *The Varsity*, the main student newspaper for the University of Toronto, reported that "a single girl in trouble often hasn't the faintest idea how to go about it [abortion] and besides, the shame [with] which society views her condition makes her afraid of confiding in anyone."[29]

Campus newspapers like *The Varsity* carried chilling tales of the tragedy of the young, single, pregnant student who, trapped by Canada's restrictive birth control laws, made a desperate journey to an abortion provider. In one example, a sobbing McGill University student confessed that on a $500 loan from a married girlfriend, she went to the United States for an illegal abortion. There she was forced to have sex with the man who performed the procedure.[30] In another, a student from an unnamed university travelled to Toronto to procure an abortion after her own doctor declined to assist her. With the help of student friends in the city, she encountered a physician who charged $300 per abortion. Suspecting he was under police surveillance, he refused to perform the operation. So too did the others she contacted. Increasingly anxious, the student travelled yet again, this time to Montreal, where she finally managed to obtain an illegal abortion for $200.[31]

These accounts challenged the sense of sexual impropriety associated with an out-of-wedlock pregnancy. Young, pregnant, single women seeking abortions were portrayed as sympathetic victims rather than as shameful criminals. Still, it can safely be assumed that the student central to these stories was white, middle class, and relatively financially privileged. The tragedy of her out-of-wedlock pregnancy signalled not only the frightening possibility of septic infection or death due to illegal abortion; it also increasingly suggested the potential derailment of professional opportunities she would experience if that pregnancy were brought to term.[32]

To counteract the problem of illegal abortion, some university students took proactive measures. They organized birth control teach-ins, insisted their campus health services prescribe the birth control pill, and developed their own educational material on birth control.[33] A committee of McGill University students compiled and published the *Birth Control Handbook* (1968). The *Handbook* was filled with accurate information about the male and female reproductive system, the mechanics of conception, and various contraceptives such as the birth control pill, diaphragm, condom, and intrauterine device.[34] The earliest editions dealt with the topic of abortion only by reproducing the section of the Criminal Code outlawing the procedure and by printing two articles, one by McGill University professor Donald Kingsbury and another by journalist Doris Giller. Kingsbury claimed to know many McGill students, the daughters of Montreal's elite, who ended up pregnant and despondent. He castigated the physicians teaching at his university's prestigious medical school, accusing them of remaining silent about Canada's restrictive birth control laws because they wanted to protect their careers.[35] Giller reported that university students had developed a network of underground contacts to abortion providers who charged from $270 to $600 for the procedure. The price, she noted, was "inflated" due to pregnant women's desperation and abortion providers' fear of imprisonment.[36]

The Legalization of Abortion

In 1969 the government, under Liberal Prime Minister Pierre Trudeau, succeeded in reforming the Criminal Code such that contraception was decriminalized and abortion was legalized. Yet even at the draft stage, the new abortion law proved contentious. Former Secretary of State Judy LaMarsh denounced it publicly as a "real namby-pamby, wishy-washy gutless kind of abortion law,"[37] perhaps reflecting the fact that abortion, for many Canadians, was far more controversial a practice than was contraception.[38]

The new abortion law formalized the medical profession's control over abortion access. Abortions were now legal under a time-consuming, complicated, stringent set of regulations. A woman could access an abortion only if she had a referral from her doctor to a TAC established at an accredited hospital. The TAC, consisting of three or more doctors (the doctor who referred the woman for an abortion could not be part of the TAC), had to rule that an abortion was necessary to preserve the mother's "life or health." The birth of babies crippled by thalidomide in Canada had sensitized the public to abortion. An Ontario businessman even offered $1,000 to any woman who had consumed thalidomide and wanted to terminate her pregnancy.[39] However, in making the mother's life or health a criterion, as opposed to the condition of the fetus, the government intended that TACs reject solely "eugenic, sociological, or criminal offense reasons for abortion." Unfortunately, the new abortion law did not define what was meant by health. Doctors serving on TACs were, therefore, at liberty to apply arbitrary medical, psychological, or sociological interpretations of the word.[40] In addition, no hospital was obligated to strike a TAC, accredited hospitals were concentrated mainly in cities, Catholic hospitals rejected abortion services entirely, and there was no mechanism to appeal a TAC's ruling. Finally, doctors could refuse to perform abortions; many were divided over the morality of the procedure.[41]

Cross-Border Abortions

Grace MacInnis, the only female member of parliament, initially welcomed the reform of the Criminal Code, arguing that wealthy women could skirt Canada's restrictive birth control laws by paying for an illegal abortion within Canada or by travelling to another country where the procedure was legal. Poor women could not. Yet she too alleged that the new abortion law was misguided because abortion, like contraception, also needed to be decriminalized.[42] Indeed, the new legislation did little to stop illegal abortion. Nor did it end abortion tourism; in fact, Canadian women journeyed for abortion services in even greater numbers. The edition of the *Handbook* that appeared after the passage of the new abortion law affirmed that the legislation "will help almost no one," noting that women around the world travelled in droves to England, Israel, and Japan to take advantage of their liberal abortion laws.[43]

Due to the efforts of Dr. Henry Morgentaler, the city of Montreal soon became a major player on the international and domestic abortion scene. A Holocaust survivor from Poland, Morgentaler immigrated to Canada in 1950 and established a medical practice in Montreal. After he took a public pro-abortion stance at the hearings of the House of Commons Standing Committee on Health and Welfare—a committee to which individuals and organizations presented submissions on the reform of the country's birth control laws—his office was flooded with private requests for abortions. A year later, in defiance of the Criminal Code, Morgentaler limited his medical practice to family planning and abortion.[44]

After the Criminal Code reforms of 1969, Morgentaler flouted the new abortion law. He performed abortions full-time at his clinic, bypassing the legal need for a TAC. Using a sliding payment scale, he charged approximately $300 per abortion, $200 if the patient was a student, and $25 to $30 if she was a single or welfare mother. Some patients paid nothing at all. To Morgentaler, clinic abortions meant that women "could go in, have the operation under minimal anesthetic, and leave in about an hour."[45] Most of his patients were francophones living in the province of Quebec. However, the speed of clinic abortions was a boon to out-of-province Canadian women and to American women sent to Montreal by abortion referral services in New York, Boston, and Minneapolis. Most of Morgentaler's patients had their abortions the day after a scheduled consultation. When women who travelled long distances could not arrange to stay overnight in Montreal, the consultation and abortion took place on the same day. A tip from the Federal Bureau of Investigation (FBI) led Quebec police to arrest Morgentaler on 1 June 1970, after he performed an abortion on a seventeen-year-old patient who had travelled to Montreal from Minnesota. His arrest launched a series of legal attacks against the new abortion law that were fought all the way to the Supreme Court.[46]

Cross-border abortion tourism accelerated when, a month after Morgentaler's arrest, New York State drastically reformed its abortion law. The United States government had criminalized abortion in several statutes between 1860 and 1880. Doctors could legally perform therapeutic abortions only if they were intended to save the woman's life. From the 1940s onward, the introduction of hospital TACs greatly reduced the number of therapeutic abortions performed. Women of colour and poor women were disproportionately negatively affected; because of their race and class privileges, white middle-class women were much likelier to have access to therapeutic abortions. Women of colour and poor women were also more likely to be sterilized after the procedure. Some doctors performed abortions in exchange for sterilizations; these surgeries were known as a "package deal."[47]

The burden American TACs imposed on women seeking abortions led activists in the early 1960s to form groups like the Society for Humane Abortion. The society distributed pamphlets with information on abortion providers in Mexico, Japan, and Sweden, and helped send a substantial number of American women to other countries for abortions.[48] As in England and Canada, eugenic concerns played a role in the legalization of abortion. Because the Food and Drug Administration (FDA) did not approve the use of thalidomide, only a few American women, like Sheri Finkbine, took the drug. The popular host of a children's television program, Finkbine's personal travails brought abortion tourism to international prominence when, refused an abortion in the United States, she journeyed to Sweden to obtain one.[49]

In 1970 Alaska, Hawaii, Washington, and New York each reformed their abortion laws. Whereas the first three states required a residency period of at least thirty days before an abortion could be performed, New York opened the procedure to non-residents. It is estimated that out-of-state American women travelled anywhere from five hundred to two thousand miles to reach New York for an abortion.[50] Between 1970 and 1971, a total of 4,437 Canadian women had abortions in New York alone. The next year, five thousand Canadian women did the same.[51] In 1973 the American Supreme Court ruled in *Roe v. Wade* that a woman's decision to have an abortion in consultation with her physician within the first trimester of pregnancy was a protected constitutional right. This landmark ruling gave Canadian women even more access to abortion south of the border.

Carceral Space

Dissatisfaction with the 1969 abortion law in Canada generated more real-life accounts of abortion tourism, spurred feminists to organize around abortion access, and led the government to commission a formal review of abortion practices in the country.

After the passage of the legislation, accounts of abortion tourism began to appear in mainstream publications and in women's magazines. The university student press had concentrated on the tragedy of the young, single, pregnant student seeking an abortion. Now mainstream publications and women's magazines spotlighted the efforts of pregnant married women who sought abortion services. Significantly, post-1969 accounts erased the sexual impropriety gap between the pregnant single woman and the pregnant married woman by positioning *all* women wishing to terminate their pregnancies within the same carceral space:

> So, under the new law, if you are pregnant and your health is in the balance, and you know you can't face the likelihood of bearing a deformed child, that you cannot care for another child in an already overburdened and underprivileged family, or

that you will live embittered by shame and resentment and lost opportunities for the rest of your life, or that your health may be impaired to the point of canceling your enjoyment of living, you won't be allowed a personal choice. Your whole future way of life will be decided not by you, but by a committee of three or more doctors, who will assume that they know much better than you do what your own needs and capabilities are. The abortion board [TAC], with this power, will satisfy its own conscience without any regard for yours.[52]

Mainstream publications and women's magazines held that the new abortion law was unworkable for three main reasons. The first reason implicated doctors' dubious interpretation of the legal requirements involved. In one account, a gynecologist told his thirty-six-year-old married patient and mother of one child that it was pointless to refer her to a TAC because her past history of breast infections would not be considered suitable legal grounds for a therapeutic abortion in Toronto. Whether or not his assessment was correct was unclear: the patient did not seek a second opinion. Determined to have an abortion, she flew to England. At the London Harley Street office, she found a "foyer already lined with suitcases bearing tags from Pan Am, TWA and Air France." The nurse grumbled about Canadians who "think they can come in here at any time," but scheduled the woman's abortion for the next day. After the procedure, the patient returned for a follow-up examination, only to observe that the foyer was once again filled with overseas luggage.[53]

The second reason encompassed the personal beliefs of physicians about abortion. A thirty-two-year-old married mother of two discovered she was pregnant. She suffered from health and financial problems, yet her doctor refused to refer her for an abortion, saying: "It's nice to have three children, you know." The woman investigated going to England but ended up in Montreal at an abortion clinic she did not identify. When her doctor eventually discovered she was no longer pregnant, he admitted that he had in the past sent women to Japan for abortions, depending on the dictates of his conscience. Another woman, twenty-five years old and single, suspected she was pregnant but was too embarrassed to consult her own family doctor because she feared his disapproval. She sought out another physician, only to have him castigate her about her immorality. He refused to refer her for an abortion. She then travelled 1,200 miles to an underground abortionist, who tried to abort her with knitting needles. This attempt failed. The woman eventually flew to England, where she obtained an abortion from medical staff who treated her well and did not judge her.[54]

The third reason—women's uneven access to abortion due to socio-economic disparities—received the most prominence. Financially privileged women could travel to terminate their pregnancies. Women with few monetary resources were forced to go into debt to finance the cost of travel, accommodation, and abortion, or had to forgo the abortion altogether.[55] Some women could escape the carceral space demarcated by the abortion law while others remained trapped within it. In one such instance, a twenty-five-year-old married woman became pregnant because of contraceptive failure. Fearing a TAC would turn down her request, she decided to seek alternatives. Her own doctor recommended a legal abortion in London, but the cost was prohibitive. Unable to come up with the $800 a London abortion would cost, she arranged for an illegal abortion in Montreal. However, the unnamed doctor (possibly Morgentaler himself) was arrested just before her arrival, stranding her and the other women who had come to the same clinic from various parts of North America. The woman headed back to Toronto to a women's birth control centre that made abortion referrals. She finally ended up at the Toronto General Hospital. The doctors serving on the hospital's TAC questioned her about her sex life, her contraceptive use, her marriage, and her reasons for the abortion. Only then did the TAC grant her request, ending, as she put it, her "exercise in anguish."[56]

Feminist Activism and Abortion Law Repeal

Spurred by that anguish, some fledgling women's liberation groups determined that the new abortion law constituted a weighty infringement upon Canadian women's rights. Poor and working-class women were affected even more severely because they could rarely afford a legal abortion inside or outside Canada.[57]

The Vancouver Women's Caucus (VWC) organized an Abortion Information Service (AIS) in December 1969. The service provided married and single women with referrals to abortion providers across the border in Washington. The AIS also helped women to navigate the complex requirements of the new abortion law. During the first four months of its existence, the AIS counselled three hundred women. Only ten of these women managed to obtain an abortion through a TAC. In test cases, the AIS discovered that TACs were most likely to grant abortions to women who were married, middle class, and white, confirming the impact of socio-economic disparities on abortion access.[58]

The VWC proposed that women who wanted the new abortion law repealed travel en masse to the capital of Canada for a Mother's Day protest in an "Abortion Caravan."[59] The Caravan's main feature was a coffin filled with coat hangers, representing symbolically women who had died of illegal abortions. Once the Caravan arrived in Ottawa in early May 1970, women from the West met up with those who had journeyed from the East. On Parliament Hill, a visibly pregnant Doris Powers, a member of a grassroots group for the rights of the poor, addressed the crowd. She informed the women present that a Toronto hospital TAC had rejected her request for an abortion. Powers proclaimed that had she consented to sterilization, she may have been granted an abortion. She closed her rousing speech by insisting that the ability to travel to access abortion services had life or death consequences: "We, the poor of Canada, are the dirt shoved under the rug of a vicious economy. In obtaining abortions, we pay a price second to none, *our lives*. We can't afford to fly off to England for a safe, legal abortion. We have to seek out the back street butchers."[60]

Rallied, the crowd marched to the prime minister's residence and dumped the coffin on the grounds. The next day, about thirty women involved in the action entered the House of Commons as visitors. They chained themselves to seats in the visitors' galleries and stood up to denounce the new abortion law. In the ensuing pandemonium, the women were cut loose and dragged out by security guards. Although popular media reaction was generally derisive,[61] some quarters acknowledged that the new abortion law was unworkable. Echoing the now-familiar theme of the impact of socio-economic disparities on abortion access, the *Toronto Star* opined that the legislation had not reduced illegal abortion because "affluent women can get safe, legal abortions outside the country. Back-street butchery or self-inflicted torture is often the result for the poor mother."[62] The federal government was unmoved. When VWC members met with Trudeau a few weeks after the Ottawa protests to discuss repealing the new abortion law, he suggested unrepentantly that Canadian women seeking abortions could always travel to the United States.[63]

The Caravan drew the attention of Canadian feminists to the need for the repeal of the new abortion law. But while some insisted that abortion law repeal should remain the central focus of the women's movement, others argued that women's concerns were too diverse for such a singular agenda. By the mid-seventies, the Canadian Association for the Repeal of the Abortion Laws, later the Canadian Abortion Rights Action League (CARAL), made abortion law repeal its main goal. To that effect, the national organization became involved in fighting Morgentaler's legal battles and in assisting abortion referrals inside and outside Canada.[64]

Assessing the Impact of the New Abortion Law

Rather than repealing the new abortion law, the majority opinion of the *Report of the Royal Commission on the Status of Women* (1970) envisioned amending it. The federal government struck the Royal Commission in 1967 to conduct public hearings from coast to coast on the economic, legal, and social position of women in Canadian society.[65] By the time the Royal Commission released its report, the abortion legislation had been in operation for only one year. The commissioners were themselves conflicted about the morality of abortion. Still, the majority of them found that the new abortion law made access to legal abortion in Canada very difficult. In addition, the legislation was discriminatory because poor women, unlike women with economic security, did not have the option of leaving the country for a legal abortion. The majority of the commissioners recommended amending the new abortion law to "permit abortion by a qualified medical practitioner on the sole request of any woman who has been pregnant for 12 weeks or less." In keeping with statutes enacted by other jurisdictions that had legalized abortion, they further recommended broadening this time frame should the pregnancy threaten the physical or mental health of the woman or lead to the birth of a severely disabled child.[66]

The Canadian Medical Association (CMA) took another route. Under the leadership of Bette Stephenson, physicians asked the government to define for TACs the meaning of "health." In response, Justice Minister Otto Lang, a devout Catholic and ardent opponent of abortion, commissioned a formal review of abortion practices in the country.[67]

The upshot of the review was the *Report of the Committee on the Operation of the Abortion Law* (1977). It was known colloquially as the *Badgley Report* after the committee chair, Robin Badgley, a University of Toronto sociologist. Commissioners Badgley, Denyse Fortin Caron, and Marion Powell concluded that since the passage of the 1969 abortion law, deaths from illegal abortions had decreased. Yet only 20.1 per cent of hospitals in the country had established TACs, leading to serious regional variations in abortion access. An average eight-week interval elapsed between a woman's first contact with her doctor and her abortion. Finally, the lack of uniform interpretation of the law meant that "the procedure provided in the Criminal Code for obtaining therapeutic abortion is in practice illusory for many Canadian women."[68]

The *Badgley Report* expressly established why the abortion legislation had failed to eliminate illegal abortion and how it had stimulated abortion tourism simultaneously. Badgley, Caron, and Powell treated abortion tourism as fundamental to their enquiry, even excerpting testimonials from women who had travelled to procure an abortion before and after the passage of the law. Their data showed that Canadian women's voyages to Britain for abortion services slowed after 1969. The new abortion law was one contributing factor. But so too was the emergence of "abortion referral pathways" to the United States.[69] According to the commissioners, these pathways came into play once "some women could not meet the requirements of hospital therapeutic abortion committees, did not wish to do so, or were not referred to hospitals with committees by their physicians."[70]

Doctors, non-profit organizations, and commercial abortion referral agencies directed Canadian women to American abortion services. Some of these abortion services were housed in stand-alone clinics or in clinics attached to hospitals in states close to the Canadian border. Women from the Maritime provinces went to New England for abortions; Quebec women turned to Vermont; Illinois, Michigan, and New York attracted women from Ontario. Manitobans crossed into Minnesota and North Dakota, while California and Washington drew women living in Western Canada.[71] Some women resented having to go to the United States because they felt entitled to receive reproductive health care in their own country. As one woman told the commissioners: "My faith was shattered, and when it was suggested in my search to find a doctor that I go to _____, I was tempted to pay the $200 and go. But now it became a matter of principle. I pay my premiums, I rarely use the services I am supposed to be insured for and now I had a real need and I was being advised to go the States, pay out of pocket, act like a criminal, sneaking over the border."[72]

Cross-border abortion became a profitable business benefiting owners of abortion clinics, commercial abortion referral agencies, and the transportation industry. Available figures indicated that abortion clinics could make a profit of $80 per operation, while the referral agencies could gain an additional $75 per client. The cost of a return bus ticket to a clinic ranged from $11.20 to $20.55. It was calculated that between 1970 and 1975, from 45,930 to 50,106 Canadian women had gone to the United States for abortions. These numbers meant that during this period between 15.9 and 23.5 per cent of Canadian women obtaining abortions had their abortions in the United States.[73]

On the Road, Again

By 1980 Toronto had outpaced Montreal as Canada's "veritable mecca for abortions."[74] Although Ontario's largest city served thousands of local women as well as women from other communities, it still could not meet the demand. When the Ontario Ministry of Health asked Powell, a commissioner for the *Badgley Report*, to evaluate hospital abortion access in the province, she delivered a stinging assessment in her *Report on the Therapeutic Abortion Services in Ontario* (1987). Because she included the demand for and availability of abortion services by geographic area as one of her four main terms of reference, Powell was able to track the abortion tourism of Ontario women. She found that abortion services were much less available in smaller centres. One in five women who obtained a hospital abortion had to leave her county of residence. A minimum of five thousand women per year had abortions in freestanding clinics in Canada and the United States. Those women who did leave their counties of residence had to travel repeatedly for each step in the referral process, paying out of pocket for transportation and accommodation. The lengthy delays TACs caused led to a high rate of second-trimester abortions in the province, especially among teenagers. Those requiring second-trimester abortions could obtain them in only eight of the province's counties or in the United States.[75]

The following year, the Supreme Court struck down the 1969 abortion law as unconstitutional. In rendering the decision of the majority, Chief Justice Brian Dickson recognized that as a result of the legislation, many women were forced to travel to other jurisdictions to procure an abortion.[76] Despite the fact that abortion has been legal in Canada since that 1988 decision, is deemed a medically necessary service under the *Canada Health Act*, and occurs in hospitals as well as in non-profit and for-profit abortion clinics, abortion access remains grossly uneven across the country. Differences in provincial health insurance plans to fund abortions have eroded some women's ability to access an abortion. A few provincial governments refuse to fund abortions that take place outside hospitals. Medical institutions may impose TAC-like requirements or gestational limits for granting an abortion. The pool of abortion providers has shrunk due to ageing and lack of training at medical schools, as well as threats, harassment, and violence from anti-choice forces. Finally, fewer hospitals across the country are doing abortions; recent statistics show that only 15.9 per cent of general hospitals perform abortions, down from the 20.1 per cent figure recorded in the *Badgley Report*.[77]

Such extra-legal impediments perpetuate the need for Canadian women to travel to access abortion services.[78] Before and after abortion was legalized in

1969, white, middle-class, and relatively financially advantaged women *could* travel to access abortion services inside and outside Canada. Today the reverse is true. Now marginalized women—Aboriginal women on reserves, teenagers, women from the North, women from rural areas, and women from Atlantic Canada—*must* travel to access abortion services. Canadian women seeking late-term abortions still often journey to the United States.[79] Unlike the publicity attending real-life accounts of Canadian women's abortion tourism that appeared in the university student press, mainstream publications, women's magazines, and government-commissioned reports between 1960 and 1980, the travels of this population are cloaked in silence. Although a very public debate over two-tier health care, wait times, and privatization of medical services rages, it may well be that the same socio-economic disparities that earlier prevented marginalized women from travelling to access abortion services currently force them to journey to hospitals and clinics outside their home communities without the benefit of media hue and cry. The lack of attention paid to these journeys not only highlights the vulnerability of this population but also provides confirmation that abortion need not be illegal in order to be inaccessible to many women.

Notes

I thank the Social Sciences and Humanities Research Council of Canada and my research assistants for their contributions.

1 David Lodge, *A David Lodge Trilogy: Changing Places, Small World, Nice Work* (London: Penguin Books, 1993), p. 25.
2 Alyssa Best, "Abortion Rights along the Irish-English Border and the Liminality of Women's Experiences," *Dialectical Anthropology* 29 (2005): 425. As an example of how the term "abortion tourism" is used by anti-abortion forces, see the comments made by a blogger, "Swedish Tourism Fears Grow as Sweden Fights for Late Term Abortion," http://swenglishrantings.com/entry/?tag=stockholm (accessed 22 August 2008).
3 James D. Shelton, Edward A. Brann, and Kenneth F. Schulz, "Abortion Utilization: Does Travel Distance Matter?" *Family Planning Perspectives* 8.6 (1976): 260–2; Stanley K. Henshaw, "The Accessibility of Abortion Services in the United States," *Family Planning Perspectives* 23.6 (1991): 246–52; and R. Todd Jewell and Robert W. Brown, "An Economic Analysis of Abortion: The Effect of Travel Cost on Teenagers," *Social Sciences Journal* 37.1 (2000): 113–24.
4 *The Irish Journey: Women's Stories of Abortion* (Dublin: Irish Family Planning Association, 2000). See also Ann Furedi, ed., *The Abortion Law in Northern Ireland: Human Rights and Reproductive Choice* (Belfast: Irish Family Planning Association Northern Ireland, 1995). My thanks to Marie Hammond-Callaghan, Sandra McAvoy, and Carolyn Phillips for these references. Some additional sources are Siobhan Mullally, "The Abortion Debate in Ireland: Repartitioning the State," in Vijay Andrew, ed., *Women's Health, Women's Rights: Perspectives on Global Health Issues* (Toronto: York University Centre for Feminist Research, 2003), pp. 27–49; Ruth Fletcher, "'Pro-life' Absolutes, Feminist

Challenges: The Fundamentalist Narrative of Irish Abortion Law 1986–1992," *Osgoode Hall Law Journal* 36.1 (Spring 1998): 1–62; Abigail-Mary E.W. Sterling, "The European Union and Abortion Tourism: Liberalizing Ireland's Abortion Law," *Boston College International and Comparative Law Review* 20.2 (Summer 1997): 385–406.

5 For examples of abortion tourism in academic literature, see Bill Rolston and Anna Eggert, eds., *Abortion in the New Europe: A Comparative Handbook* (Westport, CT: Greenwood Press, 1994), and Gail Pheterson and Yamila Azize, "Abortion Practice in the Northeast Caribbean: 'Just Write Down Stomach Pain,'" *Reproductive Health Matters* 13.26 (2005): 44–53. For some examples of abortion tourism in popular culture productions, see Lynda S. Myrsiades, *Splitting the Baby: The Culture of Abortion in Literature and Law, Rhetoric and Cartoons* (New York: Peter Lang, 2002).

6 Angus McLaren and Arlene Tigar McLaren, *The Bedroom and the State: The Changing Practices and Politics of Contraception and Abortion in Canada, 1880–1980* (Toronto: McClelland and Stewart, 1986); Janine Brodie, Shelley A.M. Gavigan, and Jane Jenson, *The Politics of Abortion* (Toronto: Oxford University Press, 1992); Gail Kellough, *Aborting Law: An Exploration of the Politics of Motherhood and Medicine* (Toronto: University of Toronto Press, 1996); Sanda Rodgers, "Abortion Denied: Bearing the Limits of the Law," in Cynthia Flood, ed., *Just Medicare: What's In, What's Out, How We Decide* (Toronto: University of Toronto Press, 2006), pp. 107–36.

7 For anecdotal evidence of Canadian women travelling for abortions, see Childbirth by Choice Trust, *No Choice: Canadian Women Tell Their Stories of Illegal Abortion* (Toronto: Childbirth by Choice Trust, 1998). I am currently principal investigator on a Social Sciences and Humanities Research Council of Canada grant to study the topic of abortion tourism to abortion clinics in Canada.

8 I am indebted conceptually to the work of Michel Foucault as utilized by Mona Oikawa, "Cartographies of Violence: Women, Memory, and the Subject(s) of the 'Internment,'" in Sherene H. Razack, ed., *Race, Space and the Law: Unmapping a White Settler Society* (Toronto: Between the Lines Press, 2002), pp. 73–98. I also acknowledge the influence of Sheryl Nestel, "Delivering Subjects: Race, Space and the Emergence of Legalized Midwifery in Ontario," in Razack, ed., *Race, Space and the Law*, pp. 233–55.

9 Angus McLaren, *Our Own Master Race: Eugenics in Canada, 1885–1945* (Toronto: McClelland and Stewart, 1990).

10 Childbirth by Choice Trust, *No Choice*, pp. 13–14.

11 Constance Backhouse, "The Celebrated Abortion Trial of Dr. Emily Stowe, Toronto, 1879," *Canadian Bulletin of Medical History/Bulletin canadien d'histoire de la médecine* 8 (1991): 159–87.

12 Jane Jenson, "Getting to *Morgentaler*: From One Representation to Another," ch. 2 in Brodie, Gavigan, and Jenson, *Politics of Abortion*, pp. 24–5.

13 McLaren and McLaren, *Bedroom and the State*, pp. 20–53.

14 Eleanor Wright Pelrine, *Abortion in Canada* (Toronto: New Press, 1972), p. 58.

15 Patricia Jasen, *Wild Things: Nature, Culture, and Tourism in Ontario 1870–1914* (Toronto: University of Toronto Press, 1995), pp. 3–20.

16 Taras Grescoe, *The End of Elsewhere: Travels among the Tourists* (Toronto: McFarlane Walter and Ross, 2003), pp. 69–70, 80.

17 Julia Harrison, *Being a Tourist: Finding Meaning in Pleasure Travel* (Vancouver: UBC Press, 2003), p. 13. See also John Urry, *The Tourist Gaze: Leisure and Travel in Contemporary Societies* (London: Sage Publications, 1990).

18 House of Commons Standing Committee on Health and Welfare, Minutes of Proceedings and Evidence, 3 October 1967, p. 4.

19   Debbie Nathan, "Abortion Stories on the Border," in Maxine Baca Zinn, Pierrette Hondagneu-Satelo, and Michael Messner, eds., *Gender through the Prism of Difference,* 2nd ed. (Needham Heights, MA: Allyn and Bacon, 2000), p. 123.

20   House of Commons Standing Committee on Health and Welfare, p. 9.

21   Robin F. Badgley, Denyse Fortin Caron, and Marion G. Powell, *Report of the Committee on the Operation of the Abortion Law* (Ottawa: Minister of Supply and Services Canada, 1977), p. 64.

22   Simon Lee, "Abortion Law in Northern Ireland: The Twilight Zone," in Ann Furedi, ed., *The Abortion Law in Northern Ireland: Human Rights and Reproductive Choice* (Belfast: Family Planning Association Northern Ireland, 1995), pp. 20–2. See also Dilys Cossey, "Britain," in Furedi, ed., *Abortion Law in Northern Ireland,* pp. 56–62.

23   Jasen, *Wild Things,* pp. 5–7.

24   Harrison, *Being a Tourist,* p. 35.

25   Raminder Kaur and John Hutnyk, eds., *Travel Worlds: Journeys in Contemporary Cultural Politics* (London: Zed Books, 1999), p. 1.

26   Annie Phizacklea, "Women, Migration and the State," in Kum-Kum Bhavnani, ed., *Feminism and "Race"* (Oxford: Oxford University Press, 2001), pp. 319–30, and Sonita Sarker and Esha Niyogi De, eds., *Trans-Status Subjects: Gender in the Globalization of South and Southeast Asia* (Durham: Duke University Press, 2002).

27   Christabelle Sethna, "The Cold War and the Sexual Chill: Freezing Girls Out of Sex Education," *Canadian Woman Studies/les cahiers de la femme* 17 (1998): 57–61.

28   Christabelle Sethna, "The University of Toronto Health Service, Oral Contraception and Student Demand for Birth Control, 1960–1970," *Historical Studies in Education/ Revue d'histoire de l'éducation* 17.2 (2005): 265–92.

29   Tony Bond, "Conception and Birth: Birth Control ... a factual survey ... Abortion," *Varsity: Review* (12 March 1965): 2. I thank Catherine Gidney for this reference.

30   Donald Kingsbury, "We Send Her to the Butcher Shop," *McGill Daily* (30 October 1967): 5.

31   "What Does a Girl Do If She's in the Middle of the School Year and Suddenly Discovers She's Pregnant?" *Varsity* (6 March 1968): 6–7.

32   Kristen Luker, *Abortion and the Politics of Motherhood* (Berkeley: University of California Press, 1985), p. 118.

33   Sethna, "University of Toronto Health Service."

34   Christabelle Sethna, "The Evolution of the *Birth Control Handbook*: From Student Peer Education Manual to Feminist Self-Empowerment Text, 1968–1975," *Canadian Bulletin of Medical History/Bulletin canadien d'histoire de la médicine* 23.1 (2006): 89–118.

35   Donald Kingsbury, "Pregnancy and Social Action," in Donna Cherniak and Allan Feingold, eds., *Birth Control Handbook* (Montreal: Student's Society of McGill University, 1969), pp. 33–4.

36   Doris Giller, "Abortion in Montreal," reprinted from the *Montreal Star* in *Birth Control Handbook,* p. 34.

37   "Judy: Reaction to Book Surprised Her," *Vancouver Sun* (25 January 1969): 6.

38   McLaren and McLaren, *Bedroom and the State,* pp. 132–8.

39   Childbirth by Choice Trust, *No Choice,* p. 127.

40   Maureen Muldoon, *The Abortion Debate in the United States and Canada: A Sourcebook* (New York: Garland Publishing, 1991), pp. 173–4.

41   Gerald Waring, "Report from Ottawa," *CMAJ* 98.8 (28 February 1968): 419.

42   Ian Macdonald, "House Told Money Governs Abortion," *Vancouver Sun* (28 January 1969).

43 *Birth Control Handbook* (September 1969), p. 40.

44 Catherine Dunphy, *Morgentaler: A Difficult Hero* (Toronto: Random House of Canada, 1996), pp. 61–6.

45 Thinly disguised as "Dr. C.," Dr. Henry Morgentaler is quoted in Pelrine, *Abortion in Canada*, p. 77.

46 Dunphy, *Morgentaler*, p. 89.

47 Leslie J. Reagan, *When Abortion Was a Crime: Women, Medicine, and the Law in the United States, 1867–1973* (Berkeley: University of California Press, 1997), p. 208.

48 Leslie J. Reagan, "Crossing the Border for Abortions: California Activists, Mexican Clinics, and the Creation of a Feminist Health Agency in the 1960s," in Georgina Feldberg, Molly Ladd-Taylor, Alison Li, and Kathryn McPherson, eds., *Women, Health, and Nation: Canada and the United States since 1945* (Montreal and Kingston: McGill-Queen's University Press, 2003), pp. 355–78.

49 Faye D. Ginsburg, *Contested Lives: The Abortion Debate in the American Community* (Berkeley: University of California Press, 1989), pp. 35–7.

50 Rachel Benson Gold, "Lessons from before Roe: Will Past Be Prologue?" *The Guttmacher Report* 6.1 (March 2003), http://www.guttmacher.org/pubs/tgr/06/1/gr060108.html (accessed 12 July 2006).

51 Cope Schwenger, "Abortion in Canada as a Public Health Problem and as a Community Health Measure," *Canadian Journal of Public Health* 64.3 (1973): 223, 225. See also "Abortions up 25.6 percent," *Canadian News Facts* (16–30 November 1973): 1113.

52 Mollie Gillen, "Our New Abortion Law: Already Outdated?" *Chatelaine* (November 1969): 102.

53 "Toronto Mother Tells of Her Experiences in Having a Legal Abortion in London," *Toronto Star* (13 June 1969), reprinted in *Pro-Choice Forum* (September 1999): 8.

54 Mollie Gillen, "Why Women Are Still Angry over Abortion," *Chatelaine* (October 1970): 34–5, 80–4.

55 Nanette J. Davis, "The Abortion Consumer: Making It through the Network," *Urban Life and Culture* 2.4 (January 1974): 450.

56 Roberta Squire, "I'm Married, Happy, and Went through Hell for a Legal Abortion," *Chatelaine* (October 1970): 51.

57 "Women Declare War," *Pedestal* (March 1970): 2.

58 "Women Declare War," p. 18. See also Ann Thomson, *Winning Choice on Abortion: How British Columbian and Canadian Feminists Won the Battles of the 1970s and 1980s* (Victoria, BC: Trafford, 2004), pp. 19–30.

59 Frances Jane Wasserlein, "'An Arrow Aimed at the Heart': The Vancouver Women's Caucus and the Abortion Campaign, 1969–1971," unpublished MA thesis, Simon Fraser University (1990).

60 Doris Powers, "Statement to the Abortion Caravan," in *Women Unite! An Anthology of the Canadian Women's Movement* (Toronto: Canadian Women's Educational Press, 1972), p. 124.

61 Simon Fraser University Archives, F-73, Item 1, Douglas Fisher, "This Noise of Women Gags Voice of Reason," *Vancouver Sun* (May 1970).

62 "Law's Choice—or Girls'?" *Toronto Star* editorial, reprinted in *Vancouver Sun* (26 May 1970): 5.

63 Judy Rebick, *Ten Thousand Roses: The Making of a Feminist Revolution* (Toronto: Penguin Canada, 2005), p. 46.

64 Dunphy, *Morgentaler*, p. 127.

65 Barbara M. Freeman, *The Satellite Sex: The Media and Women's Issues in English Canada, 1966–1971* (Waterloo, ON: Wilfrid Laurier University Press, 2001).

66 *Report of the Royal Commission on the Status of Women* (Ottawa: Information Canada, 1970), pp. 284–5.
67 Dunphy, *Morgentaler*, pp. 156–7.
68 Badgley, Caron, and Powell, *Report of the Committee*, p. 28.
69 Badgley, Caron, and Powell, *Report of the Committee*, p. 74.
70 Badgley, Caron, and Powell, *Report of the Committee*, p. 19.
71 Badgley, Caron, and Powell, *Report of the Committee*, pp. 76–8.
72 Badgley, Caron, and Powell, *Report of the Committee*, p. 194.
73 Badgley, Caron, and Powell, *Report of the Committee*, pp. 381–4.
74 Dunphy, *Morgentaler*, p. 183.
75 Marion Powell, *Report on Therapeutic Abortion Services in Ontario: A Study Commissioned by the Ministry of Health* (27 January 1987): 6–7, 23–5, 34–6.
76 *R. v. Morgentaler*, [1988] S.C.J. No. 1 (S.C.C.).
77 See Nancy Bowes, Varda Burstyn, and Andrea Knight, *Access Granted: Too Often Denied: A Special Report to Celebrate the 10th Anniversary of the Decriminalization of Abortion* (Ottawa: CARAL, 1998); CARAL, *Protecting Abortion Rights in Canada: A Special Report to Celebrate the 15th Anniversary of the Decriminalization of Abortion* (Ottawa: CARAL, 2003); Jessica Shaw, *Reality Check: A Close Look at Accessing Abortion Services in Canadian Hospitals* (Ottawa: Canadians for Choice, 2006).
78 Christabelle Sethna and Marion Doull, "Far from Home? A Pilot Study Tracking Women's Journeys to a Canadian Abortion Clinic," *Journal of Obstetrics and Gynaecology Canada* (August 2007): 640–7.
79 Les Perreaux, "6-month Abortion Option in Wings," *Montreal Gazette* (11 September 2004).

Controlling Cervical Cancer from Screening to Vaccinations: An American Perspective

Kirsten E. Gardner

In the United States, contemporary conversations about cervical cancer are informed by a rich history of cancer awareness efforts that target female audiences. Since at least 1913, women have been encouraged to consult physicians at the first sign of irregular vaginal discharge, which is an early warning sign for cervical cancer.[1] Beginning in 1957, many American women began participating in cervical cancer screening. This mid-century innovation allowed for earlier detection of cervical cancer via a vaginal smear, more popularly referred to as a "Pap smear."[2] Most recently, in 2006 the U.S. Food and Drug Administration (FDA) approved Gardasil, a vaccine that promised to prevent infection from significant human papillomaviruses (HPVs), thereby interrupting cervical cancer.[3]

The twentieth-century history of cervical cancer in the United States illustrates the change and continuity evident in public awareness about women and cancer. Specifically, for nearly a century, cancer-awareness materials for women have emphasized that cancer poses a particular risk to females, especially due to the susceptibility of female reproductive organs to cancer. Additionally, women have worked conscientiously to inform one another about the risk of cancer and have frequently cooperated with the medical profession in emphasizing the importance of early detection.[4] Finally, early detection has been proven successful when applied to cervical cancer cases. Since the advent of the Pap smear, cases of cervical cancer in the United States have consistently declined, with the highest incidence in populations that have not been screened.[5]

The 2006 announcement of a cervical cancer vaccine created public excitement about advancements in cancer research.[6] Popular newspapers, magazines, and media sources covered the story and suggested that the vaccine had potential to nearly eliminate cervical cancer in the United States. Although many women had a general knowledge about cervical cancer, its risk, and the recommendations for routine screening via Pap smears, few had knowledge about the nearly two decades of research on HPV. Therefore, when Merck began an advertising campaign to teach American women about the vaccine, it also fostered scientific literacy about HPV—a sexually transmitted virus with a high incidence in the United States, identified as a cause of cervical cancer and genital warts. Story after story explained that the vaccine would block four strands of the virus that have been linked to as many as 70 per cent of American cervical cancer cases.[7]

In its efforts to sell a new product, Merck became the leading public authority on HPV and the benefits of a cervical cancer vaccine.[8] Equally significant, it assumed a role in public education, translating scientific and clinical findings into accessible language that would capture the public imagination. Merck's central role in the HPV conversation that emerged in 2006–07 demonstrated the impact of private industry on cancer education in the twenty-first century.

Today, private industry plays an ever-increasing role in American health education campaigns. Comparing the announcement of Gardasil's FDA-approved vaccine (2006) to the announcements promoting the Pap smear and cervical cancer screening (1957) clearly makes this point. In the former, the FDA made its approval announcement, the media offered coverage, and then Merck launched an aggressive advertising campaign. The marketing strategies of the Merck Gardasil campaign likely taught many more women about HPV than any contemporary public health campaign might have accomplished. Merck embraced print, media, and Internet advertising and quickly informed the country about the medical impact of the discovery of HPV. It emphasized that the vaccine could interrupt the virus, thereby preventing the potentially fatal impact of cervical cancer. The vaccine was championed as a scientific breakthrough, promising to impact cervical cancer mortality throughout the world. As John Niederhuber, acting director of the National Cancer Institute (NCI), explained, "This represents a triumph of basic science and of molecular biology research."[9] In the 1957 educational campaign, on the other hand, the American Cancer Society (ACS) co-operated with government agencies to coordinate awareness efforts, open detection centres, and encourage women to comply with screening guidelines, but there was little, if any, intervention from private companies.

In addition to highlighting the centrality of private interests in contemporary cervical cancer awareness, Merck's campaign reflected important shifts in popular representations of women in the cancer-awareness campaign. For much of the twentieth century, the U.S. public learned about cancer from non-profit organizations such as the ACS and government-sponsored initiatives, including those of the NCI and the U.S. Public Health Service. After nearly a century of awareness campaigns that typically depicted women as a homogeneous group represented by white, middle-class females, Merck launched awareness campaigns defined by diversity and multiculturalism. The Gardasil campaign presented women of various races and ethnicities in a range of domestic and public spaces. The advertisements adopted language and images of empowerment, depicting the women as potential cervical cancer patients who could confront the dreaded disease on their own terms.[10] Merck promised American women that its vaccine could eliminate a large proportion of cervical cancers.[11] In image after image, audiences saw a variety of women of colour from a wide range of racial and ethnic backgrounds espousing the belief that they could be "one less" statistic, "one less" woman battling cervical cancer, thanks to Gardasil.[12]

This essay offers a comparative examination of cervical cancer-awareness initiatives in the United States launched in the mid-twentieth and early-twenty-first centuries. Since the American Society for the Control of Cancer (ASCC) launched popular cancer-awareness campaigns in 1913, women have been taught that lumps in the breast and irregular vaginal discharge could be early indications of cancer. This emphasis on early detection taught the public that patients play an important role in cancer detection. In 1957 the promotion of the Pap smear was facilitated by an already entrenched message that early detection saves lives. Women learned that annual Pap smears reveal precancerous indications and thereby facilitate effective treatment. In 2006, when women learned about the value of a cervical cancer vaccine, especially if administered before the start of sexual activity, the message of early detection and prevention once again resonated. This chapter compares these two educational efforts while highlighting the transformations that have occurred in popular cervical cancer-awareness efforts and the continued emphasis on women's responsibility in cancer-detection models.

History of the Pap Smear

Mid-century Americans believed that science and technology offered solutions to many vexing problems, and with this cultural backdrop, the ACS turned to cancer research as a venue for cancer cures.[13] Cancer-research funding had typically given priority to cancer treatments and detection through biopsy rather than prevention. In the late 1940s, however, after decades of investigation of cervical cells, Dr. George Papanicolaou gained ACS attention and support for his research on cervical cancer screening.[14]

Papanicolaou, born in Greece in 1883 and the son of a physician, earned a medical degree from the University of Athens in 1904. Uncertain about pursuing medicine, he went to the University of Munich to study philosophy and received a PhD six years later. Described as a "gentle, modest man," he emigrated to the United States in 1913 with his wife, Maria Mavroyeni. He then directed his energy to scientific research that would prove critical to cervical cancer screening in the United States and around the world. He spent his first years in the United States studying pathology at New York Hospital.[15]

His early work at New York Hospital focused on guinea pig egg cells, likely inspiring his interest in cytology. In collaboration with Charles Stockard, Papanicolaou launched a large study of vaginal fluids (collected from ill and healthy women at New York Hospital beginning in 1923). Perhaps the most lasting outcome of these studies is Stockard and Papanicolaou's recognition of precancerous cells in vaginal fluid. Years later, Papanicolaou would still vividly recall his realization that he could identify a precancerous cell, describing it as "one of the greatest thrills I ever experienced in my scientific career."[16]

Although he realized the significance of his discovery almost immediately, his preliminary reports generated little enthusiasm in the scientific community; physicians and scientists remained partial to biopsy for cancer detection. Papanicolaou recalled, "I failed to create much faith among my colleagues in the practicability of this procedure."[17] He subsequently abandoned this research for the next decade.

In 1938 his interest was renewed when he developed a partnership with Dr. Herbert Traut.[18] For the next several years, he, Traut, and fellow gynecological pathologist Andrew Marchetti worked on staining, identification, and diagnostic principles. In 1943 Papanicolaou and Traut published their findings in *Diagnostic Principles of the Vaginal Smear*.[19] With this publication, the research community and others began to appreciate the potential of cellular examination and early cancer detection. "This may be compared to an avalanche," recalled Papanicolaou, "which, once started rolling, constantly kept gathering speed and more strength."[20]

The ACS directed interest and funding to research on cancer screening with increased frequency after World War II, in part because ACS medical and scientific director Charles Cameron supported the idea and in part because postwar culture believed in science and technology. But most significantly, the ACS had redefined its mission to centre on research.[21] Advances in cervical cancer-screening research seemed a perfect fit with this mission. Journalist W.L. White tapped into the excitement surrounding smear technology and its potential impact to reduce cervical cancer mortality. White wrote in 1947: "[A] test has recently been devised, a test which is quick, cheap, painless, and simple, 96 per cent accurate, a test which any country practitioner can give in his office, the results of which he can send for interpretation to a properly trained expert."[22] White's assurance about the potential, accuracy, and efficiency of the test was premature; however, his tone captured the hopefulness surrounding a new medical breakthrough in cancer diagnosis and detection.

In 1948 the national ACS cytology conference marked the beginning of a clear commitment to exploring the feasibility of cervical screening throughout the United States. But unlike White's summation of the test as quick, easy, and painless, the ACS and others recognized the expense of the test, the huge demand for specialists to read cancer smear slides, and the necessity of influencing human behaviour (in this case, the behaviour of women over the age of thirty-five) to comply with invasive and routine medical testing. For the next decade, the ACS, NCI, and other organizations would encourage additional research in the field, launch clinical trials of vaginal smear testing, and plan a national education and awareness campaign. But between 1948 and 1957, as cervical cancer studies and trials continued, the public learned little about this technology. Cancer organizations did not want the public to learn about the test too early, when gaining access to the technology was still difficult. At the end of the 1947 cytology cancer conference, in spite of the desire to celebrate the medical advances discussed, the ACS and others agreed to deliberately halt the public and popular promotion of early detection of cervical cancer through cell examination. White's 1947 promised "test which is quick, cheap, painless" was not ready.

Although Papanicolaou recognized the merits of screening, he continued to promote the more traditional message that cancer diagnosis required biopsy. He emphasized that the smear offered merely an indication of cervical cancer. Like many ACS officials, Papanicolaou appreciated the labour-intensive nature of any system of universal cancer screening. Cervical cancer screening would require a huge transformation in the medical field:

clinics and other medical spaces would need to accommodate new staff with expertise in cancer detection via pathology.[23] In spite of these practical limitations, the notion of an effective cancer screening test appealed to many. Undoubtedly, Papanicolaou (and other scientists) benefited from the ACS's increased support of research in the postwar era. As ACS president David Wood explained, the ACS wanted to increase "availability of funds for research."[24] And as research confirmed the diagnostic capability of this test, its popularity only increased.

Promoters of universal cervical screening claimed that the incidence of death from uterine cancer could decline by as much as 75 per cent with early cell diagnosis and prompt treatment.[25] Although significant barriers to universal screening still existed, Americans embraced the idea. However, obstacles such as the dearth of trained American pathologists and women's ignorance about the exam persisted. If thirty million American women over the age of forty were to participate in cervical cancer screening, a professional revolution would need to take place—the number of pathologists would have to increase exponentially and quickly. Alternatively, as Charles Cameron, the former medical and science director of the ACS, proposed, a new category of "screeners" or "cyto-technicians" could fill this medical gap. Monica Casper and Adele Clarke have astutely analyzed why and how this new professional category emerged.[26] They argue that the Pap smear emerged only after great "tinkering" and renegotiation of labour, technology, expectations, and political pressure. Instead of an immediate success, the Pap smear gradually assumed its role as the "best tool" for screening. As Casper and Clarke note, "In short, the Pap smear served as a symbol of the 'new' cancer research, and offered a 'cheap' means of importing prevention and early intervention into routine clinical practice."[27]

Educational Agenda

For many years, at least beginning with the creation of the American Society for the Control of Cancer (ASCC) in 1913, cancer awareness advocates worked to include cancer discussions within popular culture. Throughout the twentieth century, Americans learned about cancer through posters and bulletin boards, health pamphlets, lecture series, and community viewings of cancer films. Perhaps most importantly, cancer educators successfully encouraged journalists to direct attention to the cancer problem. Readers of popular women's magazines such as *Ladies Home Journal* and *Good Housekeeping* learned about women's risk of cancer, as did readers of popular health journals such as *Hygeia* and *Today's Health*.[28] A concise article entitled "Cancer Facts for Women" surmised in 1946, "Cancer could not kill nearly as many people as it does today if everybody knew the first and most important fact about this disease—that it can be cured IF it is caught in time."[29] The article further illuminated the contemporary advice about the dreaded disease: a woman must visit a physician immediately if she notices either a lump in her breast or irregular vaginal discharge. Women learned about the importance of reproductive health and consistently heard that physicians could only cure cancer if the disease was detected in its earliest phase.

Although Papanicolaou and his colleagues had begun publishing their findings about the potential of smear technology as early as the 1920s, the public did not learn about it until the 1940s. Even then, the conversation evident within popular culture (especially within women's magazines) suggested a cautious optimism about the applicability of this technology to cancer prevention programs. In short, patient vigilance was consistently encouraged and praised, and early detection was placed squarely in the hands of women.

For well over a decade, American cancer educators negotiated the boundaries between verifying medical discoveries, planning screening programs, and informing the public about new technology. Finally, in 1957 the ACS and others initiated a major educational campaign. The ACS marked this moment with the release of its educational and dramatic film *Time and Two Women*.[30] This short film, which featured gynecology expert Dr. Joseph Meigs, traced the story of two white, middle-class women diagnosed with uterine cancer.[31] Meigs offered background to each case as the scene went back and forth between the two women, with Meig's oral narration in the background. One woman routinely participated in cervical screening: she was diagnosed with cancer and treatment was effective. The second story featured a woman who ignored her reproductive health. By the time she visited a doctor due to irregular vaginal discharge, it was too late. The physician could not cure the cancer. This woman "failed" to practise preventative health screenings and unfortunately died from cancer.

Multiple copies of *Time and Two Women* travelled throughout the United States, spreading the clear message that early detection saved lives, and that a woman's duty to herself, her family, and American society included her commitment to early detection of cancer. Women's clubs and other organizations throughout the United States, ranging from the National Council of Negro Women to local ACS chapters, hosted film screenings and information sessions about cervical cancer. These programs encouraged women to alert their neighbours and women within their communities to respond to the risk of cervical cancer and engage in the life-saving practice of early detection and cervical screening.

A concerted effort to convince women over the age of thirty-five to participate in cervical cancer screening was initiated in 1957. As public discussions of uterine cancer screening expanded, concern lingered that "even where physicians and pathologists are ready, an immense program of public education is needed."[32] In addition to the new film that was circulating throughout the country, the ACS introduced the idea of cervical cancer screening in multiple venues. It participated in health fairs and speaker series, and encouraged popular magazines to tell women about this diagnostic tool. The educational message tended to reflect dominant norms in American culture: for example, the campaign conscientiously catered to notions of femininity, initially opting for the term "cell examination for uterine cancer" because "vaginal smear" and "Pap smear" sounded too "unpleasant."[33] Over time, the common adoption of terms that included "smears" and "tests" would prove unavoidable. By the time U.S. public health policy included cervical screening, the goal of the ACS had become ambitious. It's message was that "*all* adult American women must be screened every year. A big job."[34]

Educators relied heavily on the early detection rhetoric that promised the public that the key to curing cancer was early detection. Once the public became convinced of this point, advances in early diagnosis technology proved all the more compelling. Long before launching the 1957 cervical cancer-awareness campaign, women had been told about healthy cancer-prevention habits. For decades, and especially since the creation of the ASCC in 1913, popular messages about cervical cancer prevention and early detection had encouraged women to visit physicians routinely (advice varied from annually to every six months), especially after the age of thirty-five. As early as the 1930s, medical advice suggested that any tears and injuries in the cervical area needed prompt treatment as a preventative to cervical cancer. And of course, any irregular vaginal discharge should cause women to seek immediate medical consultation. For educators, the mission was clear: "The American Cancer Society's research, service, and education program are spearheading a nation-wide effort to save the women of America from death by uterine cancer."[35]

The education campaign that began in 1957 experienced some success in teaching the public about the exam; it had less success in changing the behaviour of the majority of American women. In 1961, the ACS returned to one of its most useful allies in early-twentieth-century cancer awareness campaigns, the General Federation of Women's Clubs (GFWC). Throughout the 1920s and 1930s, the GFWC had encouraged its affiliates to teach women about the importance of early detection. The ACS now turned to this umbrella organization with hopes that it would encourage women to have routine cervical cancer screening. The "Conquer Uterine Cancer Program" emerged at the same time that Gallup polls and other surveys indicated that many women had heard of the Pap smear, but fewer had gone to a clinic or office for the exam. Moreover, the ACS noticed that even when women participated in cervical screening, they rarely returned for the advised subsequent annual exam. The data suggested that at a time when approximately fifty-seven million women lived in the United States, approximately sixteen million women had heard of the test but only five million women per year had a cervical screening. Moreover, approximately 40 per cent of American women remained unaware of the test, and approximately nine million women were due for repeat examination.[36]

When a Gallup survey asked women in 1964, "Have you ever heard or read about the 'Pap Smear' examination used to detect the presence of uterine cancer?" seventy-seven per cent of respondents replied in the affirmative. When those who responded affirmatively were further asked if they had had the examination, only 48 per cent replied "yes."[37] The National Council of Negro Women (NCNW) took note of this disparity and quickly mobilized within the black community to promote cervical screening.[38] In 1963 it sent information to members that read, "Twice as many Negro women as white women fall victim to uterine cancer." It further urged all NCNW members to participate in and to promote cervical screening. As Estelle Osborne explained, the objective of the NCNW was no less than "to reach as many Negro women as we possibly can—through our organizations and within the communities in which we live—to urge that they begin a life-time habit of annual physical check-ups including the 'Pap' test."[39] The NCNW's commitment to cervical cancer screening was further pronounced by its drive to tally the number of members who participated in cervical screening. It sent forms to each chapter and member requesting that women report their participation in cervical screening. The NCNW maintained confidentiality but was concerned with collecting the number of participants. Routinely, chapters sent postcards to the NCNW leaders reporting that they were "happy to take part in the CONQUER UTERINE CANCER PROJECT sponsored by the NATIONAL COUNCIL OF NEGRO WOMEN and the AMERICAN CANCER SOCIETY." Further, chapter presidents promised, "I will report, quarterly, to the local unit of the ACS the number of our members who have had checkups and

Pap smears."[40] The educational leadership of the NCNW was remarkable on several fronts, perhaps most noticeably in its willingness to co-operate with the ACS, an organization that at the time did little to respond to the evident and emerging disparities in cancer care.

Since 1957, pamphlets, films, and educational programs have emphasized the need to educate all women in the United States about uterine cancer screening. As *Negro Digest* wrote about the ACS's participation in this effort, "Their goal is to encourage every woman, regardless of race, to get an annual medical examination from her own doctor, which will include the cell examination for uterine cancer."[41] But although the ACS created alliances with African-American physicians and ministers, and with such groups as the National Association of Colored Women, Alpha Kappa Alpha Sorority, and the National Beauty Culturist League, the promotional material it created and distributed offered no representations of women of colour. Throughout the 1960s, black organizations sponsored film viewings of *Time and Two Women*—a film that featured white women, white physicians, and white audiences throughout. Although it conveyed an important message, it offered no multicultural representation of the United States and instead relied on pervasive images of a dominant American culture based on a white, middle-class family model.[42]

As early as 1963, notable African American community leader Dorothy Height responded to the ACS call, considering ways in which she could transmit the ACS message to African American women.[43] She wrote, "We have shown different cancer films at our meetings and the members have become more aware of the job being done by the American Cancer Society."[44] Recognizing black women's health as a priority, Mrs. Albert K. Kight, the president of the National Congress of Colored Parents and Teachers, explained, "The educational aspect of the program enables us to help protect ourselves and our families against the disease. We find it deeply gratifying to disseminate this information to our neighbors and to assist with raising funds to continue the educational program of the society." The co-operation evident between the ACS and African American women signified black women's desires to reduce cancer in the community, as well as a need for health material that would help achieve this goal.

For black activists, the higher rate of uterine cancer among African American women (approximately twice the incidence as in the general population) made uterine cancer a particular problem. In addition to sponsoring programs within women's clubs, black journals devoted articles to the issue. In 1961 *Negro Digest* printed very clear instructions for African

American women. First, black women should participate in prevention programs. Second, women should commit to early detection procedures. Finally, women should seek treatment immediately. Implicit in these messages were instructions not to delay, ignore, or avoid cancer diagnosis and treatment. Moreover, these messages echoed the dominant messages evident in popular culture that targeted white audiences. Curiously though, some educators inserted additional issues of sexual behaviour into uterine cancer education for African American female audiences. This trend was not paralleled in the popular press, which tended to target general audiences.

"Through understanding of the necessity and importance of personal hygiene and periodical medical examinations for uterine cancer, many lives can be saved," wrote Vincent E. Saunders, the chief health educator of the Chicago Board of Health.[45] Pitching his article to both men and women, he emphasized that poor sexual hygiene could cause uterine cancer. He encouraged men to be circumcised and to ensure that their sons were circumcised. He also urged both men and women to be tested for venereal disease as part of routine health care. Whether these assertions were included to advance an anti-venereal disease campaign or because of the entrenched racist stereotypes about black sexuality is not clear, but likely both motivations influenced his impulse to link venereal disease education and cancer.

For the next several decades, the ACS, NCI, and other health advocates continued to encourage women to have Pap smears and incorporate cervical screening into routine health care. Although community and local efforts such as the one launched by the NCNW responded to particular needs within a community of women, more times than not the cervical screening campaign envisioned a singular category of women. By focusing on women as a singular category, education campaigns frequently marginalized those who did not see themselves represented in dominant American culture. Since the creation of the ASCC, many of the educational campaigns had relied on images of white, middle-class, educated, and urban women as a model for all women in the United States. Around the turn of the century, however, the ACS, NCI, and others recognized the shortcomings of this programming and shifted tactics to direct more cancer messages to women of colour within the United States.

Impact of Race and Ethnicity

In 1996 the U.S. government published a landmark report entitled *Racial/Ethnic Patterns of Cancer in the United States: 1988–1992*. Collecting data on racial and ethnic disparity and cancer, this report, created by SEER (Surveillance, Epidemiology and End Results) exposed the disparity evident among different communities of women in the United States. Vietnamese women had a higher incidence of invasive cervical cancer than Hispanic women, who had a higher incidence than Chinese women. Moreover, African American women experienced the highest age-adjusted mortality, while Hispanic women ranked second. The report detailed risk factors, including early age of sexual intercourse, multiple sexual partners, viruses, and cigarette smoking. It also emphasized two prevention strategies: behaviour modification and screening technology. Modifying risky sexual behaviour promised to lessen the risk of cervical cancer, as did smoking cessation.[46]

In 1998 the NCI issued a pamphlet entitled "El papanicolaou! i un habito saludable, para toda la vida!" ("The Pap smear! A healthy habit for life!"). The accompanying image—a women curled in a chair, reading, with a cat by her side—blurred racial categories. The message continued, "El papanicolaou puede ayudar a detector el cancer del cuello del utero en su etaga temprana, cuando todavía es fácil de curar" ("The Pap smear can help detect cancer of the cervix in its early stage, when it is still easy to cure").[47] Another popular health education pamphlet, also printed in Spanish, informed women about the definition of cervical cancer, the necessity of vaginal smears, details about the frequency of the test and where it is performed, how to understand results, potential diagnosis, and treatment options. At last, as health advocates recognized the diversity of Americans, turn-of-the-century cervical cancer-awareness efforts began to include pilot educational programs that targeted Chicana, African American, and other under-represented audiences.

A 2001 pamphlet entitled "Pap Tests: A Healthy Habit for Life" features an African American woman consulting a female doctor whose racial/ethnic identity seems to be Latina.[48] In subsequent pages of the pamphlet, women of various races and social strata are shown learning about cervical cancer. In addition, the pamphlet employs the power of *testimonios*, sharing such sentiments as "If I start to feel embarrassed, I take some deep breaths, and then I feel better." A nurse offers advice to a patient that she should avoid exams during her period, soon after douching, or within twenty-four hours of sexual intercourse. In addition to increased racial diversity, turn-of-the-century pamphlets also targeted older American women. "Pap Tests for Older

Women: A Healthy Habit for Life" lists ten common questions that elderly women confront regarding cervical cancer screening.[49]

By 2006, the year the FDA approved Gardasil, cervical cancer-awareness campaigns were dramatically different than those that were launched in 1957 with the announcement of the Pap smear. Gardasil represented women from a variety of racial, ethnic, and class backgrounds. It placed women of colour at the centre of its advertising campaigns, and it used feminist language to assure women that they remained the most important agents in their health care decisions. Informed by the history of several powerful political movements (including the civil rights movement, the Chicana movement, the black women's health movement, and the feminist movement), the publicity campaign to promote Gardasil indicated that a transformation had occurred in cancer awareness. First, women were no longer represented as a homogeneous group dominated by representations of white, middle-class mothers. Instead, advertisements included dozens of faces and multiple voices, all female and all working to spread a message of cancer control via vaccination. In addition, private industry displaced non-profit and governmental agencies as the purveyors of cancer-awareness information.

Conclusion

In recent decades, the role of women in American cancer politics has evolved significantly. Cancer survivors have formed political coalitions demanding more research funding directed to women's cancers and health disparities. Women have gained coveted and prestigious positions as members of scientific funding review boards, asserting the importance of lay representation within professional gatherings. Publishers have supported the genre of cancer *testimonios*, providing an increasingly rich and diverse library of cancer narratives.[50]

Cervical cancer screening has exponentially reduced the incidence of uterine cancer in the United States. The promise and excitement surrounding screening in its early years proved well founded. The remarkable decrease in reproductive cancers since the mid-twentieth century suggests that the technology worked. Yet a closer look at cervical cancer screening, incidence, and treatment among various groups of American women reveals that cervical screening has had the greatest impact on privileged citizens—white women with health insurance.[51] Data suggest that the impact of cervical cancer screening could be even more pronounced if it were universally applied. Economic disparity continues to play a significant role in women's health, long after technological solutions emerge.

Reviewing this history suggests the important role that popular culture plays in perpetuating ideas about health, prevention of disease, and treatment. Influencing health behaviour, beliefs, and practices takes place within a broad cultural setting. To have the greatest impact, all women need to identify with the messages espoused. Within the United States, a variety of educational campaigns that directly respond to women's concerns regarding age, race, ethnicity, language, and class seem to guarantee more success in encouraging healthy behaviour. Merck has addressed many of these cultural issues in its marketing campaign; however, its high price tag indicates that it may face the same fate as the Pap smear—limited applicability among populations that are economically oppressed. Commitment to cancer prevention and women's health, whether led by public or private initiatives, must confront technological, cultural, and economic barriers. As Merck and other companies confront these barriers, their marketing initiatives reflect a long history of women's participation in cancer awareness.

Since 1957, women have learned about early screening for cervical cancer. Although its application has been far from even, it has successfully reduced American cervical cancer and promoted a model of early intervention against cancer. The introduction of an HPV vaccine builds on this history, relying on the public perception that early intervention works and that cancer can be interrupted. Although the Gardasil campaign reflects a multicultural America, and perhaps even feminist voices that empower women to confront cancer with this innovative vaccination, its universal potential remains elusive. Most notably at this point, the vaccine is expensive and legislative efforts to mandate the vaccine seem to be failing on a systematic basis.[52] This vaccine may have the potential to transform cervical cancer incidence in the United States in a parallel fashion to the transformations ushered in with the Pap smear in mid-century. However, the lessons of the past suggest that universal screening requires more than technological innovation. Cultural expectations, economic resources, and faith in the product will need widespread acceptance and support to ensure that all American women can indeed be "one less."[53]

Notes

1 *History of the American Society for the Control of Cancer, 1913–1943* (New York: New York City Cancer Committee, 1944).

2 Named after its creator, George Papanicolaou, also known as "Dr. Pap." See Harold Speert, *Obstetric and Gynecologic Milestones: Essays in Eponymy* (New York: Macmillan, 1958).

3 Jennifer Corbett Dooren, "Merck Cervical-Cancer Vaccine Is Approved for Use in Women: Gardasil Could Sharply Cut Key Viruses behind Disease," *Wall Street Journal* (9 June 2006): 16.

4 Kirsten E. Gardner, *Early Detection: Women, Cancer, and Awareness Campaigns in the Twentieth-Century United States* (Chapel Hill: University of North Carolina Press, 2006).

5 "How Many Women Get Cancer of the Cervix?" American Cancer Society website, http://www.cancer.org (accessed 11 April 2009);   Roger W. Rochat, "Pap Smear Screening: Has It Lowered Cervical Cancer Mortality among Black Americans?" *Phylon* 38.4 (1977): 429–47.

6 "FDA Licenses New Vaccine for Prevention of Cervical Cancer and Other Diseases in Females Caused by Human Papillomavirus," press release (8 June 2006), http://www.fda.gov/bbs/topics/news/2006/new01385.html (accessed 26 October 2009).

7 For example, see Jane Brody, "HPV Vaccine: Few Risks, Many Benefits," *New York Times* (15 May 2007): 7; Peter Sprigg, "A Promising Vaccine…," *Washington Times* (17 July 2006): A17; "Medical Edge: Ask the Mayo Clinic," *Seattle Post Intelligencer* (17 December 2007): F3.

8 Merck & Co., Inc. is a global pharmaceutical company founded in the nineteenth century with headquarters in New Jersey.

9 Angela Zimm and Justin Bloom, "FDA Approves Merck's Cervical Cancer Vaccine," *Boston Globe* (9 June 2006; accessed online 26 October 2009).

10 James T. Patterson, *The Dread Disease: Cancer and Modern American Culture* (Cambridge: Harvard University Press, 1987). Patterson offers a foundational examination of cancer in modern America, and as his title suggests, the disease has evoked fear and dread throughout the twentieth century.

11 To be sure, many women's groups had launched educational efforts that promoted transformative education, already disrupting the dominance of a white, middle-class model. However, unlike many successful local initiatives, Merck's campaign penetrated dominant American culture, normalizing transformative models.

12 "TV Commercial for GARDASIL [Quadrivalent Human Papillomavirus (Types 6, 11, 16, 18) Recombinant Vaccine]," http://www.Gardasil.com/tv-commercial-for-Gardasil.html (accessed 15 January 2009).

13 See chapter 6, "Hymns to Science and Prayers to God," in Patterson, *Dread Disease.*

14 Rochat, "Pap Smear Screening," and Mike Quinn, Penny Babb, Jennifer Jones, and Elizabeth Allen, "Effect of Screening on Incidence of and Mortality from Cancer of Cervix in England: Evaluation Based on Routinely Collected Statistics," *British Medical Journal* 318 (3 April 1999): 904.

15 Donald G. Cooley, "Men behind the Medical Miracles—Part II," *Today's Health* 37 (February 1959): 24–5, 66–7; Esther Allegretti, "Dr. George N. Papanicolaou: Profile," *Cancer News* (Summer 1957): 13–15.

16 Cooley, "Men behind the Medical Miracles," p. 66. See also Harold Schmeck, Jr., "Cancer Pioneer Nears Age of 75," *New York Times* (11 May 1958): 65.

17 Allegretti, "Dr. George Papanicolaou," p. 14.

18   Cooley, "Men behind the Medical Miracles," p. 66.

19   George N. Papanicolaou and Herbert F. Traut, *Diagnosis of Uterine Cancer by the Vaginal Smear* (New York: Commonwealth Fund, 1943).

20   Allegretti, "Dr. George Papanicolaou," p. 14.

21   Monica J. Casper and Adele E. Clarke, "Making the Pap Smear into the 'Right Tool' for the Job: Cervical Cancer Screening in the USA, circa 1940–95," *Social Studies of Science* 28.2 (1998): 255–90. Casper and Clarke offer an excellent background on the historical circumstances that ushered in the Pap smear as the best cervical cancer detection tool in mid-century. See pp. 259–62.

22   W.L. White, "Killer of Women," *Ladies' Home Journal* 64 (November 1947): 51, 108, 110. Quotation on p. 51.

23   Cooley, "Men behind the Medical Miracles," p. 66.

24   David A. Wood, "Looking ahead in Research," *Cancer News* (Winter 1957): 16.

25   "16,000 Women," *Cancer News* 11.1 (1957): 2–9. See p. 3.

26   "16,000 Women," p. 3.

27   Casper and Clarke, "Making the Pap Smear," p. 276.

28   *Ladies' Home Journal* and *Good Housekeeping* targeted middle-class white women readers, while *Hygeia* and *Today's Health* offered lay explanations of professional research and medical issues.

29   Jerome S. Peterson, "Cancer Facts for Women," *Hygeia* 24 (June 1964): 416.

30   Joe V. Meigs, *Time and Two Women* (Audio Productions, 1957; distr. American Cancer Society).

31   Dr. Meigs was the author of several books on cervical cancer including *Surgical Treatment of Cancer of the Cervix* (New York: Grune & Stratton, 1954). Along with Somers H. Sturgis, he also edited the four-volume *Progress in Gynecology* (London: William Heinemann Medical Books, 1947–64).

32   George N. Papanicolaou, "Cancer That Can Be Cured," *Today's Health* 36 (May 1958): 64.

33   "16,000 Women," p. 4. Educators considered the term *cytological studies* but dismissed this as too "complicated."

34   "16,000 Women," p. 4.

35   Papanicolaou, "Cancer That Can Be Cured," p. 64.

36   "Launch Drive to Wipe Out Uterine Cancer," *Today's Health* 39 (September 1961): 69.

37   George H. Gallup, *The Gallup Poll: Public Opinion 1935–1971* (New York: Random House, 1972), p. 1874.

38   The NCNW was founded by Mary McLeod Bethune in 1935 to represent the concerns of black women. It tapped into a tradition of club work and community activism and also offered a home to black women's clubs often excluded from the GFWC. It actively engaged in health issues and supported cancer awareness.

39   Records of the NCNW, letter by Estelle Osborne to "Friends" (16 April 1963), series 10, box 19, folder 13. Estelle Osborne served as the Vice President of the NCNW. She was a nurse, an assistant professor of nursing at New York University's School of Nursing, and a community leader. See "Estelle Obsorne, 80, Is Dead: Leader in Nursing Profession," *New York Times* (17 December 1981): D23.

40   Records of the NCNW, "Conquer Uterine Cancer: An American Cancer Society Project in cooperation with the National Council of Negro Women," series 10, box 19, folder 13.

41   Vincent E. Saunders, "A Memo to Negro Women: Uterine Cancer Can Be Reduced," *Negro Digest* 10 (August 1961): 27.

42   Saunders, "A Memo," p. 28.

43 Among many other achievements, Height served as national president of NCNW between 1957 and 1998. See Dorothy I. Height, *Open Wide the Freedom Gates: A Memoir* (New York: Public Affairs, 2003).

44 Saunders, "A Memo," p. 28.

45 Saunders, "A Memo," p. 30.

46 B.A. Miller et al., eds., *Racial/Ethnic Patterns of Cancer in the United States 1988–1992, National Cancer Institute*, NIH Pub. No. 96-4104 (Bethesda, MD, 1996).

47 National Cancer Institute, *El papanicolaou! i un habíto saludable, para toda la vida!* (Bethesda, MD: Oficina de Comunicación sobre el Cáncer, Instituto Nacional del Cáncer, 1998).

48 National Cancer Institute, "Pap Tests: A Healthy Habit for Life" (National Institutes of Health, Public Health Service, NIH Publication No. 96-3213, updated July 2001).

49 "Pap Tests for Older Women" (Washington, DC: NIH Publication No. 01-3213, September 2003).

50 Betty Rollin, *First, You Cry* (New York: Harper Paperbacks, 2000); Sandra Butler and Barbara Rosenblum, *Cancer in Two Voices*, 2nd ed. (San Francisco: Spinsters Ink Books, 1996); Rose Kushner, *Breast Cancer: A Personal History and an Investigative Report* (New York: Harcourt Brace Jovanovich, 1975); Audre Lorde, *The Cancer Journals*, special edition (San Francisco: Aunt Lute Books, 2007 [1980]).

51 Quinn et al., "Effect of Screening," p. 904.

52 Gardiner Harris, "Panel Unanimously Recommends Cervical Cancer Vaccine for Girls 11 and Up," *New York Times* (30 June 2006): A12. At $360 for a series of three shots, the vaccine is one of the most expensive in the medical market.

53 "TV Commercial for GARDASIL."

The Challenge of Developing and Publicizing Cervical Cancer Screening Programs: A Canadian Perspective

Mandy Hadenko

C ervical cancer is one of the few cancers that with early detection, can have a 100 per cent cure rate. By the mid-twentieth century, medical communities in Canada, the United States, and the United Kingdom understood cervical cancer as a potentially preventable disease, if properly organized screening programs were in place. Once knowledge about the disease was established, a prompt response on the part of health and government officials in the development of screening programs might have been expected. This was not the case in several Canadian provinces, even with a screening model in British Columbia (B.C.) as early as the 1950s. As Gardner demonstrates in the previous chapter, the Canadian experience with cervical cancer screening was very different from the American experience. Gardner argues that early in the twentieth century, women actively sought screening for this disease and "worked conscientiously to inform one another about the risk of cancer."[1]

This chapter focuses on early Canadian responses to cervical cancer screening, with particular attention given to Ontario and B.C. Within these provinces, there was a greater increase in knowledge on a more public level, both via print and film, than in other provinces, and in this chapter, I argue that print and film were integral places for women to seek knowledge about this disease. As Barbara Clow argues in *Negotiating Disease: Power and Cancer Care, 1900–1950*, in the early twentieth century, the Canadian public and medical professionals were largely invested in dealing with cancer treatment options rather than prevention. While science and technology took a powerful hold of Canadian society in the 1950s and 1960s, there was little focus on prevention. Even though scientists wanted to prove they could "cure" any disease, cervical cancer was still not on the radar of concern for the Department of Health in Ontario, Canada's most populous province.[2] Furthermore, prior to the mid-1960s and the advent of medicare, Canadian women had to pay for preventive health care. It was extremely difficult for health officials to convince women who felt perfectly healthy to pay for cancer screening. For centuries, women had been held responsible for the health of their households, but women resisted seeking screening, attempting to avoid a diagnosis of cancer even though it usually ended in death.[3] Once a fully funded health care system was in place in the 1960s, the prevention of cervical cancer seemed easier and more financially feasible for all Canadian women. Yet women were still reluctant to be screened, physicians were not active in educating and encouraging their female patients to be screened, and follow-ups were difficult to obtain. In Ontario, without government-funded and -monitored programs specifically devoted to screening, quality laboratory screen readings could not be guaranteed.

The founding of the Canadian Cancer Society in 1938 and the National Cancer Institute of Canada in 1947 increased cancer research and public awareness of both cancer and the lack of screening-program funding. Both the United Kingdom and the United States showed real initiative in funding and focusing on cancer research. In Canada, national conferences were held as early as the 1940s to discuss cancer research, mortality and morbidity rates, and, eventually, the prevention of cancer. However, as will be shown in this chapter, there was very little focus on cervical cancer until as late as the 1960s, except for the particularly early development of a central cytology laboratory and screening program in B.C. in the late 1940s and 1950s. Various discoveries, such as the understanding of the human papilloma virus (HPV) in the early 1980s, eventually moved cervical cancer awareness in the right direction. In 2007 both the medical community and the general public alike were openly discussing a "cancer vaccine," Gardasil, which purported to eliminate HPV from the cervical cancer equation completely. However, this type of vaccine has not come without criticism, as issues of sexuality, religious morality, and political motive surrounded its release.

The postwar transition of focus from a curative to a more preventive approach proved that prevention was on the minds of medical officials and researchers, but effective screening would require recall/follow-up systems, the monitoring of laboratory technicians and screening techniques, and increasing public awareness of the disease. In the 1990s, Ontario released a proposal for a cervical cancer screening program that appeared likely to succeed. This chapter demonstrates that even though the greater medical community in Canada was on board with the international movement to "conquer" cancer, it was much slower to organize fully funded public education programs focused on cervical cancer. This chapter also shows that women had to move beyond their physicians' offices to seek information about their cervices and how to protect them from cancer. Women consulted popular sources, including *Chatelaine*, the *Toronto Star*, and various films produced by the National Film Board.

Professional Development, Cancer Conferences, and Symposia

The twentieth century was a ripe time for progress in both medical understanding of cervical cancer and national bodies dedicated solely to the treatment and education of the public about cancer. Two societies were established that would prove to be instrumental in cancer care, research, and prevention in North America: the Canadian Cancer Society (CCS) and the American Cancer Society. Both entities developed from separate earlier groups that focused primarily on cancer research and treatment. Once each society was developed, there was more focus on raising money for cancer care and prevention programs to screen and educate the public than on research. As Kirsten Gardner argues in the previous chapter, the American Cancer Society was active in the development of public education programs on cancer very early in the twentieth century, leaving Canadians to wonder why the CCS waited until much later to invest in such initiatives. However, like the American Cancer Society, the CCS, along with Health and Welfare Canada, sponsored several conferences that would prove to be vital to the state of cancer care in Canada and the further evolution of cervical cancer screening programs later in the twentieth century.

While research was changing medical understanding of cervical cancer, the international medical community was responding to the cancer "epidemic" via conferences and symposia. Beginning in the 1920s, cancer was discussed in terms of bacteriology. This was a reflection of the medical community's recent success at curing tuberculosis. Borrowing from this success, the medical community spoke about cancer in terms of it being curable, similar to tuberculosis, which "rendered the disease less mysterious and suggested it would be as easy to conquer as an infectious disease."[4] In 1926 a key symposium marked the international agreement that "human society needed to mount a response to cancer."[5] Delegates from around the world, including Canada, arrived in Lake Mohonk, New York, to organize a "war against cancer."[6] Points of discussion were issues surrounding public education and treatment facilities with adequate equipment and staff.[7] This symposium in New York only started the ball rolling. Key addresses at the Toronto Academy of Medicine in 1929 and a lead editorial in 1930 in the *Canadian Journal of Medicine and Surgery* represented a call for a "national effort to combat cancer."[8] An additional response to the symposium in 1926 was the various provincial cancer programs that were established across Canada, starting in Saskatchewan in 1929.[9]

On the heels of these groundbreaking professional symposia, CCS was formed in 1938 with "the mandate to spread important information about the early warning signs of cancer to the Canadian public."[10] Its objectives included coordinating efforts to reduce cancer mortality, disseminating information on cancer, aiding in the investigation of cancer cures, supporting research, and raising funds to meet all of its objectives. The mission statement of the CCS (as updated in 1989) was "the eradication of cancer and the enhancement of quality of life of people coping with cancer."[11] The CCS headed most Canadian cancer-related public health initiatives and received a considerable amount of funding from the King George V Jubilee Cancer Fund to aid in its work. Despite national support from National Health and Welfare and the CCS, each province was responsible for creating its own public health education.[12]

The National Cancer Institute of Canada (NCIC) was created in 1947 through a joint initiative of both the CCS and National Health and Welfare. The NCIC focused on supporting cancer research through grants and other mechanisms, offering programs for training and development of personnel in cancer research, disseminating information relating to cancer research and control, facilitating and participating in activities sponsored by related agencies, and acting in concert with the CCS.[13] The development of the NCIC encouraged researchers to focus on cervical cancer. For example, Ernest Ayre, a Canadian medical doctor and researcher, applied for a Grant-in-Aid from the NCIC in 1947. He needed funding to further validate the use of the Pap smear in the battle against cervical cancer. He proposed to "investigate squamous carcinoma of the cervix in an effort to accumulate correlated evidence regarding cell metabolism, cell behaviour, and cell morphology."[14] He wanted to set up an extensive laboratory with expert staff to study cell behaviour and cell metabolism from cytology smears and scrapings. Furthermore, he hypothesized that "a vitamin B deficiency factor in uterine cancer cases coupled with intensive nutritional and hormonal studies in this disease" could be proven.[15] The total request of funds for Ayre's proposal was $14,800.[16] Although this research was important to validate the Pap smear, money was also needed to conduct more exploratory research in this area. Evidence of researchers needing money is apparent; whether or not these individuals received continued funding from national health agencies is another question. Health Canada records do not provide the answer.

Also in 1947, a cancer conference, sponsored by the NCIC and the CCS, and clearly part of the much larger medical "war against cancer," was held in Ottawa. It was understood that "for the person that has cancer today the greatest hope lies in early accurate diagnosis and treatment by an expert."[17] Although cancer prevention and cervical cancer were not a focus at this particular cancer conference, even though the Pap smear was well known in the medical community, the conference moved the national dialogue on cancer forward.

In 1967 NCIC sponsored another cancer conference focusing on prevention and control in Montreal. This meeting, directed by B.C. doctors with input from Ontario, focused on cervical cancer screening options and the impact of mass screening on incidence and mortality rates. Since B.C. was the first jurisdiction to develop a central cervical cytology lab and province-wide screening program, its representatives were instrumental in educating and convincing other provinces of the need for organized screening programs. The "meeting [was deemed to have been] worthwhile in that it stimulated frank and informal discussion of certain aspects of the problem of cancer. It was hoped that the conference might stimulate interest in this area on the part of younger members of the medical staff of teaching hospitals."[18] An open discussion about the importance of cervical cancer screening had finally occurred. This helped bring about change in other provinces by forcing evaluation of their poorer responses.

During this conference, Dr. D.A. Boyes of B.C. reported on the impact that a mass screening program had had on cervical cancer rates, stating that "the fall in morbidity from invasive cervical carcinoma in [his] Province was shown to be about 50% when two thirds of the female population 20 years and over had been examined."[19] Mortality rates from cervical cancer had shown little change in the rest of the country—a result, Dr. Boyes believed, of a lack of organized screening programs. He also discussed the benefits of having a central laboratory as opposed to several private labs, as "the large volume of specimens also keeps down the cost per specimen."[20]

The idea of self-sampling Pap smears was also discussed. Dr. Anderson of the Ottawa Civic Hospital announced that the "accuracy of the resulting screening was lower than for cervical scrapes."[21] Although the technique was questionable, it was agreed at the conference that it might have potential success in communities where medical personnel were available to take specimens during a pelvic examination. It was, however, concluded that self-sampling had no place in an area where appropriate medical personnel were available.[22] Self-sampling had been proposed previously in 1964 by Ontario Minister of Health Dr. M.B. Dymond as a less costly option than tests done in the physician's office. He advocated its cost-cutting potential, even though the procedure resulted in a higher rate of false negatives. In a 1964 memorandum to Dymond, Deputy Minister Dr. W.G. Brown concluded that any shift to a do-it-yourself examination program would be a mistake and would hinder the progress of an organized provincial screening program.[23] This may have also reflected desires of the medical community to contain cancer research and treatment (and indeed authority) within their profession.

Other provincial governments established task forces reporting to their ministers of health following a Charlottetown, P.E.I., conference of provincial ministers of health. The Quebec minister proposed the establishment of several expert task forces to study the various provincial screening and therapeutic programs useful in battling cervical cancer. Each task force had specific instructions, and in their June 1976 report, the NCIC made the following recommendations:

- Health authorities should encourage and support screening programs for cancer of the cervix;
- women should be informed of their degree of risk of developing cancer;
- a schedule of screening should be designed according to degree of risk;
- quality control in laboratories should be encouraged; and
- registries should be maintained for follow-up, and designed to permit inter-registry comparison.[24]

Yet these recommendations were not implemented in Canada, or in many other countries, for a number of years. As the establishment of task forces in the 1970s indicates, it took a few decades for this cancer to make it onto the radar of national and provincial health concerns. Ontario saw a few incidences that gave hope that perhaps a screening program was in the works; however, it was some time before a funded, organized program would be successfully put into place. Even without an organized screening program, though, many women in Ontario found other ways to educate themselves about cervical cancer prevention.

Developments in Cervical Cancer Screening and Public Information

There is a significant difference between cervical cancer screening and an organized cervical cancer screening program. Since the inception of the Pap smear in 1928, screening has been in place in many countries, as doctors started to use the technique to screen women for cervical cancer. However, without proper recall systems, consistency in reading of smears, laboratory quality assurance, and monitoring of public information, screening did not reach its full potential. In the United States, as Gardner argues, since the early part of the twentieth century, women have been encouraged to seek medical help at the first sign of irregular discharge. And as early as 1957, American women actively participated in cervical cancer screening. Contemporary discussions of cervical cancer in the United States are sensitive to issues of race and class, and new public awareness campaigns (such as the one for Gardasil) are encouraging women's awareness through a focus on risk factors such as HPV. Gardner also notes that the American Cancer Society invested in smear technology as early as the 1940s, encouraging a much earlier initiative to cancer prevention for women. Conferences, clinical trials, and media campaigns all successfully moved the United States through the twentieth century toward a very proactive approach to cervical cancer screening.

Unlike the American story, organized screening in Canada originated in one province and eventually, over several years, spanned the entire country. In the late 1940s, B.C. became the frontrunner in developing Canada's earliest cervical cytology lab and organized screening program. Other provinces in Canada were slow to follow B.C.'s initiative. Provincial governments were aware that proper screening and organized programs were necessary in battling cervical cancer rates, but they did not react with the necessary organization and funding. Dr. Ernest Ayre, a dominant figure in cytological work in the mid-twentieth century, informed clinics across Canada of the importance of cervical smears in decreasing the incidence of cervical cancer. For example, in 1948 Ayre informed Dr. A.W. Blair, director of the Regina Cancer Clinic, that routine cervical scrapings were necessary in all clinics. Dr. Ayre showed that five hundred routine scrapings "in the free gynaecological clinics [had led to the detection of] 11 cancers ... missed by routine examination."[25]

In the early years, Ontario was not as focused on cancer prevention as was B.C.; however, it did establish a cancer clinic in an urban centre, opening a cancer detection clinic in Toronto's Women's College Hospital in 1948. The idea was to examine "well women" in order to detect cancer. Although the clinic was geared toward diagnosis and not necessarily prevention, it was an important part of Ontario's activity in cancer control.

Funded at first by the province and then by the Ontario Cancer Research and Treatment Foundation (OCRTF), the clinic examined and treated both asymptomatic and symptomatic women and men within two decades of its establishment.[26] The onus was still on primary care physicians to recommend such examinations; the clinic did not simply "take patients off the street."[27] After a short while, the OCRTF could no longer subsidize the clinic, and fees were required of all patients. Eventually the cost per patient reached as high as $19.13. This fee included the doctors' fees, X-ray, laboratory fees, a nurse, supplies, and administration.[28] This clinic was reaching only a small portion of Ontario's female population—Torontonians able to pay for such a health service. Clearly, issues of class and location limited the demographic of women who could attend this clinic.

During the 1960s, the Ontario government was pressured to develop a funded, organized cervical cancer screening program. For example, the Municipality of Kitchener-Waterloo requested financial assistance for a program. In 1963 Health Minister Dymond denied the request, stating that he was "becoming steadily and increasingly befuddled about the place and function of municipal government."[29] He similarly refused other municipal requests, advising Minister of Municipal Affairs J.W. Spooner,

> Commenting on the resolution, I would say that city councils know nothing about this. Historically, Ontario has done more in this field than all the rest of Canada put together, and, indeed, when people need the latest treatment for cancer, they come to Ontario. I don't know if you ever have an opportunity to tell municipal councils in a kindly but firm way to "tend to their knitting," but it seems to me they need to be told this, and soon, I realize it is a difficult matter but, then, I never underestimate your powers![30]

Apparently Dymond believed that because Ontario had a prestigious cancer clinic in Toronto, there was no real cancer problem. He did not acknowledge the limited regional availability of screening, hence the outcry from other municipalities, who were lobbying for prevention services, not increased cancer treatment services.

Physicians also pressured the provincial government to establish organized screening. In 1965 Dr. Erwin A. Crawford submitted a proposal entitled "A Cytology Screening Programme for Cancer of the Cervix in the Province of Ontario," which included extensive statistical data regarding mortality and morbidity rates and the state of cervical cancer screening procedures in Ontario up to 1965. According to the proposal, Ontario had 1,244,000 women between the ages of twenty-five and fifty-four. Assuming that about one-sixth of these women had had hysterectomies, the study isolated one million women susceptible to cervical cancer in Ontario who should be screened. About 2.2 per cent of this group would develop carcinoma of the cervix, and half of those would die if they developed invasive cancer of the cervix.[31] The proposal then stated, "If all of these cases could be detected in the stage 1 cancer of the cervix, 80% could be cured, but if they all could be detected in the pre-invasive stage and treated, the deaths from cancer of the cervix could virtually be reduced to a zero quantity."[32] Not long after these localized attempts to pressure the provincial government in Ontario to create more organized screening opportunities, a more national response erupted via a conference focused on cancer treatment and prevention services.

The Walton Report arising from the 1973 conference in P.E.I. emphasized the desperate need for cervical cancer screening programs across Canada. The report publicized not only the serious nature of cervical cancer but also the importance of regular screening. Despite the publicity surrounding the Walton Report, however, government-funded screening programs were still not initiated. Two and a half years after the report's publication, Health and Welfare Canada sent out a questionnaire to health departments, agencies, and affected associations.[33] The initial questions asked about the report's effect upon policy: for example, "in the last two years, has your health department, agency, or association instituted ways to: i) inform women of their degree of risk of developing carcinoma of the cervix ... [or] ii) persuade women at risk to participate in the screening program?"[34] The questionnaire also asked whether physicians had increased their recommendations for smear examinations and how many local laboratories were responsible for processing the smears.[35] The authors of the Walton Report were hoping for substantial results with its publication. Not only were changes hoped for in the efficiency of laboratories and data collection, but also in the incorporation of the report's recommendations into the curricula of local training institutions.[36] These hopes were dashed as reports surfaced that few of the recommendations were being implemented.

Only thirty questionnaires were sent back, and every province and territory was represented by at least one respondent. The results in each province were interesting. Newfoundland, Nova Scotia, Quebec, and B.C. had "instituted concrete modifications in their official screening programs."[37] Such modifications included notifying physicians if a patient's smear was out of date, introducing a province-wide central cytology registry, and altering the recommended frequency of smear examination.[38] In Ontario, sporadic press releases were created to persuade assumed high-risk women to be screened. Despite a few small changes, Ontario did not institute enough changes within their screening practices to greatly affect mortality and morbidity rates. Ontario also reported that "a registry did not exist in a completely provincial sense and ... it had no plans to set one up" in the future.[39] In addition to individual provincial responses, the federal government attempted to inform women of their degree of risk by inserting an information pamphlet in the envelope accompanying family allowance cheques. With the addition of the pamphlet and the distribution of the Walton Report, the federal government felt they were sufficiently informing women of their inherent cervical cancer risk.[40]

Shortly after the Walton Report and the resulting questionnaire, Health and Welfare Canada launched a public education program called "Operation Lifestyle." This program comprised several different aspects, with cervical cancer playing a small part. In the fall of 1978, Health and Welfare Canada created a small pamphlet encouraging women to have annual Pap smears and educating women very generally about the risks of cervical cancer. Key risk factors such as age, previous health, and sexual activity were all mentioned.[41] Where this pamphlet was distributed and how many were printed at the time is unknown, but it can be assumed that it was primarily made available in clinics, sexual health centres, and other public health offices.

Some other limited measures were taken to educate the Ontario public about Pap smears and cervical cancer during this time. In an Ontario Medical Association Report to Council in 1984, clinical recommendations were made to pressure physicians to provide screening services to young women seeking contraceptive guidance.[42] There were also recommendations to encourage responsible sexuality through school curriculum, to provide barrier contraceptives in 75 per cent of all schools and universities by 1992, and to identify and assess methods to recruit high-risk women into regular screening by 1994.[43]

However, there were more easily accessible sources for women beyond formal government and medical publications. Without formal involvement in the medical community, laywomen found popular ways to communicate awareness and access information about cervical cancer. Until the mid-twentieth century, women relied on medical professionals to provide current understandings of the disease. As we know, power dynamics between doctor and patient often did not make the sharing of information particularly democratic. Neither were all physicians, or their patients, always fairly or thoroughly informed about the disease and its prevention. As a way of breaking through this dynamic, popular sources of information such as *Chatelaine* magazine and the *Toronto Star* empowered some women to learn and make educated choices about their own health. Parallel movements in the early 1970s—such as second-wave feminism, the women's health movement, and the self-help movement—finally created a climate conducive to open discussion surrounding cancer and its prevention. By bringing cervical cancer out from the vault of physicians' offices to the forefront of public discussion, women could take greater ownership of their bodies and their health.

Well before the women's health movement and the 1970s, the self-proclaimed feminist publication *Chatelaine* frequently published articles focusing on women's health. During the 1950s and 1960s (and as early as the 1930s and 1940s), arguably the peak of *Chatelaine*'s existence, the editors and publishers focused on catering to a "mass, national audience of women because television did not offer much programming specifically devoted to women's issues."[44] It is not surprising that during the early years of television, cervical cancer did not even grace the minds of television producers and writers. Cervical cancer was hardly talked about within the private confines of the physician's office, let alone on nationally broadcasted television.

Despite *Chatelaine*'s underlying feminist agenda at the time, it seems as though in regard to cervical cancer, the editors played it safe and focused on the voice of the all-knowing physician. For example, in a November 1930 article, Dr. John W.S. McCullough discussed cancer prevention. He attempted to quell generalized fears of the disease and provided ideas on prevention. Since it was too early for Dr. McCullough to mention the Pap smear, he wrote about preventing cancer (mouth cancer, in particular) by way of avoiding such "irritants" as some types of oils, jagged teeth, and a rough pipe stem.[45] He only mentioned cancer of the womb once: he stated that "the absence of irregular bleeding from the womb implies the absence of cancer of the womb," suggesting that if women could remember this simple fact, "much ungrounded fear would be prevented."[46] He also briefly mentioned breast cancer but offered little more than suggesting that women palpate their own breasts on a regular basis.[47]

By the 1940s, *Chatelaine* was publishing numerous features relating to cancer. For example, in November 1945, Adele Saunders wrote an article entitled "Plain Talk about Cancer," which argued that it was the fear of cancer that was more "treacherous" than the disease itself.[48] Bolstering twentieth-century medical triumphs in the understanding of cancer, Saunders clearly wanted people to believe that "cancer caught in its early stages is the most curable of all major causes of death, yet is the second greatest killer of our time. If prompt and adequate treatment is carried out, 70 to 80% of all early cancer is curable."[49] She noted that at that time, cancer of the uterus was responsible for nine hundred Canadian deaths a year. She further reinforced the medical understanding of the time that women who had many children were more susceptible to cancer of the neck of the womb. She believed, as is still believed today, that any abnormal bleeding should be a clear danger sign to all women.[50]

Although physicians wrote many of the earliest cancer articles in *Chatelaine*, a new voice was emerging by the late 1950s. Women began to speak out about their own experiences with cancer and their medical practitioners. This was the first real shift from general public cancer discussions to more publicly shared intimate experiences with cancer. This against-the-grain approach to editorials, according to Valerie Korinek, was *Chatelaine*'s 1950s mantra. In contrast to its American counterparts, *Chatelaine* challenged stereotypes of suburbia and "uncritical portraits of domestic bliss."[51] These portraits not only discouraged women of the 1950s and 1960s from talking about the taboo of cancer, but encouraged women to focus on postwar "affluence and good times of breadwinning dads and fulltime moms." Canadians of the 1950s and 1960s were not necessarily experiencing "good times" but were pressured to live "modern" during a time of extensive, and often devastating, socio-economic changes.[52] Contemporary medical opinion began to co-exist with women's voices and experiences, further validating personal experience. Through personal testimonies, women were validating themselves as experts of their own bodies, proving that they no longer required a physician to authenticate their experience or their knowledge.

One of the earliest articles in *Chatelaine* about a woman facing cancer was published in 1954. Dorothy Sangster told the story of Torontonian Jean Shaw, mother of six, and the strength of her and her family in the face of a diagnosis of cervical cancer. By the end of the article, the main themes are clear: medical science treated and cured Jean of cancer, and Jean suddenly realized the joys in motherhood, housework, and grocery shopping. Although written by another woman, much of Jean's voice and personal experience were present throughout: she was a woman who loved her family, who was determined to have everything in order in case she died, and who "never found crying a solution to anything."[53] She was a strong woman and never accepted any pity from anyone, including her husband and physician. Jean demanded honesty early in her relationship with her physician, especially if the diagnosis was cancer. Even so, the physician "softened the blow by declaring the disease was still in an early stage, and that early diagnosis and treatment resulted in many a cure."[54] Jean also claimed that it was the trauma she experienced with her numerous childbirths that caused the development of cancer. Voicing these conclusions to her physician, Jean was met with the opinion that there was no medical explanation for her diagnosis and, up to that point, no conclusive evidence to prove that childbirth trauma led to the development of cervical cancer.[55]

Another example of patient experience, published in 1959, is Kathleen L. Nouch's story about her experience with breast cancer. She explained how, after three different doctors insisted she had "imagined" the lump she had found, she desperately tried to forget it. After fourteen months, she discovered a noticeable abnormality in her breast, and after one visit, it was confirmed as breast cancer.[56] This article, and others similar to it in *Chatelaine*, reveal the breakdown of the medical community's monopoly on cancer discourse and authority over women's bodies.

While newspapers such as the *Toronto Star* did not necessarily focus on personal experiences with cancer, they also contributed in the 1950s to the new popular discourse on cancer prevention. Articles encouraging the public to validate the Pap smear were further reinforced by statistical data and professional opinion, all in accessible language. These articles provided women with the tools to engage in their own preventive health care. In 1955 a news brief entitled "Women! You Need No Longer Die from Your No. 1 Cancer Killer" (the full article was soon released in *Journal*, another popular publication at the time) discussed the Pap smear and its success in detecting cervical cancer not only in its early stages but also in its precancerous stages. This news exclusive mentioned key risk factors understood at the time, including women's greatest "burdens"—motherhood and marriage—and even suggested a male role in cancer development.[57] Also in 1955, another article was printed doubting the "cancer test." At this time, it was considered an American-born test that was not economically practical for provinces such as Ontario. Concerns about reliability and economics for Ontario health care providers seemed to outweigh the benefits of the test. One doctor stated, "[C]ancer of the cervix makes up less than 15% of the total cases of cancer in women in Ontario," implying that 15 per cent was simply not enough to invest in a mass screening program. The article criticized a program launched in Memphis, Tennessee, where women walking down the streets were bombarded with signs encouraging them to take a voluntary ten-minute screening test for cancer of the neck of the womb. While the Memphis project claimed to have had a screening success rate of 100 per cent, Ontario medical leaders were skeptical that investing in a test that only focused on one site was worth it. At this time, the Women's College Hospital was still running its well-women cancer clinic, but for $15, women were screened for numerous diseases, including tuberculosis and various sexually transmitted diseases. It did not seem practical to the medical officials at the time to invest "$1000s of public funds to uncover any unexpected cases of cancer early enough that the chances of cure rise from one out of five to three out of four."[58]

By the mid-1960s, the *Toronto Star* was publishing a few cervical cancer articles every year. The articles discussed key risk factors such as early marriage, early sexual activity, and multiple births, and continued to endorse the Pap smear as the most efficient tool in detecting this cancer early. In June 1967, the *Toronto Star* even published an article discussing the "do-it-yourself" cervical cancer test. This at-home test was arguably so easy to do that any woman could give herself a Pap test at home and simply send the specimen to her physician for examination. This article, originating in Chicago, discussed the unacceptable number of American women who did not even know what the Pap smear was, much less participate in annual examinations. This do-it-yourself technique, argued four Chicago physicians, would make this test accessible to all women, regardless of their class and access to health care.[59]

Prior to the women's health movement in the 1970s, films also played a role in popular cancer education. Cervical cancer was not, however, a cancer that made an appearance in any films during the 1950s. Like state-funded periodicals during the 1950s, films focused on general technological advances in understanding cancer, but did not discuss cervical cancer and its prevention. The 1950s were still early in terms of general understanding of the prevention of cancer. For example, the serious medical implications of smoking on the development of lung cancer were not yet fully understood. These films were a novel way for cancer experts to educate the public by breaking down literacy and class boundaries and reaching a more diverse population.

In 1951 the National Film Board of Canada produced *A Progress Report on Cancer*, directed by Morten Parker. This film attempted to chronicle the progress science had made in the "fight" against cancer. Using a villainous theatrical mode, this film portrayed cancer as something that science needs to "attack" and "conquer." The language used by the narrator focused on creating a dichotomy between science and disease: in this case, cancer. This militaristic language fit the time period, as the Second World War was just over and images of war were still fresh in the minds of Canadians. Countries were focusing on restructuring, recovery, and rebirth. Canada was no different, as many historians have argued; in the 1950s, the government focused on modernity and a return to normalcy, the family and repopulation, reviving lost industry, and the rebirth of the Canadian economy.[60]

One of the main purposes of *A Progress Report on Cancer* was to educate the public about science's progress in the fight against the disease. While the film used one case study of a man with a cancerous sore on his cheek, there were few specific references to different types of cancer and ideas about prevention. This film focused on treatment and cures of a disease that continued to kill people every day. Similar to the articles published in *Chatelaine* and the *Toronto Star* in the 1940s and 1950s, the public discussions of cancer were attempts to quell people's fears of dying from this often-incurable disease. However, these public discussions were often accused of "fanning cancerphobia."

Despite the potential for criticism and open concerns for creating a culture of "cancerphobia" in North America, the National Film Board of Canada produced a few other cancer-related films in the 1950s, such as *Report on Cancer* (1959), directed by Julian Biggs, and *Cancer Clinic* (1954), directed by Allen Stock. In the late 1960s and 1970s, public access to cancer information changed dramatically. Not only was cancer information released to the public in more accessible ways, but there was a direct focus on prevention of illnesses such as cervical cancer.

In Canada, the 1970s was a very radical time for women's health. The women's health movement, the self-help movement, and the much larger second-wave women's movement all demanded changes in both society and health care, and fought to bring cervical cancer out from the vault of physicians' offices to public forums for discussion. But one question always looms: how many women actually had the opportunity to access the resulting information? Class and literacy were two obstacles women may have faced when attempting to learn more about cancer, and even more specifically, cervical cancer. This all began to change in the 1970s. *Chatelaine* and the *Toronto Star* published more articles drawing attention to the systematic barriers to health care and bodily knowledge that women were experiencing. Not only did medical opinion now co-exist with women's voices and authority over their own bodies, but a new language of prevention was emerging, especially for cervical cancer, and access to knowledge about cancer was finally opening up. It also became clear to those involved in the women's health movement that change in the way health care and health care knowledge was delivered had to come from the bottom up. Some examples of attempts to achieve this goal are the creation of the Vancouver Women's Health Collective and the attempt by relatively conservative periodicals to discuss women's health more candidly. The 1970s also saw women critiquing the government's lack of movement on combatting cervical cancer.

Chatelaine played a role in disseminating ideas of the Women's Health Movement in the 1970s. Just as Korinek argues that *Chatelaine* furthered the march of "feminist awareness and organizing in Canada,"[61] I would argue that it did the same for women taking back the power to manage their own health and health care opportunities. This is demonstrated by *Chatelaine*'s shift from simple ads for the "fight against cancer" to more editorials and multi-page features focusing on cervical and breast cancer. Many of these articles emphasized preventive health and women's self-management of health care. In 1973, for example, *Chatelaine* published an article introducing the "breast Pap" smear and how it was able to find "cancers as small as rice grains."[62] A controversial article was published, also in 1973, on male chauvinist gynecologists. The article, entitled "Your Gynecologist: Show Me a Gynecologist and I'll Show You a Male Chauvinist (Even If She's a Woman),"[63] sparked much discussion and many letters to the editor. Most women enthusiastically supported *Chatelaine*'s publication of the article, as they could relate it to their own terrible experiences with their gynecologists, but others were appalled that it was even published. Dr. Charlotte S. Dafoe of Edmonton could not believe *Chatelaine* would publish such an "utterly sick article." She believed that it was a true "disservice to women" and argued that "the vast majority of gynecologists [were] intelligent men and women who [were] doing their best to practice their profession in a satisfying way."[64] In 1975 features continued to focus on breast cancer and began critiquing the growing number of unnecessary hysterectomies performed by doctors.[65]

The introduction of a regular "Health" column demonstrated a keener awareness of women's health care needs in the 1970s. The column disseminated the latest information from the medical community but also communicated prejudices held by medical professionals. In 1972 Dr. Robert Kistner stated that cervical cancer was more common among promiscuous "hippy type" women on oral contraceptives "who have coitus four or five times a day with different partners when they are using drugs." While this may not paint a very nice picture of women of the "hippy type," Dr. Kistner was emphasizing the link between sexual activity and cervical cancer. He added that cervical cancer was rare in nuns and Jewish women because of a strict or abstinent sexual lifestyle.[66] Also in 1972, the "Health" column discussed how often adult women should have Pap smears. Gynecologist J. Edward Hall believed that women up to thirty-five should have an annual Pap smear, and after thirty-five, they should undergo the procedure as often as every six months.[67] In 1974 Dr. John Wakefield, a renowned British gynecologist, claimed that the occupation of the husband might be a risk factor to the wife for developing cervical cancer. He argued that women married to miners, quarrymen, and other labourers "had the highest incidence of cancer of the cervix, while those married to artists, technical workers or professional men, had the lowest." The conclusion that blue-collar families produced higher incidences of cervical cancer drew out the disease's class dimensions.[68] These professionals often disseminated health knowledge coloured by classist, sexist, and racist suppositions.

In the early 1970s, the *Toronto Star* publicized several articles focusing on cervical cancer. In 1971 Marilyn Dunlop discussed Dr. Carl Burton French's organization of several cancer detection clinics in Toronto. French, who had been a campaign chair for the CCS, later created similar clinics in the Caribbean and South and Central America.[69] Other articles discussed various "new" causes for cervical cancer such as diethylstilbestrol (DES) and a virus carried by men. This was the herpes type-2 virus carried by both men and women, but the article focused on the man passing this virus on to his female partner.[70] These concerns about virus and cervical cancer risk eventually led to the discovery in the 1980s of the clear connection between HPV and cancer.

During the 1970s, Dr. Lindsay Curtis, the *Toronto Star*'s health expert, answered many questions on cervical cancer. In 1973, for instance, she responded to a woman who had asked for advice after receiving a positive smear test.[71] In 1974 Dr. Curtis wrote an article about a seemingly healthy young woman in the early stage of her second pregnancy whose Pap smear came back positive. Dr. Curtis discussed options with this young woman, who at first was in complete denial. The key lesson of the story was that this type of cancer, if caught early enough, was very treatable, so all women should have annual examinations.[72] Other "Your Health" columns in the *Toronto Star* included "Pap Test Reveals Cancer" in 1974 and "Routine Checkup Showed Women Had Cervical Cancer" in 1976. In the later 1970s, the health columns focused on the herpes type-2 virus and cervical cancer, in addition to genital warts. In 1978 Dr. Newman dealt with one woman's concerns that her husband thought she was "loose" because she had genital herpes (*not* contracted through intercourse). Dr. Newman reminded readers that up to 20 per cent of genital herpes cases are contracted in swimming pools and from public toilet seats.[73] These columns revealed that one obstacle to women's maintenance of regular Pap smears was its association with morality issues.

Films further provided viewers in the 1970s with visual examples of a disease they might read about. The National Film Board of Canada produced films focusing on breast and cervical cancer. *Still a Woman* (1973), directed by Dina Lieberman, openly discussed post-mastectomy experiences of women, and in 1974 Cheryl Wright produced *Cancer in Women*, which not only demonstrated various preventive procedures but also brought the brutality of cancer to the screen. Focusing on the prevention of breast and cervical cancer, the film showed very graphic images of cancerous cervices, filmed an entire pelvic exam, and demonstrated how to perform a breast self-examination. Wright, a medical photographer at a large Nova Scotia hospital, argued that the majority of the cancer cases she had seen were cancers restricted to women. She was appalled by how many women chose to neglect their health and simply did not participate in routine screening procedures. Many women, she argued, simply knew nothing about any of the pelvic cancers or breast cancer, or about how easy it can be to prevent and even treat them.[74] Both in print and in film, the onus remained on women to know their bodies and to know cancer.

The central visual experience in *Cancer in Women* is the instructional session of breast self-examination. The image is of a woman's bare chest (her head is not part of the shot so as to depersonalize this procedure) with a male physician instructing the viewer how to examine one's own breasts. His movements are relatively quick and firm, and his examination is followed by the headless woman performing the examination herself using a much softer technique. This instructional session is followed by very graphic images of breast cancers with various quotations from women who chose to neglect their breast health (even if a lump was present) playing in the background. These quotations include "I'm too old," "My husband doesn't make very much money," and "I've nobody to watch the children."[75] Although at times more visually graphic when discussing pelvic cancer, the film takes a similar approach to cervical cancer as it does to breast cancer.

The section on pelvic cancer focuses on the Pap smear, its preventive qualities, and how simple the procedure really is. After listing the various pelvic cancers, including cervical cancer, the film shoots an entire pelvic exam, including a Pap smear. The footage starts with a view of a woman's vagina with both her legs in stirrups. A male physician then narrates and performs a pelvic exam, including both sample-taking and a rectal exam. The physician only has one of his hands gloved; the other, used to separate the vaginal lips in order to insert the speculum, is not gloved. Like the breast exam, the physician is quick and fairly rough in his technique, and the woman's face is never shown. After the exam is finished, images are shown of various types of pelvic cancers while quotations of women giving excuses for not participating in routine pelvic screening play in the background. These quotations include "I thought it was just my age, with menopause and all,"

"Being examined is so humiliating," "I don't have time," and "I feel fine."[76] The film closes with Norma Mosier, executive secretary of the Women's Institutes of Nova Scotia, stating that while this film is difficult to watch and very graphic at times, all women need to see the ramifications of "neglecting their health."[77] This film is representative of the cancer awareness campaign of the 1970s. Recognition of high rates of incidence and deaths as a result of preventable cancer such as cervical cancer pushed health advocates to demand that women take more ownership of their own health and routinely participate in screening programs.

Conclusion

With the development of publicly funded health care in Canada in the 1960s, interest in cervical cancer mortality rates peaked. There were numerous attempts to survey and discuss the situation (for example, the Walton Report and various cancer conferences), but few seemed to solidify into a workable solution. B.C. spearheaded screening programs by developing its program for all women in the province as early as the 1950s. Other provinces were much slower in responding to cervical cancer mortality rates within their own jurisdictions. Ontario realized only in the 1990s that an organized screening program was much more successful than leaving screening to family physicians and patients themselves. Remote areas, such as Thunder Bay, were hardest hit by the lack of provincial support of screening programs as late as the 1980s and 1990s. As Cancer Care Ontario demonstrated in the early 1990s, even an organized screening program faced challenges such as a problematic recall system, consistency within physicians' offices, and laboratory technician training. Other issues such as class, location, and race continued to plague an already strained program. As a result of these problems, Cancer Care Ontario developed media resources that were available to all women, including the Internet and information pamphlets. Since 1971, cervical cancer incidence and mortality rates have decreased by about 46 per cent; however, this decline has slowed since the early 1980s. According to a public health survey done in 1996–97, one in six Canadian women over the age of seventeen had never had a Pap test.[78] Between the years 1994 and 1998, 842 Ontario women died from cervical cancer.[79] Cervical cancer is still ranked the eighth most common cancer diagnosed among Ontario women and ranks eleventh in cancer deaths.[80] Clearly, there needs to be an improvement in the delivery of screening programs and the organization and training of technicians, a more reliable data collection system, and a recall system that consistently informs women of the importance of regular screening.

Beyond issues of program development, Ontario is now discussing the release of Gardasil, a vaccine for HPV marketed in Canada by Merck Frosst Ltd. The primary goal of this vaccine is to eliminate HPV from the cervical cancer equation, in addition to preventing the spread of genital warts. Gardasil was approved for sale in 56 countries, including Canada, in 2006.[81] In September 2007, public health officials in Nova Scotia, Ontario, P.E.I., Newfoundland, and Labrador began administering Gardasil to select groups of girls in grades six, seven, and eight.[82] Gardasil was instituted in B.C. schools in 2008.[83] These immunization programs attract intense public debate. Politicians and religious leaders have all weighed in on the debate, arguing about the impact of Gardasil on sexuality and morality. While some researchers believe that Canada's National Advisory Committee on Immunization's recommendations are premature due to lack of extensive scientific knowledge of the vaccine, it appears that cervical cancer is finally getting the public exposure it has been demanding for half a century.

Notes

Associated Medical Services (AMS) and its Hannah Senior General Scholarship funded part of the research for this chapter. AMS was established in 1936 by Dr. Jason Hannah as a pioneer prepaid not-for-profit health care organization in Ontario. With the advent of medicare, AMS became a charitable organization supporting innovations in academic medicine and health services, specifically the history of medicine and health care, as well as innovations in health professional education and bioethics.

1   Kirsten Gardner, "Controlling Cervical Cancer from Screening to Vaccinations: An American Perspective," in this volume.

2   Barbara Clow, *Negotiating Disease: Power and Cancer Care, 1900–1950* (Montreal and Kingston: McGill-Queen's University Press, 2001), p. 12.

3   Clow, *Negotiating Disease*, p. 19.

4   Charles Hayter, "Cancer: The Worst Scourge of Civilized Mankind," *Canadian Bulletin of Medical History* 2.2 (2003): 260.

5   Hayter, "Cancer," p. 260.

6   Hayter, "Cancer," p. 260.

7   Hayter, "Cancer," pp. 260–1.

8   Hayter, "Cancer," p. 261.

9   Hayter, "Cancer," p. 261.

10 Canadian Cancer Society, http://www.cancer.ca/ccs/internet/standard/0,2939,3172_149 80_langId-en,00.html (accessed February 2002).

11 *The Proceedings of Cancer 2000, April 1992. A Report on the Work of a National Task Force, Cancer 2000: Strategies for Cancer Control in Canada* (Toronto: Smithkline Breecham Pharma, 1992), p. 67.

12 Canadian Cancer Society, http://www.cancer.ca/ccs/internet/standard/0,2939,3172 _14980_langId-en,00.html (accessed February 2002).

13 National Cancer Institute of Canada, http://www.ncic.cancer.ca (accessed August 2008).

14   National Archives of Canada [hereafter NAC], Dr. Ernest Ayre, 1947–48, National Re-
     search Council of Canada—Advisory Committee on Medical Research [hereafter Advis-
     ory Committee], RG 29 vol. 1180, file 311-C1-31.
15   NAC, Ayre 1947–48.
16   NAC, Ayre 1947–48.
17   NAC, "Cancer Conference—Ottawa" (1947), RG 29, vol. 1183, file 311-C1-37.
18   NAC, "The Role of Mass Surveys in the Detection of Cancer," RG 29, vol. 1183, file 311-
     C1-8.
19   NAC, "Role of Mass Surveys."
20   NAC, "Role of Mass Surveys."
21   NAC, "Role of Mass Surveys."
22   NAC, "Role of Mass Surveys."
23   Archives of Ontario [hereafter AO], "Cancer Research—Pap Smear, 1964," RG 10, file
     1-1-3.40.
24   NAC, National Cancer Institute of Canada, "Briefing Notes for the Minister—Cervical
     Cancer Screening," RG 29, vol. 1180, file 311-C1-21.
25   NAC, RG 29, vol. 1174, file 311-C1-1 (part 1), p. 2.
26   Women's College Hospital Archives [hereafter WCHA], "History of the Cancer Detec-
     tion Clinic," N4-Container, p. 45.
27   WCHA, "History of the Cancer Detection Clinic—Women's College Hospital," N4-Con-
     tainer 59-file 1.
28   WCHA, "History of the Cancer Detection Clinic."
29   AO, personal letter addressed to Hon. J.W. Spooner from M.B. Dymond, Minister of
     Health, 23 December 1963, RG 10, file 1-1-3.40.
30   AO, personal letter to Spooner.
31   AO, "A Cytology Screening Programme for Cancer of the Cervix in the Province of
     Ontario," draft 1965, RG 10, file 71-4-5.
32   AO, "A Cytology Screening Programme."
33   NAC, Health and Welfare Canada, "Questionnaire on the Impact of the Walton Report
     on Cervical Cancer Screening Programs," RG 29, file 6030-75-1, pp. 1–4.
34   NAC, "Questionnaire on the Impact," pp. 1–4.
35   NAC, "Questionnaire on the Impact," p. 2.
36   NAC, "Questionnaire on the Impact," p. 2.
37   Eve Kassirer, "Impact of the Walton Report on Cervical Cancer Screening Programs in
     Canada," *Canadian Medical Association Journal* 122 (1980): 419.
38   Kassirer, "Impact of the Walton Report," p. 419.
39   Kassirer, "Impact of the Walton Report," p. 422.
40   NAC, "Briefing Notes for the Minister—Cervical Cancer Screening," RG 29, file 630-75-
     1, p. 2.
41   NAC, "Have You Had a Pap Test Recently?" Health and Welfare Canada, Fall 1978, RG
     29, file 6030-75-1, p. 2.
42   NAC, "In Situ Cervical Cancer in Young Women," Ontario Medical Association Report
     to Council, 18–19 June 1984—Committee on Child Welfare, RG 29, file 6760-4-3, box
     75.
43   NAC, "Control of Cancer of the Uterine Cervix: A National Health Objective," Draft—
     Surveillance and Risk Assessment Divisions, Health and Welfare Canada, 1988, RG 29,
     file 6760-4-3.
44   Valerie Korinek, *Roughing It in the Suburbs: Reading* Chatelaine *Magazine in the Fifties
     and Sixties* (Toronto: University of Toronto Press, 2000), p. 5.

45   He believed that many people working in spinning mills were often covered in oils and rubbing against the machines they were working on, thus potentially causing cancer. He was also concerned with jagged teeth causing tongue cancer and rough pipe stems causing lip cancer.

46   John W.S. McCullough, "The Prevention of Cancer," *Chatelaine* (November 1930): 15.

47   McCullough, "Prevention of Cancer," p. 15.

48   Adele Saunders, "Plain Talk about Cancer," *Chatelaine* (November 1945): 63.

49   Saunders, "Plain Talk about Cancer," p. 13.

50   Saunders, "Plain Talk about Cancer," p. 31.

51   Korinek, *Roughing It in the Suburbs*, p. 7.

52   Korinek, *Roughing It in the Suburbs*, p. 7.

53   Dorothy Sangster, "I Faced Up to Cancer," *Chatelaine* (September 1954): 51.

54   Sangster, "I Faced Up to Cancer," p. 51.

55   Sangster, "I Faced Up to Cancer," p. 13.

56   Kathleen Nouch, "I Learned to Live with Cancer," *Chatelaine* (June 1959): 30, 85–8.

57   "Women! You Need No Longer Die from Your No.1 Cancer Killer," *Toronto Star* (31 March 1955): 38.

58   "Doubt U.S. Cancer Test Economical for Ontario," *Toronto Star* (21 October 1955): 62.

59   Betsy Bliss, "Do-It-Yourself Cervical Cancer Test," *Toronto Star* (20 June 1967): 46.

60   For an interesting discussion on post–World War II society and change, see Douglas Owram, *Born at the Right Time: A History of the Baby Boom Generation* (Toronto: University of Toronto Press, 1996).

61   Korinek, *Roughing It in the Suburbs*, p. 365.

62   Derek Cassels, "Now the Good News … about Breast Cancer," *Chatelaine* (June 1973): 50.

63   Michele Lansberg, "Your Gynecologist: Show Me a Gynecologist and I'll Show You a Male Chauvinist (Even If She's a Woman)," *Chatelaine* (August 1973): 42, 64–6.

64   "The Last Word Is Yours," *Chatelaine* (August 1973): 134.

65   Jack Batten, "Is This Operation Necessary?" *Chatelaine* (August 1975): 48, 56–8.

66   "Health," *Chatelaine* (January 1972): 10.

67   "Health," *Chatelaine* (May 1972): 12.

68   "Health," *Chatelaine* (January 1974): 9.

69   Marilyn Dunlop, "Pioneer of the A-Bomb Now Making War on Cancer," *Toronto Star* (5 July 1971): 5.

70   Marilyn Dunlop, "Men May Hold Virus That Causes Cancer in Women: Scientist," *Toronto Star* (5 April 1973): 49.

71   Lindsay Curtis, "Your Health," *Toronto Star* (5 September 1973): E4.

72   Lindsay Curtis, "Your Health," *Toronto Star* (25 January 1974): D2.

73   Robert C. Newman, "Your Health," *Toronto Star* (27 July 1978): D8.

74   *Cancer in Women*, produced by Cheryl Wright, NFB of Canada – Atlantic Region (1974).

75   *Cancer in Women*.

76   *Cancer in Women*.

77   *Cancer in Women*.

78   "Effectiveness of Strategies to Increase Cervical Cancer Screening in Clinic-Based Settings," *Public Health Research, Education, and Development Program* (Toronto: Ontario Ministry of Health, December 2000), p. 1.

79   "Women over 50 Still Need Pap Tests," *Ontario Cancer Facts*, October 2001, http://www.cancercare.on.ca/reports_211.htm (accessed January 2004).

80   "Effectiveness of Strategies," p. 1.

81   Pauline Comeau, "Debate Begins over Public Funding for HPV Vaccine," *CMAJ* 176.7 (2007): 913.

82   Laura Eggerston, "Adverse Events Reported for HPV Vaccine," *CMAJ* 177.10 (2007): 1169.

83   "HPV and Cervical Cancer," British Columbia Cancer Agency, http://www.bccancer .bc.ca/PPI/Prevention/infection/HPV.htm (accessed July 2010).

II: Popular Representations of the Body in
 Sickness and Health

Hideous Monsters before the Eye: Delirium tremens and Manhood in Antebellum Philadelphia

Ric N. Caric

> "But what is the matter, Bill?" he asked, earnestly....
> "What's the matter? What's the matter?" eagerly enquired half a dozen others coming up.
> "Why, *the man with the poker is after him!*" I believe said the person who had first spoken, in a half laughing, half serious tone.
> "Poor fellow," ejaculated one. "Poor fellow indeed!" said another.[1]

In *Six Nights with the Washingtonians*, temperance novelist T.S. Arthur uses "the man with the poker" as a popular term for delirium tremens, a condition in which heavy drinkers develop hallucinations. The fictional character, Bill, a reformed drinker who is recounting the story, has an attack of delirium tremens while at work as a bookbinder. First, his hands tremble, after which an iron bar for which he is reaching "assumed the form of a serpent." Soon Bill sees "a face of horrible malignancy, just over my head, and a dozen serpents and dragons, and monsters of all shapes." Seeking relief at a tavern, Bill jumps away from a decanter and glass that "seemed instantly changed into a living monster." Advised that he is not well, Bill goes home and is haunted for two days by "awful and malignant shapes" before being taken to the almshouse.[2]

As Bill's condition becomes known, it turns out that he is the only man in the company who does not know that "the man with the poker" is a term for delirium tremens. When a friend informs others that "the man with the poker is after him," all of the men instantly recognize the term. Bill's unnamed friend is unsure whether to treat Bill's condition as an amusing spectacle or a potentially deadly problem, but the ambivalence is resolved in favour of pity as the other men in the tavern exclaim "poor fellow indeed." Perhaps somewhat disappointed, Bill's friend tells Bill that he needs to go home.[3]

Delirium tremens is a short-term hallucinatory disorder experienced by heavy drinkers who suddenly abstain from drinking or substantially lower their drinking levels. Symptoms include whole body tremors, intense fearfulness, and hallucinations of walls falling down, devils, and the like. This chapter examines delirium tremens in relation to traditional pre-industrial male leisure culture in Philadelphia in the 1830s and early 1840s. Delirium tremens primarily affected males: 68.3 per cent (723) of the delirium tremens cases and 79.7 per cent (51) of the delirium tremens deaths at the Philadelphia Alms House between 1837 and 1841 were men. Likewise, the overwhelming majority of delirium tremens cases reported in Philadelphia sources were craftsmen and labourers, with only a scattering of clerks and accountants.[4] The main point of contact between delirium tremens and traditional leisure was fear concerning male bodies. In *Manhood in America*, Michael Kimmel portrays the middle-class "self-made men" of antebellum America as "anxious" and "melancholy," while viewing "heroic artisans" as satisfied with being "deeply embedded within a community of equals."[5] However, artisans were highly anxious as well. In traditional popular culture, men portrayed everyday economic and family problems in terms of assaults on their bodies— as being pummelled by raging seas, "molested" by enemies, penetrated by devils, and the like.[6] In her chapter in this volume on the representation of AIDS, Heather Murray asserts that popular views of AIDS patients as "contaminated" were informed by twentieth-century images of an "invisible world of germs" threatening one's health.[7] In the traditional popular culture of nineteenth-century Philadelphia, men represented their environments in ways that were perhaps even more menacing, as imminent threats to invade, dismember, and otherwise destroy their bodies.

In Philadelphia of the 1830s and early 1840s, the dominant republican ideals of artisan masculinity were articulated in terms of overcoming these imagined dangers. To have "manly independence" meant to conquer apprehensions and re-establish a sense of body wholeness and security. Such conquests could be achieved through success in business or politics, but overcoming fears concerning male bodies was most often accomplished through the traditional workshop leisure of regular drink breaks, gambling, and practical jokes, tavern socializing, and holiday celebrations. The pleasures of traditional leisure were thus a necessary part of being "manly, honest, good-natured, and free."[8]

This chapter argues that the onset of delirium tremens symptoms involved two kinds of failures in the traditional culture of masculinity. First, I argue that the onset of delirium tremens meant that a patient's practical difficulties were so burdensome that he no longer had the ability to overcome the accompanying fears and identify with masculine ideals through participation in traditional leisure. As a result, such men consumed large amounts of alcohol primarily to suppress the "breast-disturbing fears" in which they represented their problems as attacks on their bodies rather than as an adjunct to tavern contests or voluntary society activities.[9] Second, the onset of delirium tremens meant that heavy alcohol consumption was also failing as a strategy for dealing with fears of bodily attack. Whether heavy drinkers developed delirium tremens because gastro-intestinal disorders kept them from drinking or because they could not tolerate lapses in alcohol use, they could no longer drink enough to suppress their sense of bodily fear. Thus, delirium tremens represented a final hallucinatory attempt to cope with bodily fears. For men who suffered from hallucinations, the culture of masculinity had failed them to such an extent that they abandoned culturally informed perception for an alternate reality.

This chapter also makes two historical arguments about delirium tremens. First, I argue that the number of delirium tremens cases rose significantly during the late 1830s and early 1840s, and that the increase was closely linked to early industrialization. The first shock of industrialization in Philadelphia magnified the practical problems of working-class men in that city to such an extent that traditional leisure no longer enabled men to overcome their fears of bodily attack and identify themselves as "independent men." In this context, a broad spectrum of men began to use alcohol primarily as a way to chemically suppress their fears, and they increased their alcohol consumption to such an extent that they became chronically heavy drinkers who could no longer work full-time. For such men, the ideal of manly independence that Kimmel identifies with the "heroic artisan" had become the reality of reduced capacity for work, a chronic craving for alcohol, and humiliating dependence on wives and children for care. As the pool of heavy drinkers grew during the 1830s and early 1840s, the number of men who developed delirium tremens increased because an increasing number of heavy drinkers could not control their bodily fears through alcohol consumption.

The second historical argument is that a decline in delirium tremens cases was made possible by the transformation of male culture during the 1840s. Where traditional masculinity was viewed in terms of overcoming imagined attacks, the new cultural institutions of the 1840s viewed masculinity in terms of "exposing" male bodies. For a whole range of new or newly prominent institutions like the Washingtonian temperance societies, rioting fire companies, and secret societies, masculine virtues like courage and honour were represented in terms of displaying their sense of vulnerability or degradation, exposing themselves to harm and representations of harm, and strongly identifying with a group.[10] Men who were oriented toward what Amy Greenberg calls "martial manhood" may have been more oriented toward fire companies and ethnic rioting, while advocates of "restrained manhood" would have been drawn to groups like the Sons of Temperance and would perhaps have attended minstrel shows. However, all of these cultural insti-tutions viewed bodily vulnerability as a starting point for articulating man-hood; participants did not view their masculinity to be as threatened by practical problems within these institutions as within traditional culture. Likewise, group identification with fire companies and temperance societies were largely separate from economic circumstances and could serve as a buffer against everyday economic anxiety.[11]

Delirium Tremens as a Medical Condition

Most medical writings described delirium tremens as having three distinct stages. Symptoms usually began to develop within one or two days after a man withdrew from alcohol, usually because gastro-intestinal disorders kept him from drinking his usual quota. The first stage was marked by pronounced anxiety and fearfulness. According to Willis Lea, one of the earliest symptoms of delirium tremens was a "countenance commonly expressive of great fear and anxiety or wild and staring though sometimes fixed and sullen." Likewise, Isaac Snowden claimed that "an attack is usually ushered in by a singular change in countenance" in which there was a "furious expression, rolling constantly with a wild glare." Patients also experienced uncontrolled trembling over their whole bodies and had difficulties standing and walking. Thus, a patient's generalized perception of danger was accompanied by a sense of his body as vulnerable, disordered, and impossible to coordinate.[12]

The focus on environmental threats bore a complex relation to traditional male leisure. In many ways, the intense fear of the environment was a continuation of threats men felt in their everyday lives. Anthony Rotundo argues that urban men identified masculinity with assertions of "independence" after the Revolution, an independence associated with representations of bodily wholeness and security. By wearing aprons and carrying tools during the Federal Procession of 1788, Philadelphia craftsmen associated their embodied craft skills with a "manly independence" in the sense that their skills enabled them to support families, fulfill business obligations, and serve the community. Male independence also implied the courage and honour needed to defy the "despotism" associated with the British.[13]

In *Masculinities*, R.W. Connell counters socio-biological arguments by claiming that all configurations of masculinity are "liable to internal contradiction and historical disruption." In the case of Philadelphia artisans, a constant source of contradiction and disruption was their experiencing the problems of their jobs, finances, families, and health in terms of assaults on their bodies. If independence was "manly," dangers to independent status like unemployment, debts, and poor health threatened to "unman" men and were represented through analogies to animals being killed, execution, or being drowned at sea. Men also opposed manliness to the feminine "other" and identified any failure to respond to insults as unmanly. Tailors were ridiculed as "the ninth part of man" because it was said that it took eight of these chronically thin craftsmen to subdue a woman.[14]

In the popular culture of mid-nineteenth-century Philadelphia, this combination of practical worries and apprehensions concerning assaults on the body was represented by terms like "care" and "ills," and most labouring men were burdened by such "cares." During the Revolutionary era, carpenters and tailors barely made enough money to cover subsistence needs; consequently, events like seasonal unemployment threw them into financial crisis where they could not discharge their debts or pay for rent and firewood. Most labouring men not only endured such problems, but they also struggled with representing their bodies. In songs like "Spanking Jack," a man's "troubles" were represented in terms of being drowned at sea, eaten by sharks, or having his head blown off. Steamboat engineer John Fitch analogized his "cares" to being lost at sea, enduring Indian captivity, and being beheaded.[15]

Participation in traditional leisure allowed men to overcome bodily apprehensions. Leisure activities were organized as "processes of recognition" in which participants either mounted exhibitions or competed before companies of other men. For participants in craft contests, drinking duels, and the like, the figure of the opponent presented a concentrated version of their practical difficulties and bodily apprehensions. When men defeated their antagonists, they experienced themselves as triumphing over threats associated with care, thus reconstituting their sense of independent manhood. Audiences were also quick to cheer the fastest eaters, best inventors, and most learned men, and participants experienced the leisure environment as mirroring their masculine accomplishments and providing extended periods of easy fellowship. Reinforced by alcohol, the "good cheer" of traditional leisure could then be transferred back to the work environment. In this way, popular leisure provided an effective counterweight to the unmanning effects of men's cares.[16] This countereffect was captured well by the sign at Warwick's Union Hotel:

> Whatever may tend to soothe the soul below
> To dry the tear and blunt the shaft of woe,
> To drown the ills that discompose the mind—
> All those who seek at Warwick's shall find.[17]

The onset of delirium tremens was an indication of a weakened capacity to overcome cares. James Washington made the connection between delirium tremens and "corroding care" in his medical dissertation: "Has the individual been driven to intemperance, in order to free the mind of corroding care and anxiety, arising out of … business or family matters, the mental disturbance will then, almost certainly be protracted to a much longer time than would otherwise have been the case."[18]

Care and anxiety resulted in delirium tremens because of two closely related failures in masculinity. The first was the failure to transform "cares" into independent masculinity through leisure participation. Business and family setbacks could be so severe that men could not effectively counteract their "cares" through normal leisure patterns. They might socialize in taverns and be acclaimed for their performances but still not be able to overcome the feelings of bodily vulnerability linked to their practical problems. In such cases, men would have a powerful sense of being unmanned or molested, and might compare their situations to being burned alive or having their bodies taken over. Men were "driven to intemperance" when they responded to failures in ordinary leisure by increasing their alcohol consumption to suppress their "cares and anxieties." Although those who were driven into intemperance still participated in the cultural practices of workshops and taverns, they now drank primarily to suppress their cares. However, heavy drinking created additional difficult problems. Although heavy drinking could temporarily "free the mind of corroding care and anxiety," it also tended to magnify practical problems with employment and families, which further increased a man's cares and the consequent fears for his body. Heavy alcohol consumption to free a man from anxiety could actually heighten his fears and make even heavier alcohol consumption necessary.

The first symptoms of delirium tremens resulted when drinking failed as a strategy for coping with heightened care. Men who were caught in this mutually reinforcing spiral of heavy alcohol consumption, heightened practical problems, and a fearful sense of care and anxiety either maintained heroic levels of drinking or fell into the first symptoms of delirium tremens. The difficulty and humiliation of this either-or situation is illustrated by an anonymous letter to the *Temperance Monitor* in 1836:

> At the present time I am in the practice of drinking three half pints a day, fearful, if I did not take my "quantum sufficit," that it would be my lot to have an attack of … delirium tremens; and from the fear of which I keep my supply of the *poison*—and frequently from dire necessity and bad feeling, both mental and bodily—oh, horrid!!! I am compelled to commence my cups at 2, 3, or 4 in the morning, and so continue until perhaps 9 or 10 o'clock, before I am able to attend to anything like business.[19]

Here, the weight of the anonymous man's sense of bodily vulnerability was so heavy that he drank solely to suppress it. Far from reconstituting a sense of independent manhood, this man drank solely to stabilize his feelings of "dire necessity and bad feeling" and to prevent himself from being completely unstrung by fear and trembling. Simultaneously, heavy drinking involved the man in further degradation of extreme dependence on alcohol, which he described as his "poor, miserable, and horrid condition." Drinking so much would have made others see the man as a "drunkard," subjected him to humiliation from local boys, and made him susceptible to vomiting, stomach distress, and painful accidents. If the man had a family, he would have been as dependent on his wife and children to procure alcohol, feed him, and clean up after him as any invalid. Moreover, deviations from his drinking routine would have been punished by tremors, paralyzing fears, and other symptoms that reminded him of his susceptibility to delirium tremens. Instead of identifying himself with republican values like independence, this man portrayed himself as a helpless and degraded slave to alcohol, almost the complete opposite of Kimmel's idea of the heroic artisan.[20]

Most medical writers argued that the initial treatment of delirium tremens should be focused on preparing the patient's stomach for renewed alcohol consumption. The usual course of treatment was to prescribe emetics to clear out the gastro-intestinal tract and then apply soothing treatments. Once the patient's stomach was prepared, most doctors recommended that he be given alcohol. One former patient reported that he was given a drink every fifteen minutes. If these treatments did not work, delirium tremens advanced and patients began to hallucinate threats to their lives and bodies, believing that they were surrounded by enemies or that snakes, vermin, and devils were crawling on their skin. Patients also saw "the motions of some hideous monster that seems approaching to devour him" and often imagined walls falling on them. Patients who had undergone business reverses continually recurred to their difficulties. Richard Henry Thomas made this point in a pithy way when he pointed out that "[s]ometimes he will be engaged in calculations[,] at others in collecting money from the bed clothes."[21]

Although physicians were intimidated by a patient's hallucinations and interpreted them as signs of danger, there are reasons to view hallucinations as offering advantages over the first stage of the illness. When delirium tremens patients hallucinated falling walls, attacks from murderers, or devils on their skin, they conjured up a definite entity as a "cause" for their intense fears. In seeing a murderer or devil attacking, patients brought their perceptions in line with their fears and provided themselves with something specific to fear. Likewise, while the first symptoms of delirium tremens involved unseen dangers, the specificity of hallucinations made it possible for patients to defend themselves. Thus, some patients pushed with "all their might against the walls" when they saw the walls of their rooms falling, while others hid under their beds to avoid attacks.[22]

If the preferred treatment for delirium tremens was to remove any barriers to resumed alcohol consumption, the immediate goal of that treatment was to induce what Charles Randolph referred to as a "critical sleep." If patients could be induced to sleep, they usually recovered and often were restored completely when they awoke. The main barrier to restorative sleep was usually the practical worries of the patient. Randolph approvingly quoted Dr. Armstrong as arguing that "those patients who have been driven to intoxication from some great affliction, are generally in imminent danger; for ... their raving turns incessantly upon the recent calamity, and produces an irritation and exhaustion most difficult to be counter-acted." When doctors could not get patients to sleep soundly, the men would exhaust themselves with paroxysms of watchfulness and hallucination. "The system is exhausted by excessive exertion, the eye will retain its restlessness and watchfulness, the voice becomes more enfeebled ... and the patient expires in a state of apoplexy, or else lingers for several days, and finally dies of effusion on the brain."[23]

Delirium Tremens in a Changing Culture

If the progress of a single delirium tremens case involved a small-scale failure of traditional manhood, then how did delirium tremens relate to the more general patterns of popular culture in Philadelphia? To explore this relationship, it is necessary to determine the scope of delirium tremens in the city. How many cases of delirium tremens were there? To what extent did the number of cases increase or decrease over time? What conditions led to increases or decreases in delirium tremens and to what extent can these increases or decreases be connected to developments in the culture of masculinity?

There are no city-wide statistics on delirium tremens cases. Likewise, there are almost no preserved accounts of the majority of cases that were self-medicated or treated by private physicians. Nevertheless, materials do exist that make it possible to investigate the relation between delirium tremens and popular culture on a larger scale. Specifically, the total number of deaths from delirium tremens and the death rate from delirium tremens cases can be estimated from extant sources. Based on these estimates, it is then possible to estimate the total number of delirium tremens cases. For example, if 10 men died from delirium tremens and the death rate in the population was 5 per cent, then there would have been 20 delirium tremens cases for every delirium tremens death, or 200 cases altogether. If the number of deaths stayed steady and the death rate fell, the estimate of cases would increase because there would be more cases per death. Conversely, an increase in the death rate from delirium tremens would decrease the number of cases for each death and thereby decrease the estimate of total cases. If there were 10 delirium tremens deaths at a 10 per cent death rate, then the estimated number of cases would be only 100.

Estimates of the number of delirium tremens deaths and the death rate from delirium tremens can be derived from the Register of Deaths and almshouse records. The Men's Register for the almshouse contains data on every man admitted to the almshouse beginning in 1828, almost always including the date of admission, ward assignment, and date of death if the patient died. The percentage of deaths among delirium tremens patients at the almshouse was probably higher than the death rate from delirium tremens in the city as a whole. One almshouse doctor emphasized that the almshouse often received cases only after they were far advanced. In other words, when the efforts of families and private physicians failed, a man suffering from delirium tremens might be taken to the almshouse. Thus, assuming that the death rate at the almshouse was the same as the death rate in the city as

Figure 1   Death Rate from Delirium Tremens at Almshouse

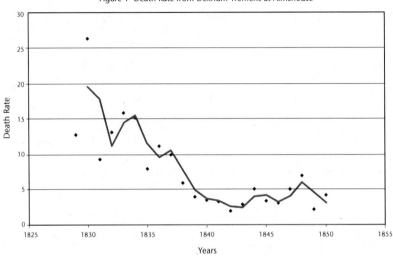

Source   Ric Caric, compiled from the Men's Register of the Philadelphia Alms House and the Register of Deaths, 1825–1860.

a whole introduces a conservative bias into calculating the total number of cases (because there would be fewer cases per death).[24]

As seen in figure 1, the death rate from delirium tremens at the almshouse went down rapidly between 1829 and 1841 before rebounding somewhat between 1842 and 1849.[25]

The primary basis for determining the number of delirium tremens cases for Philadelphia is the Register of Deaths for 1828 to 1860. Drawn from cemetery returns, the Register of Deaths includes information on the cause of death for every person listed. However, the register is very incomplete: of the 289 men who died from delirium tremens at the almshouse in 1828 and 1829, 234 were not recorded in the Register of Deaths (81.3%). Several other institutions also housed poor men, including Pennsylvania Hospital and Moyamensing Prison, and it is likely that delirium tremens deaths at those institutions were also under-recorded. It is also possible that the cemeteries failed to list all of their delirium tremens deaths. The large gap in the Register of Deaths records can be corrected somewhat by adding in the delirium tremens deaths from the almshouse that were not originally noted in the Register of Deaths. Still, the estimate of the total number of deaths in table 1 is best considered as a minimum baseline for delirium tremens mortality in Philadelphia.

Table 1 Delirium Tremens Deaths
in Philadelphia, 1829–49

Year	Deaths
1829	83
1832	135
1833	60
1834	72
1835	65
1836	100
1837	78
1838	64
1839	48
1840	51
1841	53
1842	39
1843	44
1844	58
1845	50
1846	38
1847	82
1848	52
1849	69

Given the conservative bias in the data on deaths from the Register of Deaths, there is a good likelihood that the estimate of the total number of delirium tremens cases in table 1 is low. However, the estimate is a useful tool for identifying underlying trends in delirium tremens cases.

According to this estimate, the number of delirium tremens cases rose sharply during the 1830s and early 1840s, almost tripling from 480 in 1829 to an average of 1,314 per year from 1839 to 1843. This 274 per cent increase is more than ten times the 26.8 per cent population increase for Philadelphia County between 1830 and 1840. The total number of cases shows a strong increase even though the number of delirium tremens deaths, shown in table 1, declined from an annual average of 75.8 in 1834–38 to 45.2 in 1839–43. This is because the rapidly falling death rate (from 9% in 1837 to less than 3% in 1843) means that there were more delirium tremens cases per

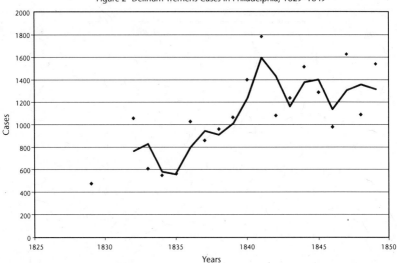

Figure 2   Delirium Tremens Cases in Philadelphia, 1829–1849

Source   Ric Caric, compiled from the Men's Register of the Philadelphia Alms House and the Register of Deaths, 1825–1860.

death. The peak in the number of cases in 1840 occurred during the depths of the 1837–43 depression. In the context of 25 per cent unemployment, the continual danger of bankruptcy, and the cultural maelstrom of evangelical revivals and fire company rioting, the estimated number of male delirium tremens cases more than doubled from 864 in 1837 to 1,784 in 1841. Delirium tremens had been recognized as a social problem as early as 1825. Fifteen years later, the problem was considerably worse.[26]

The rise in delirium tremens cases during the 1830s and early 1840s was closely linked to industrialization. Early industrialization in Philadelphia involved a mixture of large-scale factories producing coarse goods, small to medium-sized shops producing specialty goods, and the traditional trades. Most economic sectors were subject to intense competition, and levels of anxiety and uncertainty were high as a result. Journeymen faced strong downward pressures on their wages, periodic uncertainties over wage payments, longer work hours, and intensified efforts by employers to control work conditions. Spokesmen for the saddlers union reported in 1836 that employers sought to match the prices of saddlers in other cities by forcing wages down and flooding workshops with apprentices. As a result, journeyman saddlers were forced to accept significantly less than the "living wage" of $7.00 per week, if they could find work at all. Similar wage pressures could be seen in shoemaking, tailoring, and glassmaking. Wages and job opportunities declined dramatically during the 1837–43 depression. Handloom weavers only made $2.50 per week.[27]

With declining wages, paying rent and feeding children became much more difficult. As a result, men felt such an intensified sense of bodily vulnerability that they could no longer represent themselves in terms of republican values like independence and images of bodily wholeness. Instead, sources in popular culture were filled with images of vulnerable, distorted, and tormented male bodies. In burlesque militia parades, poor militiamen satirized their vulnerable and subordinate condition by parading as cornstalks, wearing female dress, or putting on blackface. Popular music mirrored men's inability to cope with business circumstances through songs representing the loss of bodily control, such as "The Steam Arm." The *Mechanics Free Press* protested strenuously against "mercenary and imperious" employers but also represented workers themselves as degraded, enslaved, or drifting down streams of pollution. Thus, artisans and factory workers found themselves unable to assert a traditional sense of manhood.[28]

As their corroding cares and anxieties grew more intense, artisans and labouring men began to emphasize heavy alcohol consumption as a strategy for coping with their anxieties concerning their bodies. In *The Alcoholic Republic*, Rorabaugh argues that drinking levels during the 1820s and 1830s increased among urban craftsmen because of their inability to save capital and become masters. The frustrations of uncertain employment, longer working hours, problems in paying debts, and bankruptcies also provided immediate motivation for artisans to "drown their cares." A letter to the *Pennsylvanian* stressed that Philadelphia journeymen would "crowd around the bar or the gaming table" after work and by "drinking to excess … thus drive away the horrors of mind occasioned by excessive toil." In this sense, men drank heavily solely for the purpose of suppressing their "cares and anxieties" instead of reasserting traditional manliness. Sprees in which participants drank very heavily for long periods of time became a preferred mode of intemperance. For example, George Dormont had been "drinking very hard for two weeks, and [had] not slept for the last three nights" before developing delirium tremens in May 1829. George Escol Sellers wrote in his memoirs about the sprees that resulted in his uncle Nathan's death from delirium tremens in 1826. Traditional holidays like Christmas had definite beginning and end points, but sprees could start at any time and last as long as a man's funds and endurance held out.[29]

The widespread increase in drinking resulted in a growing pool of heavy drinkers because of the difficulties brought on by using heavy drinking as a primary strategy for controlling the anxieties of care. According to Bruce

Laurie, Philadelphia employers in the late 1830s "expected journeymen to lose time because of excessive drinking and holidays—official and unofficial—and endured them as long as they showed up 'tolerably regularly' and avoided getting 'absolutely drunk' as a matter of habit." However, the growing number of men who took long stretches of time off from work for sprees or spent large parts of each day in taverns could not make full wages (inadequate as they were). If they had families, heavy drinkers would have struggled even more to pay rent and deal with aggrieved spouses than they would have otherwise. In this sense, heavy drinking further intensified the difficult problems that men had to cope with as a result of industrialization and would have increased a man's sense of bodily vulnerability as a result.[30]

As a broad spectrum of labouring men increased their drinking, a significant portion of those men fell into chronic drunkenness after they continually increased their alcohol consumption to suppress the additional vulnerability connected to their heavy drinking. For example, a moderately successful butcher lost his business and fell into homelessness when heavy drinking kept him from functioning. The same was the case with Robert Peacock, who slept outside during a month-long debauch that landed him in the almshouse. While tavern-keeper Joseph Parham was drinking, he broke his arms or legs five times while handling kegs and barrels, and abandoned his family three times. Far from fulfilling their obligations to families and friends, men caught in such a downward spiral depended heavily on wives and children for basic functions like preparing for work.[31]

The pool of heavy drinkers produced cases of delirium tremens because these men could no longer sustain the high levels of drinking required to suppress their overwhelming fears. Isaac Snowden stressed that "this species of insanity [delirium tremens] is mostly to be met with in habitual confirmed drunkards." Because the pool of heavy drinkers increased rapidly during the 1830s and early 1840s, the number of delirium tremens cases also increased rapidly. For the growing number of men who developed delirium tremens, heavy alcohol consumption had failed as a strategy for coping with the intensified sense of bodily vulnerability.[32]

During the early and middle part of the 1840s, the incidence of delirium tremens generally declined. The average annual number of delirium tremens cases fell slightly from 1,314 in 1839–43 to 1,300 in 1844–48. Because the number of delirium tremens cases only held steady in Philadelphia despite a population growth of 37 per cent in 1840–50, delirium tremens was significantly less pervasive in Philadelphia at the end of the 1840s than at the beginning of the decade.[33]

Several factors combined to produce the decline in delirium tremens during the 1840s. The first was the Washingtonian temperance movement, which began in Philadelphia in April 1841; more than 70 neighbourhood Washingtonian societies were formed in the city and its working-class suburbs within the next year. In 1842 delirium tremens declined, with the number of deaths listed in the Register of Deaths decreasing to 30 from an annual average of 50.3 in 1839–41, and the number of cases at the almshouse declining from 239 to 201. One would expect that drinking levels would have continued to increase because of the ongoing economic depression; however, by inducing thousands of men to join temperance societies, the Washingtonians prevented men from becoming heavy drinkers and reduced the pool of heavy drinkers out of which delirium tremens developed.[34]

While a thorough analysis of the Philadelphia Washingtonian movement is beyond the scope of this article, two points can be made. First, the "experience speeches" given by former drunkards at Washingtonian meetings involved "displays of degradation" rather than efforts to overcome dangers to the male body. Speakers like Lewis Levin talked about the all-consuming character of their drinking, the suffering of their families, and their impoverishment, bloated faces, and humiliating experiences. Washingtonians were especially keen to illustrate their helplessness as drinkers and their inability to exercise self-control with alcohol. Whereas traditional masculine culture viewed helplessness and lack of self-control as feminine weakness, the Washingtonians created a ritual process in which a man's acknowledgement of helplessness was seen as liberating. When men signed the pledge and joined a Washingtonian society, they crossed over from a cultural logic dominated by the effort to overcome bodily threats to a cultural logic in which the acknowledgement of degradation was a sign of new integrity. The Washingtonians also encouraged men to strongly identify themselves with the temperance movement as a whole and see themselves as part of the ongoing "war" between temperance and "Old King Alcohol." For many of those who joined the Washingtonian societies, signing the pledge marked the final failure of the traditional culture of masculinity and the beginning of their participation in a different kind of male culture, one in which displaying rather than overcoming vulnerability was the lynchpin of masculinity.[35]

After the end of the depression in 1843, the number of delirium tremens cases briefly rose again but then levelled off for the rest of the decade, despite rapid population growth and the decline of the Washingtonian temperance movement. Much of this relative decrease seems to have been associated instead with broad changes in popular culture. Historians of masculinity like Michael Kimmel, Eliot Gorn, and Amy Greenberg mistakenly view the more violent and hard-drinking cultural activities of the 1840s as holdovers from traditional popular culture. However, the traditional popular culture of the post-Revolutionary era was not characterized by the pervasive rioting that erupted in Philadelphia, beginning with the anti-black riot of 1834 and continuing with the burning of Pennsylvania Hall (an abolitionist meeting place) in 1838, the pervasive fire company rioting that began in the late 1830s, and the major anti-Catholic riot of 1844. Likewise, contemporary work on masculinity underestimates the overlap among the violent and the more respectable elements of popular culture during the 1840s. For example, two of the most famous rioting fire companies in Philadelphia, the Good-Will Engine Company and the Fairmount Engine Company, were closely associated with the Washingtonian movement, and one of their biggest riots was over the visit of another temperance fire company from Baltimore. Washingtonian societies also held several events with the fire department as a whole. In a similar way, Washingtonian activists like Lewis Levin were also prominent in the anti-Catholic agitation leading to the Kensington Riot of 1844, while the racial hostility of anti-black and anti-abolitionist rioting clearly informed the more sedentary entertainments of the blackface minstrel performers.[36]

What the cultural developments of the late 1830s and 1840s all shared—including the rioting fire companies, gangs, blackface minstrel entertainments, and new temperance societies like the Sons of Temperance—was a strong emphasis on group identity and displaying one's acceptance of vulnerability. Whereas traditional male culture had been organized around individual performances, the dominant cultural activities of the late 1840s were group performances designed to create representations of the characteristics, virtues, and value of Good-Will Engine, the Sons of Temperance, or whites in general. Rioting firemen represented the bravery with which they faced their enemies, but more as a group characteristic of companies like Fairmount Engine than as an individual quality. At the same time, the willing exposure of men to bodily harm and degradation became a central part of group ritual and identity. Like the Washingtonians displaying their degradation as drunkards, the volunteer firemen rioters directly exposed themselves to the weapons, injury, and possible death at the hands of their enemies. Displays of degradation were also the focus of minstrel shows in which white performers dressed in blackface, spoke in dialect, and sang songs like "My Ole Dad," in which a slave son brings up the bloated body of his drowned father while fishing. Like the fire companies, the minstrel shows were rituals in which a group's superiority was represented through images of degradation. The difference was that the white men in the audience encountered the representation of racial degradation at a distance as spectators rather than performers rather than risking bodily harm and degradation as rioters.[37]

Just because the men who participated in the cultural institutions of the 1840s shared a broadly common culture does not mean that they all embodied the same kind of masculinity. Here, Greenberg's distinction between "martial manhood" and "restrained manhood" is quite useful. Although "martial men" who participated in fire company rioting, ethnic rioting, or gang warfare might have participated in the Washingtonian temperance movement, they also rejected the domestic ideal that was promoted by the Washingtonians and accepted by "restrained men." Conversely, "restrained men" might have been more oriented toward home, church, and business, but also participated in sedentary forms of popular culture like minstrel entertainments (regularly held at Temperance Hall in the Northern Liberties) or meetings of the Sons of Temperance or other secret societies. The more sedentary activities had the same strong emphasis on group identity as did the rioting fire companies and gangs, even though they limited themselves to viewing representations of humiliation and degradation rather than exposing themselves to injury. In her book on fire companies, Greenberg indicates that fire company members changed from fire company involvement to domesticity when they got married. In this sense, there was a life-cycle transition from "martial manhood" to "restrained manhood" that could have applied broadly to the popular culture of the 1840s.[38]

Before the 1830s and 1840s, the masculine sense of independence, honour, and service to the community was threatened on a regular basis because it was so closely connected to the status of artisans as craftsmen, householders, and fathers. Men fell into the chronic drunkenness that led to delirium tremens in the course of attempting to re-establish a sense of traditional masculinity in the face of the enormous anxieties connected with making a living. In the leisure activities that dominated the later 1840s, artisans and factory workers employed leisure to articulate collective identities that were not nearly as dependent on the vicissitudes of prosperity of individual businesses, employment, and the economy. Being more separate from the immediate impact of economic contingencies, the modes of identification created by organizations like the fire companies and the minstrel shows could serve as effective buffers against the anxieties connected to the economy and make alcohol less necessary as a vehicle for combatting one's "cares." Thus, delirium tremens declined because new forms of leisure activity were more effective at combatting the severe anxieties of early industrialization than was traditional popular culture.

Conclusion

Delirium tremens was a phenomenon of cultural transformation among labouring men in antebellum Philadelphia. With the heightened sense of bodily vulnerability brought about by early industrialization, drinking practices changed from seeking to overcome a man's cares to chemically suppressing the sense of bodily apprehensions linked to those cares. In this context, men fell into long-term patterns of drunkenness that resulted in bouts of delirium tremens. The hallucinations involved in delirium tremens represented an abandonment of traditional masculinity and the adoption of direct action to combat imagined bodily threats. Thus, the increase in delirium tremens represented a failure of traditional male culture among Philadelphia workers.

The decrease of delirium tremens during the 1840s represented a further failure of traditional masculinity. The Washingtonian temperance societies appropriated mechanisms for displaying degradation from the drinking culture of the 1830s and employed them to develop new kinds of cultural practices and languages of masculinity. In the early 1840s, the success of the Washingtonian societies significantly diminished the pool of heavy drinkers out of which delirium tremens cases developed; this resulted in a decrease in the number of delirium tremens cases. Later in the decade, the development of new forms of leisure that focused on group ritual and group identity resulted in a levelling off of delirium tremens despite rapid population growth. Where the rise of delirium tremens had been a function of the failure of traditional masculinity, the decline of delirium tremens during the late 1840s was an outcome of the transition from traditional masculinity to a masculine culture better adjusted to industrialization.

Notes

This research was funded by Morehead State University.

1   T.S. Arthur, *Six Nights with the Washingtonians* (Philadelphia, 1841), p. 64.
2   Arthur, *Six Nights*, pp. 66–70.
3   Arthur, *Six Nights*, pp. 66–70.
4   Statistics on gender were compiled from the Alms House "Men's Register, 1828–1860" and "Women's Register, 1828–1860," City Archives of Philadelphia.
5   Michael Kimmel, *Manhood in America: A Cultural* History, 2nd ed. (New York: Oxford, 2006), pp. 18–21.

6   Ric Caric, "'To Drown the Ills that Discompose the Mind': Care, Leisure, and Identity among Philadelphia Artisans and Workers, 1785–1840," *Pennsylvania History* 64 (1997): 465–75.

7   Heather Murray, "'Every Generation Has Its War': Representations of Gay Men with Aids and Their Parents in the United States, 1983–1993," in this volume.

8   Caric, "'To Drown the Ills,'" pp. 465–75.

9   *Port-Folio*, 23 February 1806.

10 For Washingtonian temperance societies, see Leonard Blumberg, with William L. Pittman, *Beware the First Drink: The Washington Temperance Movement and Alcoholics Anonymous* (Seattle: Glen Abbey Books, 1991); for rioting among urban fire companies, see Amy S. Greenberg, *Cause for Alarm: The Volunteer Fire Department in the Nineteenth-Century City* (Princeton: Princeton University Press, 1998) and Ric N. Caric, "From Ordered Buckets to Honored Felons: Fire Companies and Cultural Transformation in Philadelphia, 1785–1850," *Pennsylvania History* 72 (Spring 2005): 117–58; for secret societies, see Mark C. Carnes, *Secret Ritual and Manhood in Victorian America* (New Haven, CT: Yale University Press, 1991).

11 Amy Greenberg, *Manifest Manhood and the Antebellum American Empire* (New York: Cambridge, 2005), pp. 9–12. Minstrel shows were performances in which white performers dressed in blackface and gave performances as blacks in Northern cities and Southern plantations. See Eric Lott, *Love and Theft: Blackface Minstrelsy and the American Working Class* (New York: Oxford University Press, 1995).

12 Willis M. Lea, "An Essay on Delirium tremens," Van Pelt-Dietrich Library, University of Pennsylvania (1826), p. 4; Isaac Snowden, "An Inaugural Essay on Delirium Tremens," 1817, Historical Society of Pennsylvania, p. 192.

13 E. Anthony Rotundo, *American Manhood: Transformations in Masculinity from the Revolution to the Modern Era* (New York: Basic, 1994).

14 R.W. Connell, *Masculinities*, 2nd ed. (Berkeley: University of California Press, 2005), p. 73; Francis Hopkinson, "Account of the Federal Procession of July 4, 1788," *American Museum*, Philadelphia 8 (July 1788): 63, 65, 67; Simon P. Newman, *Embodied History: The Lives of the Poor in Early Philadelphia* (Philadelphia: University of Pennsylvania Press, 2003), pp. 82–103; Caric, "'To Drown the Ills,'" pp. 465–75; *The Tickler* (17 January 1810), Historical Society of Pennsylvania. For the role of eighteenth-century medical exhibitions in defining the "other" for men, see Annette Burfoot, "From La Bambola to a Toronto Striptease: Drawing Out Public Consent to Gender Differentiation with Anatomical Material," in this volume.

15 Billy G. Smith, *The "Lower Sort": Philadelphia's Laboring People, 1750–1800* (Ithaca: Cornell University Press, 1990), pp. 116–9, 120–3; Anonymous, "Spanking Jack" in "Spanking Jack and Other Songs," in "Songs, 1805" (Philadelphia: Library Company of Philadelphia, 1805); Ric Caric, "To the Convivial Grave and Back: John Fitch as a Case Study in Cultural Failure, 1785–1792," *Pennsylvania Magazine of History and Biography* 126.4 (October 2002): 563.

16 Ric Caric, "Blustering Brags, Dueling Inventors, and Corn-Square Geniuses: Artisan Leisure in Philadelphia, 1785–1825," *American Journal of Semiotics* 12 (1995 [1998]): 323–41.

17 For sign, see John Scharf and Thompson Westcott, *A History of Philadelphia, 1609–1884* (Philadelphia: L. Ewarts, 1884), p. 989.

18 James Washington, "An Inaugural Dissertation on Delirium tremens," Van Pelt-Dietrich Library, University of Pennsylvania (1827), pp. 28–9.

19   For Robert Peacock, see "Men's Register," Philadelphia Alms House, City Archives of Philadelphia, 1828, 1829; also *Temperance Monitor*, Philadelphia: Library Company of Philadelphia (June 1836): 7.

20   *Philadelphia Gazette* (21 July 1841); also T.S. Arthur, "The Broken Merchant," in *Six Nights*, pp. 32, 43, 58. For another treatment of the body as a historical product, see Christina Burr, "'The Closest Thing to Perfect': Celebrity and the Body Politics of Jamie Lee Curtis," in this volume.

21   Charles Randolph, "Essay upon Mania á Potu," Van Pelt-Dietrich Library, University of Pennsylvania, 1825, p. 7; Anonymous, "Observations on Mania a Potu," Historical Society of Pennsylvania, 1830, p. 10; *Philadelphia Gazette* (23 February 1842); Richard Henry Thomas, "An Inaugural Essay on Mania a Potu," Van Pelt Library, University of Pennsylvania, 1827, p. 3.

22   Randolph, "An Essay upon Mania á Potu," pp. 7–8. Like AIDS, delirium tremens inspired fear in antebellum physicians. See Murray, "'Every Generation Has Its War.'"

23   Randolph, "Essay upon Mania á Potu," pp. 8–9; Anonymous, "Observations on Mania a Potu," pp. 8–9.

24   Anonymous, "Observations on Mania a Potu," p. 8; John Prosser Tabb, "Statistics of the Causes of Death in the Philadelphia Hospital, Blockley, during a Period of Twelve Years," *American Journal of Medical Sciences* 16 (1844): 365. Figure 1 was compiled from the "Men's Register" of the Philadelphia Alms House, City Archives of Philadelphia, 1828–50. Two categories of cases were counted as delirium tremens. Type I cases were "highly" likely of being delirium tremens and included diagnoses of mania a potu or delirium tremens, cases of intoxication placed in cells or Lunatic Asylum, and insanity/intemperance listings. Type II cases had a "good likelihood" of being delirium tremens and included diagnoses of intoxication with placement in the long ward or medical ward, and insanity cases where the patient was hospitalized less than a week.

25   Figure 1 was compiled from column B below.

Delirium Tremens in Philadelphia

A	B	C	D
Year	AH Death Rate	Total Deaths	Total Cases in Philadelphia
1829	0.1729	83	480
1832	0.1275	135	1,059
1833	0.1471	60	611
1834	0.1299	72	554
1835	0.1143	65	568
1836	0.0969	100	1,032
1837	0.0902	78	864
1838	0.0663	64	965
1839	0.045	48	1,066
1840	0.0364	51	1,401
1841	0.0297	53	1,784
1842	0.0277	30	1,083
1843	0.0355	44	1,239

1844	0.0383	58	1,514
1845	0.0388	50	1,289
1846	0.0387	38	982
1847	0.0505	82	1,624
1848	0.0476	52	1,092
1849	0.0448	69	1,540

Table compiled from the Men's Register of the Philadelphia Alms House and the Register of Deaths, 1825–60.

26 Figure 2 was compiled from the information in the table in note 25. The estimate for 1832 involves a correction in the data. John Prosser Tabb reported seventy-five deaths from delirium tremens at the Alms House Hospital in 1832, significantly higher than the number of deaths for any other year between 1832 and 1843. Unfortunately, the Register of Deaths has only scattered listings for 1832. Consequently, the average number of sixty-four male deaths from delirium tremens per year in the Register of Deaths for the 1830s was assumed for 1832 with a resulting estimate of 1,059 total cases for 1832.

27 For Philadelphia industrialization, see Phillip Scranton, *Proprietary Capitalism: The Textile Manufacture at Philadelphia, 1800–1885* (Cambridge: Cambridge University Press, 1983). Also see Cynthia J. Shelton, *The Mills of Manayunk: Industrialization and Social Conflict in the Philadelphia Region, 1787–1837* (Baltimore: Johns Hopkins University Press, 1986), pp. 7–25, 57–8, 61–2, and the *Pennsylvanian* (8 August 1835, 29 March 1836).

28 Susan G. Davis, *Parades and Power* (Philadelphia: Temple University Press, 1986), pp. 73–111; "Burton's Comic Songster," Van Pelt-Dietrich Library, University of Pennsylvania (1838), pp. 11–15; *Mechanics Free Press* (12 April 1828 and 13 January 1830).

29 W.J. Rorabaugh, *The Alcoholic Republic: An American Tradition* (Oxford: Oxford University Press, 1979), pp. 131–3; the *Pennsylvanian* (1 April 1836); Anonymous, "Observations on Delirium tremens," pp. 16–18; George Escol Sellers, "Memoirs," American Philosophical Society (1898), p. 21.

30 Bruce Laurie, *Working People of Philadelphia, 1800–1850* (Philadelphia: Temple University Press, 1980), p. 57.

31 *Temperance Lecturer and Almanac of the American Temperance Union* (New York: American Temperance Union, 1844), p. 23; *United States Gazette* (28 October 1841).

32 Randolph, "Essay upon Mania á Potu," pp. 1–2; Snowden, "An Inaugural Essay on Delirium Tremens," p. 192.

33 See note 25.

34 Statistics for the number of Alms House cases were compiled from the "Men's Register" of the Philadelphia Alms House.

35 Ric N. Caric, "Displays of Degradation: The Washingtonian Temperance Movement in Philadelphia, 1841–1845," *Ohio Valley History Association* (25 October 2002); *Public Ledger* (1 February 1842 and 30 April 1842).

36 Greenberg, *Manifest Manhood*, pp. 9–12; Kimmel, *Manhood in America*, pp. 20–3; Eliot Gorn, *The Manly Art: Bare-Knuckle Prize Fighting in America* (Ithaca: Cornell University Press, 1989), pp. 129–36. For rioting, see Laurie, *Working People*, pp. 61–6; for fire companies, see Caric, "From Ordered Buckets."

37 *The New Negro Forget-Me-Not Songster: Containing All the New Negro Songs Ever Published, with a Choice Collection of Ballad Songs, Now Sung in Concerts* (Cincinnati: Stratton & Barnard, 1848), pp. 12–13.

38 Greenberg, *Cause for Alarm*, pp. 57–8; Greenberg, *Manifest Manhood*, pp. 9–12.

From La Bambola to a Toronto Striptease: Drawing Out Public Consent to Gender Differentiation with Anatomical Material

Annette Burfoot

The long history of anatomical display dates back at least from the classic period when people left wax votives of afflicted body parts at Greek and Roman temples, seeking divine intervention. However, a notable development took place during the 1700s. Anatomy and its display in illustrated texts, anatomical theatres, and medical teaching museums spread throughout developed Europe as the scientific revolution settled in and modern medicine began to take shape. Within this growing visual culture, a political mediation between public and private display of the opened body heralded important gender subjectivities that persist today in the visual culture of anatomy.

This chapter compares the treatment of gender in relation to how and when the anatomical body is publicly displayed in three exhibits: the eighteenth-century exhibit at the Florentine museum commonly known as La Specola, the mid-twentieth-century Canadian gynecological collection now housed at the Kingston Museum of Health Care, and the roving, international exhibit entitled *Body Worlds II*. Despite the significant temporal and spatial settings involved, the models examined here share in the visual publication of a socially inscribed body that includes perpetuation of engendered norms. The anatomical models and their public display are emblematic of the growth in the social capital of medicine and its concomitant establishment as authority over the body throughout the time period.

Methodologically, this chapter follows what Nina Lykke describes as "feminist cultural studies of technoscience," which is an amalgamation of three key literatures and approaches: feminist studies, cultural studies, and science and technology studies.[1] The amalgamation is fluid and inter-disciplinary, "a special kind of hermeneutic tradition that can 'open up' an unlimited number of topics."[2] As a science study, we will explore how the popularization of medical anatomy from late-eighteenth-century Europe to contemporary North America played a key role in giving voice and place to modern medicine's authority over the body. A feminist analysis of the perpetuation of gender norms is core to this chapter and is based in a visual discursive interpretation of the anatomical models and their public presentation.

La Specola: Medical Science and the Gendered Body

La Specola is deemed the oldest public museum in the Western world; it is located near Palazzo Pitti, the grand former Florentine home of the Tuscan dukes. Inaugurated in 1775 as the Imperiale Regio Museo di Fisica e Storia Naturale (the Imperial Royal Museum of Physics and Natural History), the museum is found just down Via Romano from the ducal palace (Palazzo Pitti) and is connected at the back through an impressive set of gates to the palace's extensive gardens (Il Giardino Boboli). Later, the museum and the palace buildings were connected with the Poccianti Corridor, thus extending the Vasari Corridor from the Palazzo Vecchio (the seat of the ducal government) via the Uffizi, where the duchy's art treasures were stored, through the Palazzo Pitti (the ducal residence) to La Specola. These architectural details signify the important links among the government of the day, that government's prized culture, and the rising social significance of science and technology. They also echo Michel Foucault's mapping in *Madness and Civilization* of the geo-discursive pathways of civilized health a century later, as lepers were isolated from civil society in France and its colonies.[3] The body as flesh, especially obviously diseased flesh, became a social scapegoat and a useful delimiter: lepers were characterized as sinners punished by God but also served as a public reminder of the need for Christian charity. Leper colonies, along with the "saints" who worked in them, became signs of the dominant culture's benevolence and also of medicine's relatively new place as the site of salvation. Long after cures for leprosy were developed and the need for the isolation of those suffering from the disease was disputed, the social delineation between well and diseased bodies was drawn with specified roles for the sick, the physician, and the proper location for treatment: the hospital. Foucault's analysis lends itself well to the anatomical display at La Specola, which established a regime of corporeal governance that clearly educated the public on the anatomical and pathological.

The Grand Duke of Tuscany, Peter Leopold of Hapsburg-Lotharingen, is often portrayed not only as the museum's founder but also as an enlightened nobleman with a keen and unusual interest in the sciences. He gave a home to an emergent modern science as represented by dispersed collections of instruments, specimens, and teaching materials, providing the museum with the former home of the Torirgiani family. He also supplied the necessary funds to catalogue the collections according to the radical and new Linnaean system and to renovate the building to display the collections. Unlike many of his colleagues who kept their gentlemen's collections of unclassified and pseudo-scientific treasures private,[4] Leopold also stipulated that this modern scientific collection be accessible to the public. He was an early proponent of the argument that scientific knowledge contributes to overall social development: the more about science the public knows, the more advanced the society.[5] The civilizing role of science in public life is reflected in a contemporary comparison of the museum's purpose with that of fine art: "Like the art museums, the science museums [of Florence] have the triple function of preserving the collections, serving as research institutions, and aiding in the didactic process. Their educational value, not only to University students but first and foremost to the general public of all ages, is essential in creating an awareness of nature as a permanent collection."[6] And so the way was paved for the authorization of medicine as arbiter of body matters.

The public witnessing of the newly revealed human body in such a permanent collection of anatomical models reinforced the spatial control of the human body as primarily an object of the scientific medical gaze, and as gendered. The eight rooms devoted to human anatomy at La Specola were designed to be walked through in a certain order: from the outward and visual manifestations of the human body (muscles and skeleton) to the inside and functional aspects (circulatory and nervous systems, organs, and reproduction). Each room contains life-sized models, anatomical parts, and schematic drawings on the walls that refer to indices hidden in small drawers below; the indices name the parts according to what was then a relatively new system of modern medical nomenclature. Besides establishing a persistent and crucial distinction between form and function in modern medicine, this medical schooling drew significantly on dualistic gendered assumptions regarding life and death, rationality and carnality, fear and desire.[7]

Barbara Stafford demonstrates how anatomical display functions to define and limit in terms of corporeal significance as an "impulse to make public the inarticulable and the concealed." She points to how the body as space is managed through the rise of medical authority with the prolongation of scientific-led vision into the body in the wax modelling of Felice Fontana at La Specola, Florence, where models are *excatavable* or dissectible.[8] Not long before Fontana's model went on public display, Galileo upset Church dogma with his visions of Jupiter's moons as evidence of the sun and not the earth's universal centrality. What is often overlooked in the telling of this scientific revolution is that at the same time Galileo was making contentious use of the early telescope, the compound microscope was developed to look more deeply into the human body, helping to establish the process of opening up the human body to medical inspection with both public participation and approval.

Almost everyone walking into the first room of models at La Specola (skeletal and muscle systems) recoils at the almost hyper-realism of the "skinned" models that surround and fill the room. The carefully crafted and coloured wax reveals every anatomical detail and provides a constant reminder of how time will treat our bodies in the same way as death and decay will strip our mortality, layer by layer, to the bare bones. But these initial models also match perfectly Londa Schiebinger's gendered analysis of eighteenth-century illustrated skeletons.[9] Despite the difficulty in sexing the skeletal body (it is possible through minor variations in the pelvis bones), Schiebinger reveals how the illustrations were clearly sexed and stereotyped according to idealized Western European masculine traits (virtually all illustrations of the skeleton are coded male). La Specola's skeletal models represent the skeleton-as-gentleman (all are male). Skulls perch atop rather elegant figures that assume upright and animated postures. Other figures lounge horizontally in large glass cabinets, skinned faces resting on bony and sinewy hands and arms. The skeletons are followed by more male figures (genitalia as well as poses help sex the figures) with more to them, anatomically speaking. They display the circulatory, nerve, and endocrine systems so that the viewer sees the skeletal and muscular base covered with veins and arteries, glands, and nerves. Although this additional anatomical detail and more precise dissection draws us nearer to the moment of violation or the cutting into the body, these figures remain more mechanistic than organismic; of the mind more than nature.

Anatomy as an act of abstracting function from form marks the body as ready for both a newly authorized interpreter of its significance and use (historically this authority shifted to science from the Church) and as the site for mediating other social values, including those associated with social

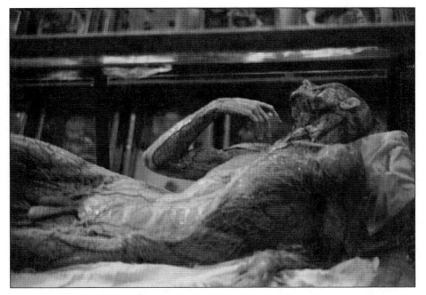

Figure 1   *Skinned Man.* Wax anatomical model from La Specola Museum, Florence. Photo by A. Burfoot, used with permission.

subjectivities, especially gender. Sexual difference—a fluid and political concept—became more marked and more common in early modern anatomical display than it had been previously.[10] Reflecting Foucault's concept of the material effects of exclusion and integration described above, Petherbridge and Jordanova speak of the denial of body integrity with its "fracturing" within anatomical display and the concurrent integration of a patriarchal politics in terms of how the parts make sense: the predominance of male parts as human parts, the growing need for sexual differentiation by body part, and the birth of obstetrics and gynecology.[11]

In contrast to the male skeletal and skinned models, a sense of the horrific is heightened as one moves into the room that follows, where three obviously female models lie prostrate in their respective glass cases. Until now, no full figure has had much in the way of skin or hair, and as such, they have appeared as distant cousins to us humans and more like some form of organic robot or cyborg: a cool caricature of a human being. Inversely, the fleshy and fulsome female figures have plenty of signs of what we hold dear in being human. They have all of their skin and most of their body hair, down to eyelashes and pubic hair. Their underarms, arms, and legs are cleanly shaven, however. Their heads are tilted backwards, exposing the neck, and their faces express a sort of drugged rapture: lips partially open and their beautiful but unfocused

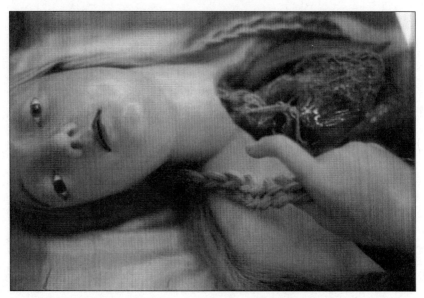

Figure 2 *Woman Holding Her Plait*. Wax anatomical model from La Specola Museum, Florence. Photo by A. Burfoot, used with permission.

eyes gazing into the distance. Their hands are gracefully posed by their sides, with one of the figures holding her own plait. These quasi-pornographic displays are ruptured, literally and figuratively, by their other role as medical illustration. Designed to exhibit the internal organs and the digestive system, the models of these young beautiful women lie with their torsos cut from clavicle to pubis and the innards pulled out and draped over both sides of their nubile bodies.

Down the corridor from this large room is a much smaller room on the way out of the museum. It is the gynecological room containing Clemente Susini's "decomposable" or modular female figure: "La Bambola," or "the Doll."[12] This is a hands-on model that is designed to have the front panel of the torso removed to reveal four successive levels of dissection until the deepest level is reached, where an opened uterus reveals a five-month fetus inside. The model in its closed form is remarkably worked in terms of rendering a beautiful and erotic female figure. The likeness is of a young woman, again supine with her head tilted back and slightly to one side as if in some state of sexual ecstasy. Her firm young breasts sport erect nipples, her lips are slightly parted, and she stares dreamily off into the distance. One leg is slightly bent allowing us to look directly at her external genitals (rendered complete with pubic hair). This model is normally displayed closed, complete with a pearly necklace designed to hide the seam of the removable front plate and to maintain the illusion of a feminine ideal as an object of masculine desire.

This "medical Venus" is surrounded by full-sized models of the female uterus (heavily pregnant, in most cases) with large amputated thigh stumps framing the external genitalia and the dissected womb. Skin, fat, and muscle are peeled back like huge oranges to reveal either a distended pregnant uterus or a well-developed fetus or fetuses inside. There are also cabinets containing a large collection of fetuses in all stages of gestation (although the earlier models illustrate homunculism—fully formed miniature humans—rather than embryology as it is understood today). There is also a choir of dissected newborns, almost all male and positioned in baby Christ-like poses with little arms reaching outwards to embrace and bless, and slightly tilted heads gazing down knowingly and forgivingly on the observer and the Doll. Within this womb-like, small, and packed room, every mystery of anatomical femininity is exposed—there are no surprises left, and the mystery of life itself glows softly in waxy realism that both shocks and delights. And off in a corner of the gynecological room is a beribboned phallus—a large penis separate from any other part of the male genitalia with a little bow wrapped around its base. It lies at the foot-end of the Doll, near her genitalia, and serves as a

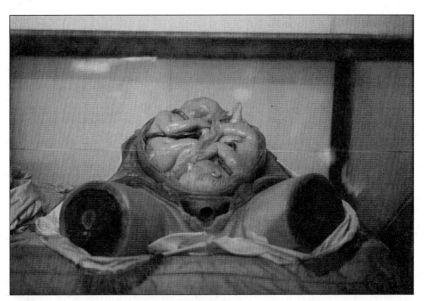

Figure 3   *Twins in Uteri.* Wax anatomical model from La Specola Museum, Florence. Photo by A. Burfoot, used with permission.

phallic pointer within a patriarchal display of curiosity and fetish. Here the female dissected body does not carry signs of social emancipation or equality in terms of a long history of the male anatomical body as the norm. A new liminal marker is made; the female dolls both embody our fears of body-based fragility (in contrast to the weakness of the soul as the central concern that precedes this era) and mortality, as their deep dissection and essentialization as agents of reproduction helps bring these same bodies into the ordered world of modern scientific rationalism. Their eroticization completes their integration as models of feminine ideals in the modern (medical) world. At La Specola, anatomy as medical ideal is youthful, female, sexually attractive, and white.[13]

Londa Schiebinger provides an excellent analysis of the integration of gender discrimination in anatomical display with the case of eighteenth-century skeleton illustrations. Since anatomical dissection to the bone renders sexual difference very subtle, anatomical illustrators used a host of design elements to indicate gender (poses, accessories, and so on) and initially used almost solely masculine models to illustrate normal skeletal structure. Between 1730 and 1790, the first female skeletons appeared in England, France, and Germany, and Schiebinger asks, "[W]as there a connection between eighteenth-century movements for women's equality and attempts on the part of anatomists to discover a physiological basis for female 'inequality'?"[14] She responds that there was indeed a connection and notes how, in this form of anatomical display, the gender of science is formed, and specific and sexual divisions of labour occur: "the feminization of feeling and the masculinization of reason."[15] Such scientifically determined sex difference was, in turn, used to advance arguments against increased social equality for women, commonly referred to as "the woman question."

From Early Modern Europe to Twentieth-Century North America

In addition to contributing to the public construction of science as social progress and the reification of engendered difference in the body's form and function, wax anatomical models served the medical profession as instructional technology for over two hundred years. They continue to serve as historical artifacts that can be used to trace how modern medicine developed its corporeal dominion with ever deeper and more involved mappings of the human body and theories of its function. By the end of the seventeenth century, anatomical wax models in medicine were well established, and this continued with at times horrific representations of gender. Abraham Chovet (1706–90) publicly displayed and charged for the viewing of his latest model, advertised as a "new figure of Anatomy which represents a woman chained down upon a table, suppos'd opened alive; wherein the circulation of the blood is made visible through glass veins and arteries; the circulation is also seen from the mother to the child, and from the child to the mother, with Histolick and Diastolick motion of the heart and the action of the lungs."[16]

Chovet was also the one who played a key role in establishing wax modelling in the United States. Because of dubious work in tracheotomies on hanging victims, Chovet ended up in Philadelphia in 1770 with wax models he had made over the past fifteen years in the West Indies. These models were used to teach medicine at the University of Philadelphia until 1884, when they were destroyed in a fire. Meanwhile other modellers went to work: Christopher Curtis of Switzerland left medical practice and modelling of anatomy to make life-sized figures of French aristocracy and notable persons. Curtis trained his niece, who became Madame Tussaud. José de Flores of Guatemala focused on completely dissectible pieces (all but one of his pieces were destroyed by fire). His incomplete masterpiece was a life-sized figure of a woman with emphasis on the reproductive organs (and interchangeable uteri and fetuses to display abnormalities and disease). Felice Fontana (1730–1805) followed and produced the Specola waxes. London's Wellcome Institute claims that some of their models are identical to those at La Specola, and both sets may have been sketched out by anatomist Bernard Albinus (1697–1770).[17]

Joseph Towne (1808–79) modelled waxes (over a thousand, and six hundred remain) at Guy's Hospital and moved into representing skin diseases with the famed Thomas Addington. Towne would occasionally sell his models, heralding a modelling business that started in the mid-nineteenth century. Many of these dermatological waxes went to the Medical College in St. Louis, Missouri. Others came to the United States via Paris's Hôpital St. Louis, ending up at Harvard for teaching cutaneous disease (including syphilis). Some of the models were also used in public health education and taken around for public display. Pictures of La Specola's models stand alongside contemporary medical illustrations and photographs in a 1939 Italian medical textbook by Vaccari. Meanwhile, a twentieth-century museum of moulages (founded in 1917) in Zurich is still being used for medical instruction. It is here that Elizabeth Stoiber continues to work. Trammond, Deyrolle, and Auzioux are commercial firms that continue to manufacture wax models of human and comparative anatomy.[18] However, throughout the twentieth century and today, anatomical modelling has largely been replaced in medical schools by dissection supplemented with medical illustrations and imaging in textbooks.

Kingston's Museum of Health Care: Closed Medical Display

An interesting exception to this trend is found in the Kingston, Ontario, wax model collection. These three-dimensional obstetrical models and somatotypes were commissioned by Dr. Edwin Robertson in the 1940s and created by a local artist, Marjorie Winslow.[19] It is possible that Robertson was first exposed to anatomical models in Edinburgh, Scotland, where he trained. He also saw the dermatologic wax models at the Johns Hopkins Department of Art as Applied to Medicine in 1940, a year following his arrival in Canada from Scotland. He commissioned the models, as he had no pathological lab for medical education purposes and because there was a "limited amount of clinical material" available in Kingston to demonstrate the array of obstetrical disease.[20] The models were completed in the early 1950s and initially displayed in a room at the Queen's Medical School in Etherington Hall, across from medical imaging. The models were not used much in medical teaching, however, partly due to shifts in medical teaching from anatomy and pathology (form) to physiology (function). In 1965 Dr. James Low took two of the models to the Queen's University medical library for display, and the rest were put into storage for about twenty-five years. Two of the stored models were lost in a fire.[21] The remaining models were recently rescued from storage and placed in the Kingston Museum of Health Care, where they can be viewed on request (they are not openly displayed).

Winslow, the artist, observed obstetrical and gynecological procedures at the Kingston General Hospital and later at the Royal Victoria Hospital, Montreal, where she was from and where Robertson also practised.[22] An unknown woman from the Johns Hopkins Medical School spent about a month teaching Winslow and Robertson how to model. Winslow was not allowed to photograph or sketch from life, and was inventive in finding ways to mimic the dimpling in skin, hair follicles, and so on.[23] The wax models were seen as a way around the scarcities created by the Second World War and as a way of presenting realistic pathologic conditions and three-dimensional models of surgical interventions in gynecology and obstetrics in a small population where patients and disease types were limited. The Kingston models consist of a series of life-sized female trunks displaying genitalia and pregnancy, some with gloved hands "in operation," and a series of smaller-than-life-sized pathological models of afflicted female reproductive parts and organs. This collection also includes about a dozen Barbie-doll-sized female somatotypes that illustrate the normal nubile, young female and a range of gross anatomical abnormalities, including anorexia, teenage pregnancy, and obesity.

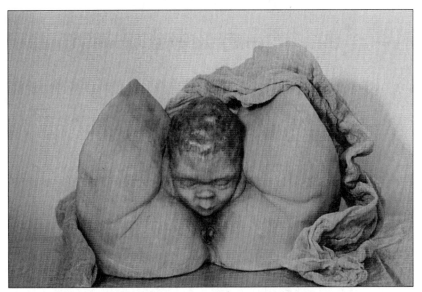

Figure 4   *Crowning — Normal Birth*. Wax anatomical model from the Museum of Health Care at Kingston, Ontario. Used with permission.

The Kingston models stand apart from other North American collections in that they include anatomical as well as pathological models, and they are obstetrical and gynecological. The somatotypes are the only known North American collection. Reminiscent of their Florentine predecessors, these models idealize the white, youthful female form for anatomical display, except in the case of the pathological somatotypes where age and body size varies and idealized forms are based in the abnormal rather than the normal. It should be noted that early modern anatomical displays, including that at La Specola, often had pathological models kept nearby but hidden from public view.[24] Although the Kingston set does not include any full-sized female models, the ones found here do resemble the truncated gynecological models surrounding the Doll at La Specola. Also, the Kingston models, like those in Florence, were meant to be used and handled by medical students but only as an emergency measure in the medical program at Queen's University. Unlike their Italian precedents, these models were never part of a careful and considered arrangement of human anatomical display. The Canadian models were pinch-hitting for the real thing usually available in local pathology (either in preserved specimens or in live patients) to which the now well-established medical profession had easy and privileged access. Although there are some similarities between the Kingston and Florence anatomical models, their roles in public display are remarkably different.

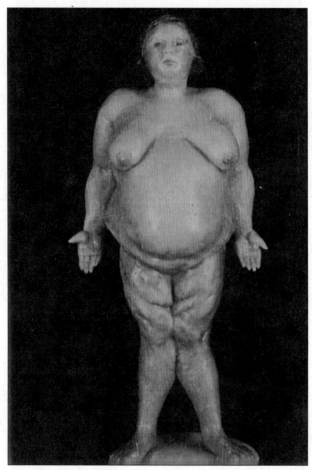

Figure 5   *Pathological Somatotype.* Wax anatomical model from the Museum of Health Care at Kingston, Ontario. Used with permission.

The Kingston models were never designed to be on public display; they reflect an important proprietal shift in terms of the body from a sharing among scientists, early physicians and midwives, and the public in the early modern anatomical display at La Specola to the restricted space of medical authority as characterized in twentieth-century medical culture. These models were housed in the hospital and were primarily available, albeit briefly, to physicians and medical students. Even though they have now been moved to the Kingston Museum of Health Care, they remain hidden from public view and are only brought out on special request. As part of the professionalization process of physicians and as the body is increasingly

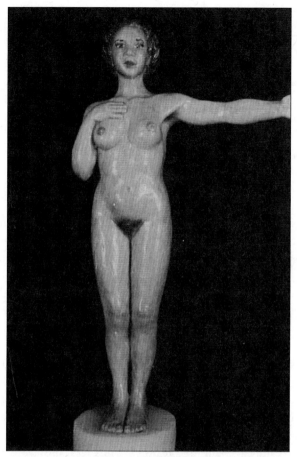

Figure 6 *Anatomical Somatotype*. Wax model from the Museum of Health Care at Kingston, Ontario. Used with permission.

drawn by and drawn into medical culture, gender discrimination intact, the dissected body remains largely hidden from public view. Until now.

Body Worlds II: The Repopularization of Anatomy

Gunther von Hagens began experimenting with the plastination process of preparing, preserving, and displaying dissected human bodies in 1977. Between then and 1982, he patented the process, and he has since made a great deal of displaying his models. Using polymers to replace bodily fluids, von Hagens is able to display what he calls "living anatomy": entire, deeply dissected corpses in a great variety of poses.[25] He prepares his bodies in atypical anatomical postures, and then opens his displays to the paying public. As of 2005, 17,203,386 visitors had been counted.[26] Also widely available are large glossy photo catalogues and DVD versions of the exhibits. Von Hagens sees himself as something of a visionary, someone akin to the Tuscan duke, Peter Leopold: he is bringing the long-hidden views of the human body under the skin to the public eye. In a brochure associated with the Toronto, Ontario, exhibit (*Body Worlds II*, 2006), a philosopher and friend, Franz Josef Wetz, describes him as "an envelope-pusher—an intellectual adventurer." In the 2005 catalogue, tables indicating increased willingness to donate bodies and body parts to science are positively correlated to attendance of the exhibits.[27] Von Hagens also associates himself with the period that gave rise to La Specola's anatomical models, claiming that "Body Worlds falls within the tradition of the Renaissance when art was a product of ability."[28] Perpetuating the aura of the Renaissance man as both artist and scientist, von Hagens is usually pictured sporting a black fedora, and he signs each anatomical display with his name.

Both *Body Worlds* exhibitions, which have toured internationally for more than ten years, feature many full-sized, dissected bodies that are real, as the public is constantly reminded. The bodies are placed in intentionally active, highly unusual anatomical positions. At the 2006 Toronto exhibit, these included a man riding a horse (also dissected), an archer in the process of firing an arrow, a swimmer, a swordsman, a jumping dancer, a skateboarder, and a soccer player. Each dissection is designed to reveal a certain set of anatomical principles, typically concerned with muscles and skeletal structure, and normally as if the person had been skinned so that eyes, lips and other readily recognizable features (rib cages, breasts, nipples, penis, scrotum) are visible. There are also deeper dissections, typically not in action poses, used to display internal organs and the nervous, respiratory, digestive, cardiovascular, and reproductive systems. One is a dissected woman who is heavily pregnant. In the Toronto exhibit, the body was hidden behind a curtained section preceded by an array of fetuses in small vials on pedestals. Lines formed for the attending crowds to look at the female body sliced open to reveal the fetus inside. The catalogue featured a different pregnant woman's body in a reclining position with an arm behind the head. More active than her Florentine counterpart, the Doll, this figure still sexualizes the mysteries of hidden human procreation and remains a powerful public draw. Most figures in the Toronto exhibit and catalogue were Caucasian (many dissections include some skin and hair). Pathology and abnormalities were displayed in terms of "obesity revealed," lung and other cancers, and abnormal fetuses (conjoined twins and so on).[29]

Conclusion

This comparison of La Specola's early modern medical imaging in wax anatomical models with two contemporary sets of anatomical models reveals an important role for the public display of the medically dissected body. Starting in Europe, anatomical display, especially the collection at La Specola, heralded a new world of medical science in which once-sacred barriers to the body were removed and entry was allowed. Mysteries, especially that of reproduction, were laid bare, with the idealized and sexualized feminine anatomical body functioning as an emblem of discovery and medical mastery. Ideal sexual orientation (the sexual economy here is heterosexually dominant), race, and ideal body types (not obese or marked by disease or deformity) are also obvious in the emerging modern anatomical body. As the medical profession became established, both in Europe and North America, the need for public display and for the anatomical body changed. Medical education and its models changed from a focus on idealized, form-based anatomy to attention to the pathological, then to physiology and a function-based fracturing of the body into components such as microbiology, endocrinology, and so on. Anatomized and pathological models of afflicted parts replaced full-sized anatomical models, and attention to artistic and idealized rendering of the body as a whole decreased. The need for public display also waned, and during the twentieth century, the models were created, used, and displayed chiefly for medical training. It is only recently that a broader interest in the historical value of the models has brought some collections, like the Kingston one, to public view. Subsequently, the collection of dissected "real" human bodies in *Body Worlds* went on public display, and the public, in large numbers, is fascinated: possibly drawn by the excitement of seeing a "real" dissected body, possibly interested in the contentious display style (the activated corpse).

Throughout all three examples of anatomical display, this peekaboo-like appearance of the dissected body also plays a highly sexualized and engendered striptease. The flaying, dissecting, and disrobing of human skin and hair (what we recognize as human) from muscle and bone structures and all else that lies beneath (the mysterious functions hidden from view) both relies on and creates gendered norms. The penetration of the body can be read as a sexual act enjoyed both privately and publicly throughout the development of modern anatomy. Early on, the obviously sexualized female body figured as a gate and invitation to all into the newly charted world of medicine. The congruence of sexual titillation and medical mastery form a powerful bond in describing and authorizing medicine's new role with the human body. This bond is echoed in contemporary displays, as reproduction and the pregnant bodies are presented simultaneously in a semi-veiled state mediating fear and desire, and as a truncated and stable obstetric object of medical study.

Contemporary medical authority over the human body no longer requires a public education in medical principles, but the publicity may be welcome. At the discursive level, much more is going on. Not only does the contemporary anatomical body on public display affirm the opened body as the proper site of medical authority, but it also illuminates continued liminal markers of ideal bodies in terms of gender, sexuality, race, and now lifestyle (eating habits, smoking, exercise, and reproduction). To see the "other" side is not difficult. Imagine a *Body Worlds III* with only the bodies of people from so-called disadvantaged societies: a body of a three-year-old child racked with rickets and weakened by chronic diarrhea and undernourishment; a pregnant body of a woman of colour with AIDs, emaciated, breasts drooping over her rib cage, with five young children nearby next to the tombstones marking her children who have died; the body of a young man with lungs blackened by the smoke from welding torches used to dismantle ocean-going liners by hand, in bare feet on the beaches of Bangladesh. He could be posed in action, hunched over a piece of mean, jagged metal. But this is not the corporeal emblem that we seek in medicine-as-social-progress. Typically, we are frightened by seeing the body laid open, whether it is real or very real looking. And the fear emanates from that which is beyond the limit, the unnamed. Femininity occupies both spaces and thus mediates the distinction. Nina Lykke refers to Donna Hraway's cyborg (a female and a metaphor for how a human being is simultaneously material and semiotic) as a "thinking technology."[29] So are anatomical models, then and now.

Notes

1   Nina Lykke, "Feminist Cultural Studies of Technoscience," in Anneke Smelik and Nina Lykke, eds., *Bits of Life: Feminism at the Intersections of Media, Bioscience, and Technology* (Seattle: University of Washington Press, 2008).

2   Lykke, "Feminist Cultural Studies," p. 12.

3   Michel Foucault, *Madness and Civilization* (New York: Routledge, 2006).

4   Paula Findlen, *Possessing Nature: Museums, Collecting and Scientific Culture in Early Modern Italy* (Berkeley: University of California Press, 1994).

5   Class division, however, was maintained at La Specola with separate opening hours, and the lower classes were only permitted entrance if they were cleanly dressed.

6   A. Berzi, C. Cipriani, and M. Poggesi, "Florentine Science Museums," *Journal of the Society for the Bibliography of Natural History* 9.4 (1980): 423.

7   Previously I have analyzed these models in terms of how they presage Freud and Lacan's interpretation of the primal scene in terms of film analyses of gender horror. The gendered analysis here is based on this work. See Annette Burfoot, "Surprising Origins: Florentine 18th-Century Wax Anatomical Models as Inspiration for Italian Horror," *Kinoeye* 2.9 (13 May 2002), http://www.kinoeye.org/02/09/burfoot09.html (accessed 7 September 2010; *Kinoeye* is an online journal of film in the new Europe); Annette Burfoot, "Surprising Origins in Italian Horror: Florentine 18th-Century Wax Anatomical Models," in Anthony Tamburri, ed., *Italian Cultural Studies 2002* (Boca Raton: Bordighiera Press, 2006), pp. 38–50; Annette Burfoot, "The Fetal Voyager: Women in Modern Medical Visual Discourse," in Bernard Lightman and Ann Shteir, eds., *Figural Vocabularies of Gender in Science, Medicine, and Technology* (Hanover, NH: University Press of New England, 2006), pp. 337–56.

8   Barbara Maria Stafford, *Body Criticism: Imaging the Unseen in Enlightenment Art and Medicine* (Cambridge, MA: MIT Press, 1994), p. 21.

9   Londa Schiebinger, "Skeletons in the Closet: The First Illustrations of the Female Skeleton in Eighteenth-Century Anatomy," in Londa Schiebinger, ed., *Feminism and the Body* (New York: Oxford University Press, 2000).

10   See Georg Bartisch's medical illustration of phallus-like reproductive organs, attributed to Bartisch's *Kunstbuche* (1575), for an example of sexual homogeneity. Brian Easlea and Carolyn Merchant, among others, have written on the history of science and sexual differentiation in terms of patriarchal politics. See also the historical and epistemological tracings of sexual differentiation in queer studies: for example, Eve Sedgwick, *The Epistemology of the Closet* (Berkeley: University of California Press, 1990).

11   Deanna Petherbridge and Ludmilla Jordanova, *The Quick and the Dead: Artists and Anatomy* (Berkeley: University of California Press, 1997), p. 63.

12   *Encyclopædia Anatomica* (Köln, Germany: Taschen, 1999).

13   In every case where it is possible to discern racial difference, the models at La Specola (and in most similar exhibitions in Bologna and Rome) are of Caucasians. There are some exceptions: for example, at the museum at Ospedale Santo Spirito in Rome, there is a preserved head of a "negro" displayed as a medical curiosity. In Bologna, there is a model of a dissected head of a "negro" displaying the brain and engaging with racist theories of cognitive capacity.

14   Schiebinger, "Skeletons in the Closet," p. 26.

15   Schiebinger, "Skeletons in the Closet," p. 52.

16   Quoted in Peachy, who is cited in Thomas N. Haviland and Lawrence Charles Parish, "A Brief Account of the Use of Wax Models in the Study of Medicine," *Journal of the History of Medicine* 1 (1970): 52–75.

17   Rumy Hilloowala, "Illustrations from the Wellcome Institute Library: The Origin of the Wellcome Anatomical Waxes *albinus* and the Florentine Collection at *La Specola*," *Medical History* 28 (1984): 432–7.

18   Haviland and Parish, "Brief Account."

19   Fiona Mattatall, "A Very Real Art," *Canadian Medical Association Journal* 164.7 (2001): 1027–8.

20   James Low, interview by Annette Burfoot at Museum of Health Care, Kingston, Ontario, 21 March 2002.

21   Low, interview by Burfoot.

22   Low, interview by Burfoot; Mattatall, "Very Real Art."

23   Marjorie Winslow, interview by Rona Rustige, former curator of the Kingston Museum of Health Care, at Belleville, Ontario, 13 July 1996.

24 An important exception is the human anatomical collection at the University of Bologna, Museo di Anatomia e Istologia Patologica "C. Taruffi," which is almost entirely made up of pathological models and is currently open to the public. However, these models were not originally on public display in the same manner as the anatomical models in Florence.

25 *Gunther von Hagens' Body Worlds: The Anatomical Exhibition of Real Human Bodies,* 7th printing, exhibition catalogue (Heidelberg: Verlagsgesellschaft, 2005), p. 33.

26 *Gunther von Hagens' Body Worlds,* p. 301.

27 *Gunther von Hagens' Body Worlds,* p. 303.

28 *Gunther von Hagens' Body Worlds,* p. 32.

29 Images from the *Body Worlds* exhibition can be found at http://www.bodyworlds.com.

30 Lykke, "Feminist Cultural Studies," p. 13.

Let Me Hear Your Body Talk: Aerobics for Fat Women Only, 1981–1985

Jenny Ellison

By 1984 aerobics, dancercise, and jazzercise were among "the most popular physical activities of North American women."[1] Aerobics emerged in the early 1980s in the wake of Title IX and the development of organizations like the Canadian Association for the Advancement of Women in Sport (CAAWS), actions that sought to advance the position of women by improving their status as athletes.[2] Due to their apparent focus on femininity and feminine display, aerobics classes have come to be seen by some sports historians and feminist theorists as a departure from the goals of liberation and equality for women. With aerobics, the potential for collective gains for women appears to have been replaced with individualistic goals; the freedom of sport co-opted for the purpose of selling a service to women.[3]

My previous research on female athletes confirmed that popular culture representations of aerobics tended to present the activity as aesthetic rather than health-promoting.[4] From the *20 Minute Workout* to Tab-Cola advertisements, an archetype of female aerobics participants emerges. Clad in high-cut pink leotards with matching leg warmers and headbands, these young, lean white women represented the self-monitoring, self-disciplining consumers of beauty culture described in Susan Bordo's path-breaking *Unbearable Weight*.[5] This chapter explores the relationship that existed between idealized images of women in popular culture and women themselves. Did such ideals and archetypes of femininity figure into women's participation in aerobics? What sort of liberation did individualized fitness activities offer to women in the 1980s?

I will address these questions through an examination of Large as Life (LaL), a Vancouver "action group" whose motto was "Stop postponing your life until you lose weight and start living now!" Formed in 1981, the group's mandate was to "promote increased self-acceptance in large women."[6] Among the first actions of the group was to hire a fitness instructor to design and teach aerobics classes for fat women.[7] Few participated in these classes until LaL members obtained Fitness Leadership training at a local YMCA. Once fat women themselves began to teach the classes, enrolment multiplied. By May 1983, the classes had expanded to ten Vancouver-area fitness centres and included weekly pool time, all exclusively for large women.[8]

To date, the focus of academic research on aerobics has been on its association with femininity rather than its relationship to health and fitness. An examination of LaL's aerobics classes shows that the boundaries between these two categories were fluid. Using personal interviews with participants and instructors, advertisements, and newsletters, this chapter provides commentary on aerobics in the 1980s. I show that LaL participants saw aerobics as a form of self-expression. The group believed that individual growth was an essential part of collective action and that aerobics would contribute to their goal of greater equality and self-esteem for fat women. This research shows that LaL's approach to aerobics was shaped by a range of discourses about femininity, feminism, and beauty. In turn, participants' understanding of themselves as fat women was shaped by the very practice of aerobics and by their interactions with one another. LaL aerobics participants were not just self-disciplining subjects: they were critical consumers attempting to carve out a space for fat women in 1980s popular culture.

The Feminist Critique of Aerobics

In order to understand aerobics for fat women only, it is necessary to understand the significance of aerobics itself to debates about women's popular culture and gender roles in the 1980s. Advocates like Jane Fonda saw aerobics as a way for women to "break the weaker sex mold," to become "strong" and "healthy," and to fulfill their "physical potential."[9] Detractors placed aerobics on an "axis of continuity" with a broader popular culture that had a negative impact on women's self-esteem.[10] Sports historian Helen Lenskyj's influential *Out of Bounds: Women, Sport and Sexuality* (1986) lays out the case against aerobics: "While its popularity signified greater female participation in regular physical activity, its association with the cosmetic and fashion industries made it, in many instances, another arena for women to compete for male attention. Like makeup and clothing, dance exercise produced more prescriptions for heterosexual appeal. The new requirements included thinness, muscularity and shapeliness, enhanced by fashionable and expensive sportswear."[11] Lenskyj's argument is that the possibilities for community among women were negated by ideals of heterosexual glamour that became attached to aerobics.[12] Consumption of women's popular culture was conflated with complicity to its messages; aerobics classes were part of a popular culture that demeaned and damaged its consumers. Popular culture representations, in turn, were seen as dangerous for women, a "psychopathology" emblematic of all that was wrong with feminine ideals.[13]

For Lenskyj, aerobics was a setback from sports feminist gains of the 1970s, which saw increased levels of participation and funding for female athletes.[14] In North America, gender equality in sport had become a mainstream issue because of the passage in the United States of Title IX of the *Education Amendments Act* (1972), which stated that federally funded schools must give girls and boys equal opportunities to play sport. This law resulted in quantifiable change in levels of participation as well as in the amount of funding girls' sport received.[15] In Canada, the "Report of the Royal Commission on the Status of Women in Canada" (1970) had recommended that the federal government take action to increase women's participation in sport. In the wake of this recommendation and Title IX, Fitness and Amateur Sport Canada sponsored a 1974 conference on women and sport, which led, after many years of lobbying, to the formation of CAAWS (Canadian Association for the Advancement of Women in Sport) in 1981. CAAWS's mandate was to "advance the position of women by defining, promoting and supporting a feminist perspective on sport and to improve the status of women in sport."[16] The organization received funding from Fitness and Amateur Sport Canada as well as the Secretary of State Women's Program, but it was run primarily by volunteers who were working in university-level sport and government sports bodies. CAAWS's initiatives tended to focus on "liberal strategies aimed at equalizing access to sport and physical activity," such as the National Coaching School for Women and a 1985 court challenge that gave Justine Blainey the legal right to play on a boys' hockey team.[17] Canadian sports were influenced by the conceptual and theoretical debates that fuelled second-wave feminism; activists believed that gender equality could be achieved by making sex differences less pronounced in all aspects of social life. Girls and women of the 1980s were benefiting from greater access to sport, thanks to the activism of this earlier generation of women.

Academic feminist critics in North America first attacked aerobics from the perspective of media effects and sex roles, arguing that aerobics (in representation and in practice) reinforced unrealistic and dangerous feminine norms. In 1987 a special issue of the feminist journal *Women's Studies International Forum* was dedicated to the subject of women and sport. What little attention was given to aerobics (also called "keep-fit") classes was not positive. Some authors perceived a conflict between the potential for collective gain that physical fitness offered to women and the individualistic practice of aerobics. Aerobics appeared to have co-opted physical fitness for the purpose of selling slenderness and colourful leotards to women. Rosemary Deem argued that "keep-fit" classes for women owed their popularity to "women's anxiety over their body weight and appearance."[18] Deem, like Lenskyj before her, felt that the purpose and meaning of physical activity determined how beneficial it could be for women. Goals such as improved strength were applauded, but women who pursued fitness for aesthetic purposes were seen as misguided and even oppressed.

Through participant observation and interviews, sociological studies of the 1990s attempted to unpack the extent to which female aerobics participants adhered to beauty norms. Pirkko Markula found that women in New Zealand were less concerned with their overall health and fitness than with so-called problem areas such as their bums and thighs.[19] Joseph Maguire and Louise Mansfield similarly concluded that aerobics was a site where "women ... sculpt their bodies in line with dominant messages about femininity."[20] Taking a somewhat different approach, Leslea Haravon Collins interviewed feminist aerobics participants to understand how they reconciled the activity with their politics. She found that these women focused on "control, competence, and stress release" in order to adjust aerobics classes to their own world view.[21] Although Haravon Collins comes close to understanding aerobics as a contested site, she is unsuccessful because her study assumes that there is something intrinsically unfeminist about aerobics. Like Mansfield, Maguire, and Markula, Haravon Collins's data are shaped by her initial problematic: aerobics itself. Attentive to the limitations of the studies cited above, this project did not assume that aerobics was either good (feminist) or bad (feminine). Nor did it assume that fat was necessarily a pejorative term or physical attribute. Participants were asked to describe their experiences in their preferred language for talking about their bodies.

Large as Life

Kate Partridge, Janet Walker, and Joan Dal Santo met for the first time on 22 October 1979, at the Cold Mountain Institute on Cortes Island, British Columbia. The women were three among twenty in attendance at a five-day workshop entitled "The Forgotten Woman: For Fat Women Only." The workshop was advertised as

> [a]n intense experiential exploration of our relationship to our body size and shape. In an effort to get at *forgotten*, unknown or unexplored material in relation to our weight, we will be on a juice fast, use journals and dream material and appropriate therapeutic techniques.
>
> This program is suitable for anyone who considers herself overweight, but may be of most use to those who are considered by others to be overweight. Medical permission required. Fee: $250.[22]

The idea for the workshop came out of an individual therapy session between Dal Santo and Miriam Ulrych, one of the leaders of the workshop. Having reached a plateau in her therapy, the recently divorced Dal Santo told Ulrych she felt it was time to work on the fact that she was fat and "seemed to be stuck with it."[23] Partridge, at the time a PhD candidate in psychology, was familiar with the work of Ellen Tallman, a Gestalt therapist who co-led the workshop with Ulrych. At thirty-two, Partridge felt it was time to deal with "the whole self-image thing."[24] Janet Walker came to Cortes at the recommendation of her therapists, who paid the workshop fee for the recently divorced mother of two. Walker was uncertain about leaving her children with a babysitter but felt that she "had to go. It was sort of like life and death, it was really important."[25] All three women described themselves as having been fat their entire lives.

Over the course of their five-day workshop, participants in "The Forgotten Woman" were encouraged to explore their feelings about fat as well as about their own fat bodies. Tallman recalled that many women had come with "a sense of shame and despair over what they hadn't been able to shift and change in relation to their body size." What she was attempting to teach the women was to "care for themselves as they were and not be their own enemy."[26] One visualization exercise began with the women lying on the floor, fully clothed. They were instructed to "feel and care" about each part of their bodies and were encouraged to "pay extra attention" to parts of their body they didn't like.[27] Another activity asked participants to "get into their bodies" and dance freely around the room. When interviewed about these exercises, only Dal Santo recalled the dance activity. She saw it as a positive one: "I just remember us dancing freely and enjoying the movement in our bodies, which is something that I think a lot of us, me for sure, and I think others too, didn't do often."[28] The workshop also changed Dal Santo and Kate Partridge's own perceptions of fat women. Both women realized that they had avoided friendships with other large women prior to the workshop in an attempt to disassociate themselves from the stigma of being fat.[29]

In an act echoing consciousness-raising activities of the early women's liberation movement, Partridge, Dal Santo, and a handful of other attendees of "The Forgotten Woman" began to meet regularly to discuss their experiences as fat women.[30] Despite the strength she found in contact with other fat women, Partridge found that talking about the problem of fat oppression was not enough. She continued to be discouraged by her own food and weight issues, and frustrated by the lack of exercise opportunities and clothing stores for large women in Vancouver. Partridge began to think that bringing fat women together to take action on these issues was the solution to her problems. In the spring of 1981, she decided to contact the fashion editor of the *Vancouver Sun* to do a story on the dearth of fashion choices for plus-sized women. Readers were encouraged to contact Partridge if they were interested in doing something about this problem. These phone calls generated so much interest that Partridge called a public meeting at a local community centre in June 1981. Fifty women attended.[31]

The membership roster and executive of LaL shifted over the course of its four-year existence from 1981 to 1985. A review of the thirty-three existing newsletters yields approximately 125 names of women who were active in LaL. Concrete information on the ethnicity, class, and sexual orientation of members is unavailable. Partridge described members as "ordinary middle-of-the-road women who were pissed off" with the clothing and fitness situation.[32] My research participants described a typical Large as Lifer as between thirty and forty years old and white. Members said that LaL attracted a mix of housewives and working women, though I encountered only the latter in the course of my research on the organization. The reach of the organization expanded beyond its official membership through its personal development seminars, fashion shows, and aerobics classes. Two hundred women attended a November 1981 fashion show and seminar at Robson Square in Vancouver.[33] Partnering with retailer Addition-Elle, LaL published, in the August 1982 issue of *Canadian Living*, a questionnaire on the fashion needs of larger women that garnered three thousand responses.[34]

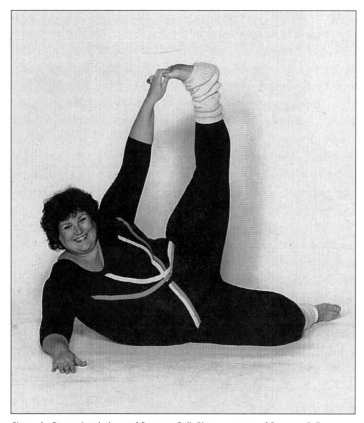

Figure 1   Promotional photo of Suzanne Bell. Photo courtesy of Suzanne Bell.

Women from across the country also contacted LaL directly after the publication of the *Canadian Living* article, which featured a profile of Kate Partridge.[35]

The politics of LaL members varied, as did their opinions on whether or not the group was itself political. This tension revealed itself in members' discussions of gender and feminism. In interviews, some members identified themselves as feminist while others shied away from such a label.[36] LaL was a women's-only group, and most members suggested that this was because fat men had an easier time finding clothes, jobs, and partners than did their female counterparts.[37] None remembered a man attempting to join the group or coming to a meeting. One of the few representations of a man in the newsletter was a cartoon depicting a man doing the dishes. The caption read: "May 19: Another LaL Meeting."[38] Although this cartoon assumed readers were heterosexual, it appears that openly lesbian women did participate. The issue was addressed early on in the "From Our Suggestion Box" section of the December 1981 issue of *The Bolster*. It read: "Question: Some of our members may be homosexual: will they be accepted here no matter what sexual preference the rest of us may have? LARGE AS LIFE is an organization *without* religious, racial or sexual bias."[39] *The Bolster* editor Ingrid Laue noted that lesbians "wouldn't have a sign on their chest saying 'I'm a lesbian,' but we knew, we knew…. It wasn't anything we objected to or found in any way odd … this [British Columbia] is lotus land."[40]

This laid-back "lotus land" approach to sexual orientation did not translate into much, if any, public discussion of lesbianism at meetings or in newsletters or workshops. Such overtly political issues, along with protest marches and lobbying politicians for fat rights, were subjects for debate at meetings, but not the focus of LaL's actions. Members generally described the group as intrinsically political rather than overtly so.[41] There are a few ways to think about this presence/absence of politics. LaL can be understood as a reformist organization; participants were critical of feminine norms but were not rejecting femininity outright. Silence about the political implications of taking action on behalf of fat women may also speak to members' sense that theirs was not a legitimate human rights issue. On the other hand, Large as Lifers may not have seen their interests reflected in the feminist movement of the day. Fashion and fitness were outside of the scope of most feminist activism in Canada at this time, and as Lisa Forman Cody's chapter in this volume suggests, feminist health advocates were no more likely to let women off the hook in the weight department than were other medical professionals.[42]

In September 1981, LaL hired "a fitness instructor from the YMCA, a little skinny thing," who taught eight women at the Canadian Memorial Community Centre.[43] Classes lasted for one hour and were offered two mornings or evenings a week.[44] During this time, Kate Partridge and Joan Dal Santo began to take a Fitness Leadership course offered through the local YWCA. Dal Santo and Partridge saw themselves as outsiders among the "30 fitness Nazis with hard bodies" they encountered every week in the course.[45] Partridge's nervousness was revealed in a note scribbled on the first page of her course package: "*Get Binder; Nametag; Be Enthusiastic.*"[46] The women may have had some reason to feel nervous. The five S's of physical fitness that the YWCA espoused on day one were "STAMINA—STRENGTH—SUPPLENESS—SLENDERNESS and SPIRIT."[47] Despite the apparent assumption of the YWCA that fat people could not be fit, Dal Santo and Partridge completed the course successfully.

LaL classes became much more popular when large women themselves began teaching the classes in 1982. Between May and September 1982, LaL's fitness classes expanded to three more Vancouver-area fitness centres.[48] By the end of 1984, LaL was operating fitness classes from ten different community centres across the Lower Mainland. This expansion was made possible by the training of additional large women as fitness leaders. Suzanne Bell regularly called for new recruits in her columns in *The Bolster*. In an article entitled "LAL Fitness Program Needs YOU!" Bell called on active women to become "role models" for fellow members: "if you are a large woman, active in sports and in good physical condition you may be interested." Addressing her comments to doubtful readers, Bell continued, "[D]on't assume you are not 'fit enough'—*speak to us first*."[49] At least seven women went on to train as LaL instructors in Vancouver and Calgary.[50]

LaL's aerobics classes began with a slow-paced warm-up, progressing through an up-paced workout, floor exercises, and cool-down. They moved at a pace suitable to absolute beginners and focused on low-impact movements suitable for de-conditioned ("out of shape") adults. The purpose of the classes was "to get healthy, to start feeling better about your body, to start understanding it, to move around more."[51] Contrary to the "feel-the-burn" and "no-pain-no-gain" stereotype of aerobics classes from this period, LaL emphasized a non-competitive environment. Suzanne Bell reminded participants that there was no shame in having difficulty keeping up. She emphasized that exercise was a group effort: "[D]on't panic—we are all in this together, and we won't be doing any Jigs ... it really is alright when we have the support of a group we feel comfortable with."[52] LaL classes offered a physically and socially safe environment for fat women. Ingrid Laue found comfort in the absence of "skinny bodies who could do all the kind of stuff that you had trouble, really trouble, doing."[53] Not all participants were de-conditioned. Some women came because they preferred working out with other large women. Janet Walker recalled that "it felt wonderful to know you had a place you could go and people weren't going to be laughing at you."[54] Part of the appeal for Walker was that she got to work out with other self-identified fat women; aerobics was a collective activity.

Although LaL gradually disappeared after 1984, its aerobics program carried on. In 1984 Suzanne Bell set up a fitness business and gradually took over LaL classes, as well as starting new classes in community centres and at her own fitness centre.[55] During this period, another Vancouverite, Jody Sandler, began to specialize in fitness for larger women. Sandler had no previous association with LaL when she took over teaching responsibilities for one of its classes in 1985. Neither the class nor the organization lasted much longer, but Sandler decided to stick with the concept of low-impact aerobics for larger women. She released her own best-selling fitness video, *In Grand Form*, in 1986, followed by *In 2 Grand Form* in 1998, and began to offer her own group fitness classes at local recreation centres.[56] Fitness for larger women was not exclusive to the Vancouver area. Kate Partridge took the concept with her when she moved to Calgary in 1982, setting up an LaL fitness program in that city through the Calgary Board of Education.[57] In 1997 Partridge launched a third chapter of LaL in London, Ontario, and the aerobics program was again successful.[58] Groups of women in Saskatchewan and Manitoba also held their own informal aerobics groups with large friends.[59] In the late 1990s, fitness classes were also offered in Toronto through Big, Bold & Beautiful, a plus-sized clothing store and modelling agency.[60] Undoubtedly, there were other similar programs and groups across Canada.

Aerobics for large women seems to have become popular in the United States at around the same time as LaL was operating.[61] Women at Large, an aerobics chain directed toward "fluffy ladies," was developed in Washington State in 1983.[62] *Radiance: A Publication for Large Women* (1984–2000) was the most significant American resource for publicizing aerobics for large women. A 1985 "Celebrate Your Body" special issue featured profiles of women in the San Francisco Bay area offering fitness classes for large women. Subsequent issues of *Radiance* featured classified ads announcing the arrival of "low impact aerobics for BBWS [Big Beautiful Women] with BBW instructors" in Illinois, New York, Texas, and Virginia.[63] The concept of "fat and fit" also gained momentum with the publication of *Great Shape: The First Exercise Guide for Large Women* in 1988. The book was co-authored by Pat Lyons and Debbie Burgard, two women who connected through *Radiance*.[64] In addition to guidance on starting a fitness program, the book included an extensive appendix listing other aerobics programs for large women, sources of fitness clothing, and exercise videos. According to Lyons and Burgard, in 1988 there were at least twenty-seven fitness programs for fat women operating in ten different states.[65]

Aerobics: Health and Popular Culture

Aerobics does not appear to have substantially altered the body shape or size of any LaL participants. Nor was it a catch-all solution to fat oppression. But its popularity suggests a much deeper and more significant phenomenon on an individual and community level than studies to date have allowed. The next section of this chapter will look at the complexity and apparent contradictions of LaL members' understanding of aerobics. The tension between aerobics as an individualized versus a group sporting practice will be explored by looking at health and beauty discourses developed within the group's newsletter, *The Bolster*. Group members' discussions about aerobics reveal that the classes were integral to the sharing and dissemination of knowledge between fat women.

The emergence of women's health centres and consciousness-raising groups in the 1960s and 1970s followed an explosion of biomedical interventions into women's lives in the post–World War II era. Responding to the lack of women-centred treatment and the perceived condescension of the medical establishment, publications like the *Birth Control Handbook* (1968) and *Our Bodies, Ourselves* (1973) sought to provide women with practical information about their bodies and the health system.[66] LaL used a similar model of consciousness raising to challenge established medical knowledge about fat people. Between facilitating the workshop "For Fat Women Only" and founding LaL, Kate Partridge worked at Vancouver's Lions Gate Hospital's weight-control program. She ran a weekly support group for outpatients who were also required to take a weekly exercise class. After conducting an outcome study, Partridge noticed that patients rarely lost weight, but most gave positive feedback about their experiences with exercise. This led Partridge to conduct her own research on fat, weight loss, and metabolism. As a PhD candidate in psychology at Simon Fraser University, Partridge had the intellectual capital to undertake such research. Nonetheless, it was a departure from her area of expertise, the use of multi-dimensional scaling in standardized psychological testing.[67]

Partridge's first line of attack was to challenge the logic of weight loss itself. As she explained to *CBC Radio Noon* (Vancouver) in 1981, "the statistics on all weight loss programs for substantially overweight people show that for all kinds of programs the success rate—and success means taking off weight to your ideal and keeping it off for two years … is about 5 per cent on average …. That means 95 per cent of people out there with extra weight aren't going to lose it permanently."[68] The statistical data on the failure rates of dieting were part of the very justification of LaL. Since most diets failed, the chances of becoming thin were … slim. It was better first, to find ways to accept and live in one's fat body, and second, to maximize the physical health of one's fat body. Armed with this data, Partridge began to investigate the relationship between fat and metabolism. Her first article on this subject was published in the December 1981 issue of *The Bolster*. "The Fat-Promoting Metabolism" suggested that "being fat is one of the factors that may keep you fat" because it is more difficult to metabolize fat tissue.[69] Early in 1982 Partridge began to prepare a booklet and an academic paper that tied her research on weight-loss physiology to the psychology of fat women. "Obesity Facts and Fiction" was published by LaL in 1982. Partridge argued that fat women's fear of potential "social rejection and humiliation" led them to reject their bodies.[70] Social stigma, rather than overeating, led to an exercise deficit and obesity.

Although her academic experience made Partridge particularly suited to this research, other LAL members used similar strategies to challenge received wisdom on dieting and obesity. Paired with their personal experiences, this newly acquired knowledge about fatness allowed members to assert themselves in areas they had not previously felt entitled to enter. Suzanne Bell's work as fitness coordinator was critical in this process. In her aerobics classes, Bell modified the five S's of physical fitness from the YWCA program and taught members the *four* major areas of fitness: "strength, stamina, stature, and suppleness."[71] Although she had no prior academic training in this area, Bell was invited back to speak to subsequent graduating classes of the YWCA's Fitness Leadership course, as well as to students at Simon Fraser University. Bell enjoyed these opportunities to challenge assumptions about fat women. She dismissed the view that fat people should be sent to the doctor before beginning a fitness program, arguing instead that a person's current activity level should be the gauge of her fitness.[72] Bell eventually published two articles on fitness for fat women.[73]

Following Bell and Partridge, other members began to attack the medicalization of fat and dieting in *The Bolster*. A December 1982 editorial cartoon satirized a common experience for fat women: being told to lose weight by a doctor. In this case, the physician, "Dr. Fullovitt, M.D.," is himself larger than his female patient (fig. 2).[74] Members also used Partridge's research to talk back to perceived assumptions about fat women—in particular, the idea that fat could not be fit. In January 1982, Barbara Berry reported, "I weigh 255 lbs. ... and I am a borderline diabetic. But I challenge anyone, slim or not, to keep up with me for even one day!"[75] The following month, Laue chastised *ParticipAction Canada* for its "Fat is NOT where it's at!" ad campaign. She charged in her February 1982 editorial that "fitness has little to do with body size, although it may take more effort, initially, to move 200lbs around the Stanley Park seawall than it takes to move 125lbs. ... [Y]our slim friend who does not believe in exercising the body beautiful may have trouble keeping up with you." Laue emphasized the physical and psychological benefits of exercise: "one FEELS so much better—not only in physical terms—when engaged in a program of regular exercise."[76] In these discussions, medical

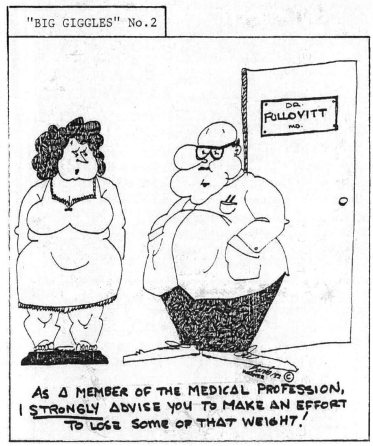

Figure 2   "Big Giggles" cartoon by Barbara Warner, of Toronto, featured in the Large as Life newsletter *The Bolster*, December 1982. Reproduced courtesy of Dr. Kate Partridge.

claims about the dangers of obesity were dismissed. The group members developed their own discourses around fat and health, and began to apply these messages to the way they thought about themselves.

LAL members' desire to improve their personal health did not preclude enjoyment of the aesthetic dimensions of aerobics. *The Bolster* became a sounding board as women sought out and tested different aerobics leotards and tights. In February 1983, Suzanne Bell published an entire article comparing different types of tights, their fit, and where to buy. Bell advised that Danskin Outsize tights were best, whereas Phantom Queen were unreliable. She listed three sources for the tights in Vancouver—"not much, but it's a start"—and noted that neither Eaton's nor The Bay had any stock. Bell further advised that her preference, Danskin style #85, was readily available in the United States in a wider variety of colours.[77] Participants, in turn, began to value their fitness clothing. Joan Dal Santo remembered "getting into" leotards "in a big way: I started getting leotards that were coloured instead of getting leotards that were all black. I'd start getting coloured leotards with black tights, and I'd get some coloured tights with other coloured leotards. And, it was fun, it got to be fun."[78] Janet Walker likewise recalled a particularly treasured pink leotard set: "I had gotten to a stage where I was exploring my body and being more bold. I loved to wear it under a black coat…. It was fun to begin to play."[79] Fitness facilitated other pleasures and forms of self-expression for participants. Aesthetics were central to, rather than separate from, LaL's understanding of physical fitness.

While members like Walker and Dal Santo were tentative in their exploration of fitness clothing, Suzanne Bell's leotards were an extension of her already

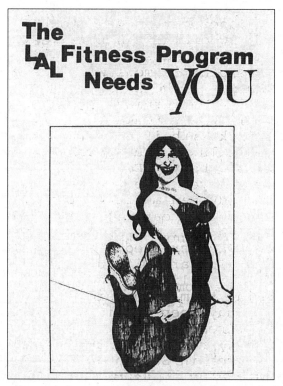

Figure 3 Large as Life fitness ad sketched by *The Bolster* editor Ingrid Laue. Laue sometimes modified clip-art drawings to make the women in them appear fuller-figured. This image appeared in an LAL pamplet. Reproduced courtesy of Dr. Kate Partridge.

confident demeanour. As Bell told one interviewer, "People notice me when I walk into a room. They can feel it: I really like me."[80] She laughed, remembering an early ensemble. "I had a purple leotard that I bought in the States and this wild top that had cut through with silver or something. I mean, I was just a sight!"[81] Bell's fashion savvy also received notice in *The Bolster*, where Ingrid Laue described her as "very trendy in peach tights, black leotards, and colour-coordinated head-band."[82] Within about a year of starting to teach fitness, Bell hit upon the idea of manufacturing fitness clothing for large women. Having done the research on finding leotards in Vancouver, she saw a space to begin her own business. She approached a company who soon began to manufacture a fitness line for larger women called the Suzanne Bell Collection. Initially, Bell sold the clothes "from the trunk of her car"; later, she held home parties.[83] Photographs from this era show women wearing coordinated leotards and tights. There was a wide range of styles in colourful fabrics. Janet Walker's treasured pink leotard was from an early Suzanne Bell collection. Walker displayed the outfit to me during a 2006 interview; some twenty-three years after its purchase, the leotard remained in superb condition.

Tie-ins like clothing and videos have been seen as evidence that aerobics was not a health-promoting activity. Mona Lloyd has compared aerobics classes to Foucault's panopticon, arguing that classes became sites for women to observe and be observed.[84] Maguire and Mansfield take a slightly different angle, suggesting that aerobics classes became hierarchies, divided along lines of fitness and beauty.[85] And, as Christina Burr's chapter on Jamie Lee Curtis (in this volume) reminds us, aerobics was thought to be emblematic of the "amplified individualism" of late-capitalist America.[86] Services developed by fat women for fat women challenge such readings of commercial aerobics culture. In the April 1982 issue of *The Bolster*, Sally Thompson described her "astonishment and delight" at exercising with "a group of my contemporaries—large women—who were starting from square one like me."[87] As her body grew larger, Evelyn Booth felt increasingly "ashamed to be seen in" regular fitness centres, "ashamed of what their attitude would be," whereas in LaL's classes, she felt "comfortable in the sense of, you're all the same."[88] The presence of a large instructor also validated participants. She was a "role model"[89] rather than a "skinny person"[90] who might potentially "talk down" to larger women.[91] Unlike popular culture representations of aerobics as a site of competition among individual women, in practice, classes became sites of mutual support where women came to see each other as allies. LaL classes showed that women negotiated and expanded the boundaries of the aerobics phenomenon in conversation with each other.

Its perceived outsider status is, however, not in itself sufficient to explain why LaL's approach appears to contradict other readings of the aerobics phenomenon. It is also necessary to understand the group as part of multiple and competing discourses of the 1980s, including the women's health and liberation movements, commercial beauty culture, and public health initiatives.

Aerobics grew out of, rather than departed from, the desire for "psychosocial freedom" of the women's liberation movement.[92] The relative silence of feminists on aerobics during its emergence in the 1970s and 1980s indicates that the phenomenon was not, initially, seen as "unfeminist." Jane Fonda, who has since become a symbol for aerobics' betrayal of feminist movements, initially saw her books as a feminist alternative for the exercise market. Her mantra, "Discipline is liberation,"[93] was meant to suggest that health, strength, and good looks were attainable for all women.[94] Like aerobic exercise itself, the apparent "tyranny of slenderness" of the 1980s was not solely or originally the product of commercial beauty culture.[95] Canadian government health messages were already disseminating the message that thin was in by the early 1980s, as Ingrid Laue's critique of *ParticipAction* ably demonstrated. *ParticipAction* was part of a number of federal government initiatives of the era, including the 1976 Survey of Fitness, Physical Recreation and Sport, and the Canada Fitness Survey of 1981, which made bodies knowable and measurable in a way that was not previously available.[96] By the early 1980s, health and fitness was a topic in which a variety of social actors had a vested interest.

Conclusion: Individualism and Collective Action

The problem of aerobics—more specifically, the problem identified in academic literature to date—has been to understand how and why women undertake such activities. Why are women apparently complicit in their own oppression? This chapter has attempted to approach this problem differently by demonstrating that LaL members did not wear one set of ideological or discursive clothing, but many. The group—its newsletter and fitness classes, and Suzanne Bell's aerobics gear—helped members to straddle the boundary between their individual differences and their collective identity as fat women. The group and its actions suggest that women's relationship to popular culture is intra-discursive and intra-subjective. Intra-discursive means that a range of discourses on femininity, fat, and feminism was influencing members of LAL. In turn, participants' understanding of themselves as fat women was shaped intra-discursively, by the practice of aerobics and their interactions with one another. Maxine Leeds Craig's study of American black beauty contests in the

1970s similarly shows that a common culture could develop around aesthetic practices. Leeds Craig argues that displays of black beauty were a way to rearticulate race and to challenge previous mainstream representations of black women as ugly and vulgar.[97] Like black beauty contests, aerobics classes became a site to solidify group identity and to rearticulate the meaning of the fat body.

Keeping this in mind, it is necessary to rethink the claim that aerobics represented a personalization and aestheticization of women's health practices in the 1980s. According to Nikolas Rose, over the course of the twentieth century, individuals came to believe that they were "entrepreneurs of themselves, shaping their own lives through the choices they make among the forms of life available to them."[98] Rose attributes this shift to the rise of psychology and the adoption of self concepts into the language and structure of everyday life. While on the surface, the notion that individuals could become "entrepreneurs of their selves" seems democratic, Rose and others argue that there were dark sides to the rise of the individual. First, psychology and concepts like self-esteem and self-worth implied that there was a healthy *normal* self.[99] Deviation from this norm was perceived as failure and threatening to the social order.[100] A second problem identified with the twentieth century's apparent focus on the self was that it privileged individualism over collective action or responsibility. People were increasingly encouraged to see their problems as personal issues rather than as part of broader political circumstances.[101]

Recent Canadian historiography has taken up the problem of twentieth-century individualism. Rather than linking individualism to psychological discourses, Ian McKay argues that the Canadian state has consistently reinforced individualism through an emphasis on preserving individual autonomy and private property rights, what McKay calls "liberal individualism." A consequence has been the development of a hegemonic liberal order wherein dissent was domesticated by the State and individualism became normalized and internalized by the citizenry.[102] Although they use different sources and theoretical frameworks in their analyses, Rose and McKay both problematize the impact that individualism had on the way people governed themselves and have been governed in the twentieth century. The questions McKay and Rose ask are not dissimilar to the questions posed about women's participation in popular culture, and aerobics specifically, in the 1980s and 1990s. Why were women apparently complicit in their own oppression? How and why do social norms develop and maintain their hegemony? This chapter does not presume to answer these questions. Nonetheless, it does suggest that answers may be found in breaking down the dichotomy between individualism and collective action; between obedience to established norms and dissent.

As Bruce Curtis and Elspeth Heamen have argued, challenges to prevailing norms were often made in terms amenable to liberal individualism.[103] Dissent does not occur separate from, but rather as part of existing discourses and frameworks for political action. For LaL, collective action was not something radically different from or hostile to individualism. The group's conception of action assumed that individual growth could contribute to broader social change. In the premier editorial of *The Bolster,* Kate Partridge wrote that "the time is ripe to change not only our own attitudes about our selves as large women, but also the attitudes of our community and society … we can no longer allow ourselves to feel like, or be treated as, second-class citizens just because we come in large sizes. Each one of us is a valuable person who deserves the freedom to express and be herself. It is the goal of Large as Life to help create this freedom, and we can only do it by working together."[104] In this narrative, Partridge wove together individual work on the self with a broader political agenda. The significance of this was not only that she used the language of individualism, but also that her dissent was couched in terms that are amenable to liberalism: citizenship and personal freedom. LaL's collective action might have challenged or attempted to rearticulate liberal individualism, but it was not necessarily adverse to it.

Terms like "complex" and "contradictory" have become truisms in the search for a language to describe historical actors who are not easily slotted into singular categories or ideological frameworks. Although LaL was complex and probably contradictory, the women who participated in the group did not understand their actions in these terms. They did not see their critique of conventional femininity—nor the mix of feminist, psychological, and health discourses that went into *The Bolster*—as part of any singular political or ideological approach to fat. Instead, this mix of narratives helped members of LaL to develop an understanding about fat that was rooted in their own experience. Psychology and self-concepts allowed members to articulate their selves in a different way. Aerobics classes contributed to this process by providing women with a space in which to explore and challenge the limitations of their fat bodies. Rather than fighting fat, the mantra "Stop postponing your life until you lose weight and start living now" was suggestive of an ethic of self-care. Being fat was not always pleasant or easy, but LaL gave members permission to treat themselves and their bodies with dignity. The notion of fat-acceptance gave these women permission to participate in health and popular culture in a way that they had not previously believed was available to them.

Notes

1 Helen Lenskyj, *Out of Bounds* (Toronto: Women's Press, 1986), p. 129.

2 Mary Boutelier and Lucinda SanGiovanni, "Politics, Public Policy and Title IX," in Susan Birrell, ed., *Women, Sport and Culture* (Champaign: Human Kinetics, 1994), p. 103; M. Ann Hall, *Feminism and Sporting Bodies* (Windsor: Human Kinetics, 1996), p. 86.

3 Susan Douglas, "Narcissism as Liberation," in Jennifer Scanlon, ed., *The Gender and Consumer Culture Reader* (New York: New York University Press, 2000), p. 267; Lenskyj, *Out of Bounds*, p. 129.

4 Jennifer Ellison, "Our Most Charming Girls: Female Athletes in Canadian Advertisements, 1928 to 2002," unpublished MA thesis, Carleton University (2002).

5 Susan Bordo, *Unbearable Weight* (Berkeley: University of California Press, 1993).

6 *The Bolster*, Vancouver (October 1981): 1.

7 The word *fat* has been adopted by many activists in Canada and the United States as a double act of politicization and reclamation of the term. About half of the women interviewed preferred the term *fat* to euphemistic and infantilizing terms like *chubby*, as well as to medical terms such as *obese*. *Fat* is a descriptive term to describe body size and it is not intended to be derogatory.

8 *The Bolster*, Vancouver (February 1983): 9.

9 Jane Fonda, *Jane Fonda's Workout Book* (New York: Simon & Schuster, 1981), pp. 45, 47.

10 Susan Bordo, "Anorexia Nervosa: Psychopathology as the Crystallization of Culture," in Irene Diamond and Lee Quinby, eds., *Feminism and Foucault: Reflections on Resistance* (Boston: Northeastern University Press, 1988), p. 90. See also Mona Lloyd, "Feminism, Aerobics and the Politics of the Body," *Body & Society* 2.2 (June 1996): 79–98.

11 Lenskyj, *Out of Bounds*, p. 129.

12 Lenskyj, *Out of Bounds*, p. 131.

13 Bordo, "Anorexia Nervosa," p. 88.

14 Helen Lenskyj, "Good Sports: Feminists Organizing on Sport Issues in the 1970s and 1980s," *Resources for Feminist Research* 20.2/4 (1991): 130–35.

15 Boutelier and SanGiovanni, "Politics, Public Policy and Title IX," p. 103.

16 Hall, *Feminism and Sporting Bodies*, pp. 96–7.

17 Lenskyj, "Good Sports," pp. 131–2, 134.

18 Rosemary Deem, "Unleisured Lives: Sport in the Context of Women's Leisure," *Women's Studies International Forum* 10.4 (1987): 427.

19 Pirkko Markula, "Firm but Shapely, Fit but Sexy, Strong but Thin: The Postmodern Aerobicizing Female Bodies," *Sociology of Sport Journal* 12.4 (1995): 434.

20 Joseph Maguire and Louise Mansfield, "'Nobody's Perfect': Women, Aerobics, and the Body Beautiful," *Sociology of Sport Journal* 15 (1998): 125.

21 Leslea Haravon Collins, "Working out the Contradictions: Feminism and Aerobics," *Journal of Sport and Social Issues* 26.1 (February 2002): 91.

22 *Cold Mountain Institute Vancouver Workshops* (September–November 1979), p. 3. Cold Mountain was a non-profit education centre that offered personal growth workshops.

23 Joan (Dal Santo) O'Brien, interview by author, Sechelt, British Columbia, 7 October 2005; Kate Partridge, "Large as Life," *The Bolster* (September 1982): 3.

24 Kate Partridge, interview by author, Crediton, Ontario, 20 September 2005.

25 Janet Walker, interview by author, White Rock, British Columbia, 6 October 2005.

26 Ellen Tallman, interview by author, Vancouver, British Columbia, 12 October 2005.

27 Eve Rockett, "Five Days on a Fat Farm," *Chatelaine* (May 1980): 42.

28 (Dal Santo) O'Brien interview.

29 Partridge interview.

30   Rockett, "Five Days on a Fat Farm," p. 178.

31   Partridge interview.

32   Partridge interview.

33   *The Bolster* (December 1981): 7.

34   *The Bolster* (September 1982): 21; Partridge interview.

35   *The Bolster* (November 1982): 17.

36   Jenny Ellison, "'Stop Postponing Your Life until You Lose Weight and Start Living Now': Vancouver's Large as Life Action Group, 1979–1985," *Journal of the Canadian Historical Association* 18.1 (2007): 254.

37   Bell interview; Booth interview; Partridge interview.

38   *The Bolster* (May 1983): 22.

39   *The Bolster* (December 1981): 4.

40   Laue interview.

41   Laura Thaw, "Political?" *The Bolster* (September 1982): 6.

42   Lisa Foreman Cody, "Eating for Two: Shaping Mothers' Figures and Babies' Futures in Modern American Culture," in this volume.

43   Partridge interview.

44   *The Bolster* (August 1981): 4.

45   (Dal Santo) O'Brien interview.

46   YMCA Vancouver and Kate Partridge, *YMCA Fitness Leadership Course Package* (Vancouver: YMCA, 1981), p. 1.

47   YWCA Vancouver and Kate Partridge, *YMCA Fitness Leadership.*

48   *The Bolster* (July 1982): 10.

49   Suzanne Bell, "LAL Fitness Program Needs YOU!" *The Bolster* (October 1982): 9.

50   Ingrid Laue, "Fitness Circuit," *The Bolster* (December 1982): 8.

51   Kate Partridge, "Large as Life," interview by Stan Peters and Ann Mitchell, *CBC Radio Noon* (Vancouver), 15 September 1981.

52   Suzanne Bell, "Fitness Anyone?" *The Bolster* (May 1982): 14.

53   Laue interview.

54   Walker interview.

55   The company has since been renamed Suzanne Bell's Fitness and Fashion Enlarged Enterprises LLP. Bell interview.

56   One thousand video sales was considered a bestseller. Jody Sandler, interview by author, North Vancouver, British Columbia, 5 October 2005.

57   *LaL Newsletter*, Calgary 1.1 (January 1983): 6.

58   Carol Peat, interview by author, London, Ontario, 17 June 2006.

59   Ruth Gillingham, interview by author, Prince Albert, Saskatchewan, 27 July 2006; Susan White, interview by author, Winnipeg, Manitoba, 11 July 2006.

60   Jackqueline Hope, *Big, Bold and Beautiful* (Toronto: Macmillan Canada, 1996), p. 83.

61   Jenny Ellison, "Aerobics for Fat Women Only," in Sondra Solovay and Esther Rothblum, eds., *The Fat Studies Reader* (New York: New York University Press, 2009).

62   Pauline Bartel, "Women at Large—Empathy Is Key to Helping 'Fluffy Ladies' Regain Esteem," *St. Petersburg Times* (5 April 1987): 6F.

63   *Radiance* (Summer/Fall 1986): 30; *Radiance* (Spring 1988): 48; *Radiance* (Summer 1991): 48.

64   Pat Lyons and Debbie Burgard, *Great Shape: The First Exercise Guide for Large Women* (New York: Arbor House–William Morrow, 1988), p. 9.

65   Lyons and Burgard, *Great Shape*, pp. 173–7.

66   Georgina Feldberg, Molly Ladd-Taylor, Allison Li, and Kathryn McPherson, "Comparative Perspectives on Canadian and American Women's Health Care since

1945," in Georgina Feldberg, Molly Ladd-Taylor, and Kathryn McPherson, eds., *Women, Health and Nation* (Montreal and Kingston: McGill-Queen's University Press, 2001), pp. 26–8.

67 Kate Partridge, follow-up interview by author, Exeter, Ontario, 16 April 2006.

68 Kate Partridge and Joan Dal Santo, "Large as Life," interview by Stan Peters and Ann Mitchell, *CBC Radio Noon* (Vancouver), 15 September 1981.

69 Kate Partridge, "The Fat-Promoting Metabolism," *The Bolster* (December 1981): 11.

70 Kate Partridge, *Obesity: Facts and Fiction* (Vancouver: Large as Life Association, 1982), p. 4. Pamphlet, personal collection of Jenny Ellison.

71 Suzanne Bell, "Before and After," *The Bolster* (September 1982), p. 7.

72 Bell interview.

73 See Suzanne Bell, "Fat and Fit: Classes for Women," *Kinesis* (May 1984); Suzanne Bell, "Fitness for Large Women," in Catrina Brown and Karin Jasper, eds., *Consuming Passions: Feminist Approaches to Weight Preoccupation and Eating Disorders* (Toronto: Second Story Press, 1993), pp. 390–9.

74 Barbara Warner, "Big Giggles No. 2," *The Bolster* (December 1982): 16.

75 Barbara Berry, "Naturally the Choice Is Up to You," *The Bolster*, Vancouver (January 1982): 11.

76 Ingrid Laue, "Editor's Sphere," *The Bolster*, Vancouver (February 1982): 1.

77 Suzanne Bell, "Clothesline," *The Bolster* (February 1983): 6.

78 (Dal Santo) O'Brien interview.

79 Walker interview.

80 Caffyn Kelley, "Talent + Skills x Action = Suzanne Bell," *Radiance* (Winter 1992): 6.

81 Bell interview.

82 Sal Thomson, "Fitness Circuit," *The Bolster* (March 1983): 16.

83 Bell interview.

84 Lloyd, "Feminism, Aerobics and the Politics of the Body," p. 92.

85 Maguire and Mansfield, "'Nobody's Perfect,'" p. 121.

86 Christina Burr, "'The Closest Thing to Perfect': Celebrity and the Body Politics of Jamie Lee Curtis," in this volume.

87 Suzanne Bell, "Feeling Great: Fitness Anyone?" *The Bolster* (April 1982): 11.

88 Evelyn Booth, interview by author, North Vancouver, British Columbia, 11 October 2005.

89 Laue interview.

90 Walker interview.

91 Suzanne Bell, "Fitness Circuit," *The Bolster* (May 1983): 23.

92 Beth S. Swanson, "A History of the Rise of Aerobic Dance in the United States through 1980," unpublished MA thesis, San José State University (1996), p. 5.

93 Naomi Wolf, *The Beauty Myth* (Toronto: Random House, 1990), p. 77.

94 Susan Willis, *A Primer for Daily Life* (London: Routledge, 1991), p. 67.

95 The term *tyranny of slenderness* is taken from Kim Chernin's *The Obsession: Reflections on the Tyranny of Slenderness* (New York: Harper & Row Perennial Library, 1981). It has been taken up in other literature; see Brown and Jasper, *Consuming Passions*; Roberta Pollack Seid, *Never Too Thin: Why Women Are at War with Their Bodies* (New York: Prentice Hall Press, 1989); and Cecilia Hartley, "Letting Ourselves Go: Making Room for the Fat Body in Feminist Scholarship," in *Bodies out of Bounds: Fatness and Transgression* (Berkeley: University of California Press, 2001), pp. 60–73.

96 Marny J. Bruce, "Physical Activity, Physical Fitness and Health: Leisure-Time Physical Activity Trends in Canada from 1981 to 1998 and the Prospective Prediction of Health

Status from Health-Related Physical Fitness," unpublished MA thesis, York University, Toronto, Ontario (2002), p. 7.

97 Maxine Leeds Craig, *Ain't I a Beauty Queen: Black Women, Beauty, and the Politics of Race* (New York: Oxford University Press, 2002), pp. 12–15.

98 Nikolas Rose, *Governing the Soul: The Shaping of the Private Self* (London: Routledge, 1989), p. 230.

99 Rose, *Governing the Soul*, p. 220.

100 Rose, *Governing the Soul*, p. 232.

101 Heidi Marie Rimke, "Governing Citizens through Self-Help Literature," *Cultural Studies* 14.1 (January 2000): 62.

102 Ian McKay, "The Liberal Order Framework: A Prospectus for a Reconnaissance of Canadian History," *Canadian Historical Review* 81.4 (2000): 617–45.

103 Elspeth Heamen, "Revisiting the Origins of the Liberal Order Framework" and Bruce Curtis, "Rural Idiocy or Agrarian Virtue? Schooling and Political Subjection in Lower Canada," papers presented at "The Liberal Order in Canadian History," 3 March 2006, Montreal, McGill University Institute for the Study of Canada.

104 Kate Partridge, "Large as Life Newsletter," *The Bolster* (August 1981): 1.

"The Closest Thing to Perfect": Celebrity and the Body Politics of Jamie Lee Curtis

Christina Burr

For the September 2002 issue of *More*, a women's lifestyle magazine targeting women over the age of forty, film actress Jamie Lee Curtis posed in a sports bra and tight spandex briefs without the aid of lights, makeup, or retouching.[1] The photograph reveals wrinkles on her face, plump thighs, big breasts, and a bulging tummy. With this image of the "unglamorous," "ordinary," and "real," Jamie Lee was intending to expose the illusion of the celebrity body. The photograph was taken at the insistence of the actress as part of a concerted effort to reinvent her celebrity status around what she claimed was a newly found self-esteem. Some in Hollywood viewed her action as a career risk, since film stars, particularly women, are not supposed to get old or fat. On the following page of the feature, a photograph of the glamorous Jamie Lee appeared. This image required three hours of primping and prepping, thousands of dollars of designer clothing and jewellery, and the work of a cast of thirteen: the magazine's creative director, a photographer and three assistants, two fashion stylists and an assistant, a hairdresser, a makeup artist, a manicurist, and a prop stylist and an assistant. The appearance of the article in *More* coincided with the publication of Curtis's children's book on self-esteem.[2] Curtis has since spoken out about the dangers of Botox and other cosmetic procedures. Yet throughout her career, Curtis's star image has been constructed in various ways around her body. In *Trading Places* (1983), *Perfect* (1985), and *A Fish Called Wanda* (1988), Curtis's star persona is defined by her lean, toned, sexy body. In *True Lies* (1994), she performs a striptease for her husband, portrayed by Arnold Schwarzenegger. More recently, in the body-switch film *Freaky Friday* (2003), Curtis played a frantic "supermom" who takes the identity of her teenage daughter.

In this chapter, I argue that Jamie Lee Curtis's star image has been fashioned out of cultural ideals about the feminine body through the use of her films and an array of textual sources including movie reviews, television interviews, and women's magazine articles. Paradoxically, the media have made use of her star image both to reinforce popular cultural ideals of the young, thin, sexy female body and to expose the illusion of the celebrity body, thus revealing to women the lie behind the ideal of female bodily perfection in Hollywood. This chapter on Curtis's star image has been influenced by scholarship in film studies and cultural studies, and by feminist writings on women's bodies, particularly on the impact of the media on women's bodies and body image. Ironically, as the chapter will demonstrate, the body politics surrounding Jamie Lee Curtis have been contradictory and ambivalent. Some feminists and journalists have applauded her outspokenness on issues surrounding the star body, suggesting that showing an imperfect body or face is an act of courage in the youth-obsessed movie industry, while others have cautioned that Curtis is only helping to perpetuate the values the gesture appears to challenge.

Women's bodies have always been, and continue to be, of central importance to feminist scholarship and politics. Since the 1970s, control over women's bodies and body image by the media and the fashion and beauty industries has been a persistent theme in feminist scholarship. Naomi Wolf and Susan Faludi stated the case, most famously perhaps, in the early 1990s in their respective bestsellers. They argue that the "beauty myth" was the most damaging aspect of a violent backlash against feminism and a political weapon aimed at women's oppression. Faludi and Wolf indicate further that women's magazines are integral to the cultural construction of the beauty myth because they perpetuate the notion that every woman can achieve the ideal feminine body (youthful and toned) through the proper regimes of dress, diet and exercise, skin care, and cosmetic surgery.[3] This has translated into the belief that by changing their bodies, women can transcend problematic social locations, thus making their lives better. In the mass media, idealized images of thin, white, youthful women are produced in what Sandra Bartky describes as the "fashion-beauty complex," largely controlled and constructed by white men.[4] The celebrity body, as feminist writers inform us, has made some women feel that they don't measure up and has impacted negatively on women's body image and self-esteem.

The problem that preoccupied many feminist theorists during the late 1980s and early 1990s was how to avoid the impasse of theories based on sex as a fixed biological essence and gender as culturally constructed. Judith Butler asserts that biological sex is not the bedrock on which gender is erected; rather, it is part of the performance of gender, and it too is culturally constructed.[5] Elizabeth Grosz and Anne Balsamo suggest that the body, as much as the psyche, can be regarded as a cultural and historical product.[6] The production of gendered bodies, these scholars argue, is a discursive as well as a material construction, within which meanings are polysemic and unstable. The studies by Butler, Grosz, Balsamo, and others provide a useful theoretical orientation for this chapter. Jamie Lee Curtis's star image has been constructed and reconstructed in film and popular media around culturally and historically specific ideals of the feminine body that have been heavily influenced by patriarchal dominance.

Film scholars were among the first to focus on the star body as a field for academic research. In two important groundbreaking books, *Stars* and *Heavenly Bodies*, Richard Dyer paved the way for the emergence of star studies as a legitimate subdiscipline within academic film studies in the 1980s.[7] He discusses film stars as industrial, ideological, and cultural products, using notions of stars as social phenomena, stars as images, and stars as signs. Star image is constituted from everything that is publicly available about a performer, which, in addition to onscreen performances, includes an extensive array of multimedia and intertextual materials, such as pin-ups, film reviews, interviews, fan magazines, music videos, public appearances, studio handouts, and more recently, the Internet. Dyer suggests that star images are not only intertextual, multimedia, and extensive; they are also mutable and unstable, and they have histories.[8] Dyer's influential notion of "the structured polysemy" of the star image, with its emphasis on multiple but finite meanings and effects, paved the way for other studies that concentrate on the instability of star images.[9]

Star image is fashioned out of a material body, or as Dyer writes, "The star is a body." Making sense of the star body is rooted in historically and culturally specific ideals about the body. For example, in *Heavenly Bodies*, Dyer considers how Marilyn Monroe was represented as a sex symbol in the context of contemporary debates over sexuality and the image of women in 1950s America.[10] The emergence of the film star is dependent on the original construction of the "physical performer," where the actor is celebrated as a "type." The progression from physical performer to "picture personality" is the subject of Richard de Cordova's study of the early history of the star system in

America. The star image was, first of all, a physical image—one that circulated through films before the publicity apparatus began to take shape that allowed for the emergence of the picture personality that extended beyond the physical image of the actor.[11] David Marshall points to the persistence and dominance of women in the category of physical performer in the film industry. An intense focus on the body and its reformulation through cosmetics, surgery, diet, and exercise is central to the construction of the female star, which Marshall suggests perpetuates an idea of female stardom stalled, since few women in Hollywood are able to make the transition to performer.[12] Women, more so than men, are star bodies rather than star performers.

Jamie Lee Curtis and the Feminine Body Ideal of the 1980s

Jamie Lee Curtis, the daughter of film stars Janet Leigh and Tony Curtis, embarked on her film career in the late 1970s with a series of low-budget teen horror films, beginning with John Carpenter's *Halloween* (1978), which earned her a reputation as the "Queen of Scream." She became a star in her own right in a series of Reagan-era films following her break-out role as the prostitute Ophelia in *Trading Places* (1983). The success of Reagan's America lay in its ability to redeploy an amplified individualism focused on the body, which masked the consequences of late capitalism, including high unemployment, poverty, hyper-industrialization, deregulation, compulsive acquisitiveness, and extensive consumer credit.[13] As Cole writes, "Physical transcendence and free will became America's hottest commodities."[14] The transformed self, equated with a lifestyle of self-improvement, success, ambition, discipline, and effort, was rendered most visible in the lean, hard, muscular body produced in fitness clubs. This body ideal became the normalizing lens through which other bodies—racialized bodies, homosexual bodies, fat bodies, and AIDS bodies—were judged and condemned.

At the centre of the plot of *Trading Places* is a debate over social Darwinism. The Duke brothers, Randolph (Ralph Bellamy) and Mortimer (Don Ameche), are a pair of wealthy commodities traders who debate the nature of man. Mortimer is convinced that genetic makeup is everything and that good bloodlines will triumph over adversity. Randolph, on the other hand, adheres to the theory that man is what the environment makes him. To put their theories to the test, they arrange to disgrace their firm's manager, Louis Winthrop III (Dan Ackroyd), and replace him with a black street hustler, Billy Ray Valentine (Eddie Murphy). Winthrop's fall from grace must not only cost him his job, but his home, all his savings, his fiancée, and the esteem of everyone he knows. The Dukes do this by framing him as a drug dealer, and they pay Ophelia, a prostitute played by Jamie Lee Curtis, to make him look like a pimp in front of his fiancée. Alan Nadel suggests that there is little to distinguish Ophelia, a hooker with a heart of gold and a lot of T-bills, from her yuppie counterparts: "like them she is entrepreneurial, upwardly mobile, and has loyalty to little beside money." In Reagan's America, upward mobility was connected to control over a woman's body. As Ophelia states, "Her body is her capital," which she emphasizes to Winthrop by appearing topless briefly in the scene where he comes to stay at her apartment. But the patriarchal authority controls her body, and by implication, her reproductive freedom as well.[15] The popular cinema's framing of sexuality as exchange has long been central to its representation of women and women's work, however. "None more so," Yvonne Tasker asserts, "than the female star, already defined in terms of the body and performance."[16]

Perfect, released in 1985, was intended to catapult Curtis into stardom. In the film, she plays Jessie Wilson, a hip, sexy, and confident aerobics instructor, alongside John Travolta as Adam Lawrence, a roving investigative reporter for *Rolling Stone* magazine. *Perfect* is based on an article that one of the film's co-writers, Aaron Latham, wrote for *Rolling Stone*. The article, entitled "Looking for Mr. Goodbody," describes the emergence of health clubs as the singles bars of the eighties.[17] In the film, Adam is sent to Los Angeles by *Rolling Stone* editor Mark Roth (played by the real editor of the magazine, Jann Wenner) to investigate the alleged framing by the State Department of a businessman arrested for drug dealing. Adam suggests to Roth that he might also investigate the boom in health clubs as the singles' bars of the eighties. Adam locates a health club for his story, The Sports Connection, which he dubs "The Sports Erection." While conducting preliminary research at the club, Adam is introduced to Jessie Wilson (Curtis), a dedicated aerobics instructor known as the "Aerobics Pied Piper." Adam asks her for an interview, but she refuses. She has a strong dislike for the press: as a teenager, she was an Olympic contender in swimming, but the media were more interested in her affair with her married coach than her athletic ability.

Jessie agrees to an off-the-record lunch with Adam, where he wins her over with his theories of popular culture. But he hides his spin on the health club story from Jessie. Instead, he proposes that it is probably no coincidence that the post–World War II baby boom generation was approaching thirty just as the health boom started in the United States. He suggests that the baby boomers were leading a physical awakening comparable to the spiritual Great Awakening that grips America every hundred years or so. Focusing on conditions in President Reagan's America, Adam proposes that individuals want to take responsibility for their bodies since the government won't do it. Thus, he concludes, the United States has come full circle back to Emerson's ideals of self-reliance, and health clubs like The Sports Connection are all-American, "little capitals of Emersonian America."

In *Perfect*, Jessie/Curtis performs a sexualized display of the body and an aesthetics of beauty derived from the body-centred ideals of Reaganism. Commenting on the "feminizing of muscle" in the 1980s, Laurie Schultz writes, "'Working out,' being 'in shape' (and possessing the capital and leisure to do so) are the new markers of feminine sexuality, desirability and status." In comparison to the 1970s "healthy" body ideal, which emphasized the "slim-lined" look, Schultz notes that the 1980s ideal body carried more muscle mass. The fit feminine body ideal of the 1980s was slim, taut, and toned, with a well-developed though not bulging musculature, as the discourses of health, fitness, and beauty became more conjoined.[18] According to the dominant cultural ideals of femininity operating in Reagan's America, a woman could have an ideal body if she worked hard enough, cared for her body, and fine-tuned it with beauty products or even cosmetic surgery. This has tended to result in a wholesale condemnation of aerobics as unfeminist, although Jenny Ellison's chapter in this volume suggests that in the early 1980s, "fat" women co-opted aerobic and popular cultural ideals of femininity and embodied them in their own ways.[19]

In the film, Adam takes one of Jessie's aerobics classes at The Sports Connection. The "aerobic curve" of activity resembles an erotic curve of sexual excitement and release.[20] The mirrored aerobic studio, where each participant follows Jessie, who directs the class from a podium, forms the backdrop for the sexual/aerobic encounter between Jessie and Adam, carried out to the disco beat of "Shock Me" by Whitney Houston and Jermaine Jackson. During the warm-up, Jessie seduces Adam with eye-to-eye contact as Houston sings "Shock me with your love / Do what you want." The lengthy film sequence is choreographed with numerous full frontal shots of pelvic thrusts and circular rotations of the hips, with the camera alternating between Jessie and Adam as the sexual tension mounts between the couple.

Jessie/Curtis's body is described using the language invoked to characterize the 1980s ideal body: she is "slim," "strong," "athletic," "confident," "sexy," "healthy." The lyrics to the film's title soundtrack reveal that she is the "closest thing to perfect":

She's the closest thing to perfect that I've ever seen,
She's an ideal lady,
She's so well defined,
She's driving me crazy,
She's got those long, lean streamlines.[21]

The role of aerobics instructor requires that Jessie/Curtis be an authority as a result of her position as leader, but, as Margaret Morse writes, "she must also physically embody as much as possible the end results of an aerobic transformation, that is bodily perfection, which is still presented as only attainable in the future by the exerciser."[22]

The plot line about health clubs as the singles bars of the eighties builds on this quest for the perfect body, following almost verbatim Latham's article in *Rolling Stone*. Sally, played by Marilu Henner and modelled after Lori Segal in the article, is big-breasted and happy-go-lucky. She met her fiancé, a Chippendale's male stripper, at The Sports Connection. Linda, played by Laraine Newman, is vulnerable, desperate, and promiscuous. In the film, one of the club's male members describes her "as the most used piece of equipment in the gym." Linda considers herself pretty, but she plans to have cosmetic surgery because she wants to be "perfect." When Jessie confronts Adam, she tells him that he will ruin Linda's life if he publishes her story. Jesse asks, "What's so wrong with wanting to be perfect?" Instead, Adam submits an article based on health clubs as a return to Emersonian ideals of self-reliance. The editor, however, decides to have another journalist rewrite the article using Adam's name and incorporating the interviews with the two women.

Several themes recur in biographies of Curtis from interviews with various popular magazines promoting *Perfect:* she is the daughter of Hollywood "royalty," her rise to stardom began with her early work in horror films, and following her break-out role in *Trading Places* she became known as a "body actress." Her star image was constructed around her physical performance and conformity to 1980s feminine body ideals. This star image, however, was multivalent, inconsistent, and contradictory. The media presented Curtis in different ways for public consumption. Over the years, Curtis has been adept at manipulating the Hollywood publicity machine.[23] She credits her parents not so much with influencing her performance but with teaching her "the business end of the business."[24]

In May 1985, two women's fashion magazines, *Harper's Bazaar* and *McCall's*, put out special "best body" issues. *Harper's Bazaar* proclaimed Curtis "The Best Body in Movies," and *McCall's* included Curtis in its list of

"America's 10 Best Bodies."[25] In promoting *Perfect, Harper's Bazaar* declared that "no element of the film is more provocative than Curtis's voluptuous figure." *Bazaar* reported that Curtis maintains her star body with a regimen of "light weight lifting, daily sit-ups and aerobics classes a couple of times a week." Curtis revealed that she began the exercise program the previous year after experiencing "D-day—the day my body started to drop," although she was only twenty-six at the time. The article suggests that maintaining the ideal feminine body requires a considerable amount of work, as well as a strict low-fat diet.[26] *Esquire* journalist Gary Kinder writes: "For eight months Jamie has eaten nothing but salads, some broiled fish and chicken, and a lot of pasta lightly seasoned with garlic and olive oil…. She wants Jessie to have 'thin skin,' the look of an athlete with no fat between the layer of skin and the layer of muscle."[27] In these popular magazine articles, Curtis's star image is built around the 1980s ideal of the body that can only be realized through strict programs of exercise and diet, and that is the purview of the young.

Paradoxically, her star image was also built around a critique of the feminine body ideal and the fitness craze, a view that perhaps more women could identify with since the ideal feminine body was beyond the reach of all but privileged young, white, middle-class, heterosexual women. In a June 1985 interview for *Vogue* magazine, Curtis criticized the body-focused popular culture. "I'm not an advocate of the health craze," Curtis stated. "It's about the physical elite rather than the brain elite. I wish it could be the other way around."[28] The *Vogue* article further suggests that part of Curtis's public appeal is her androgyny. She is "smart and sexy, funny and tough." *Vogue* remarked, "She's all woman and almost butch enough to be one of the guys."[29] While Hollywood expects actresses to have "perfect" bodies, *People* magazine declared, "Forget what the song says—don't call Jamie Lee Curtis the closest thing to Perfect." During the interview with *People*, Curtis spoke of her ongoing struggle with her body and revealed that she has never felt very comfortable with the way she looks. She criticized the photographs of women in fashion magazines, including her own in *Harper's Bazaar*. Curtis commented: "I don't look good when you put a lot of makeup on me and put those dresses on me. I look like an idiot." She criticized the fitness craze and its emphasis on the perfect body: "If you think that having a tight ass means you're going to fall in love, you're wrong." She continued, "To think that finding perfection with your body is going to make you a happy person is not true at all."[30] Curtis remarked that in Hollywood, where "everyone has a lot of great experts around—weight trainers, masseurs, dance coaches, nutritionists" and "[l]ife is timed around the trainers or the gym," she was "relatively sane" about working out until she started filming *Perfect*. "Then, suddenly, when I got the role and started to train four to five hours a day and got into Jesse's puritanical physicality, I started to notice my body ... I became obsessed with my jeans fitting to skintight perfection."[31] Although Curtis might very easily have become an "aerobics actress," following the lead of Jane Fonda, she rejected numerous offers to do exercise videos and workout books.

In a 1985 interview with Charlene Krista for *Films in Review*, Curtis stated: "I certainly hope that after all this time, I won't be known for my body."[32] Although *Perfect* was not a success either with the critics or at the box office, it cemented Curtis's reputation as a body actress. During the 1990s, Curtis played a series of eclectic roles. She developed a name as a comedic actress in *A Fish Called Wanda* (1998) and in her role as Hannah Miller in the television series *Anything but Love*, which ran for four years from 1989 to 1992. She played a gritty cop in Kathryn Bigelow's thriller *Blue Steel* (1990) and the mother figure in three movies: *My Girl* (1991), its sequel *My Girl 2* (1994), and *Forever Young* (1992). She also made a number of made-for-television movies, notably *The Heidi Chronicles*, based on Wendy Wasserstein's Pulitzer Prize– and Tony Award–winning play. Curtis played the title role of Heidi Holland, an art historian who is transformed by the women's movement but whose efforts at self-fulfillment are marred by doubts and loneliness.

In 1994 Curtis starred alongside Arnold Schwarzenegger in *True Lies*, one of the biggest action films produced to date. The film is a combination of a domestic comedy and a parody of the James Bond–style action hero, with deception and transformation as its central terms. The film revolves around Harry Request's (played by Schwarzenegger) duplicity as a husband who masquerades as a mild-mannered computer sales representative while actually leading the glamorous life of an international spy. Curtis plays his neglected wife, Helen, who becomes involved with a used-car salesman masquerading as a spy in order to attract bored middle-class women. Initially, frumpy dresses, awkward movements, and an outdated hairstyle conceal Curtis's famous star body. She is transformed when Harry tricks her into thinking she is on a government mission and must pose as a hooker. Ordered to "wear something sexy," Helen arrives in a frilly frock—the least sexy dress imaginable. Helen tears off the long, puffy sleeves, and long skirt, creating a tiny body-hugging little black dress, and performs a striptease for a "John" who turns out to be her husband. The transformation from frump to vamp begins. By the end of the film, Helen is able to demonstrate physical agility while dancing the tango, and Harry and Helen are finally united as spies located in a world of glamour and romance as Helen is transformed into a "Bond girl."

Yvonne Tasker points out that the white female star is incorporated into this white, male "fantasy land" only after a fairly thorough humiliation.[33] Feminists and some film critics panned *True Lies* for its denigration of women and declared director James Cameron's portrayal of "Bond-type bimbos a step backwards."[34] At press junkets, Curtis guided the discussion around themes of diet and exercise—specifically, about how she got her thirty-five-year-old body in shape for the striptease. She emphasized the comedic aspects of the film, whenever possible avoiding the political issues that it sparked. As for the critics who viewed the film as misogynistic, Curtis stated: "If someone wants to say that, then that's fine. I'm not going to make a case to defend it, because I frankly think it's fabulous and funny, and they should lighten up."[35]

In biographies and interviews during the 1990s, Curtis spoke of her marriage to actor-director Christopher Guest and of raising the couple's two adopted children, Annie and Tom. A recurring theme in her interviews was the importance of a "normal family" life. As Richard Dyer points out, there is ambiguity and contradiction in the star image between stars-as-ordinary and stars-as-special. There is a paradox between the extravagant lifestyles of stars and stars as ordinary people, living just like the rest of us. Stars serve to legitimate what is seen as ordinary about a society.[36] Although the daughter of famous film stars, Curtis grew up with her mother and stepfather in a Los Angeles canyon sheltered from the movie industry. In a 1998 interview for *Redbook*, a woman's magazine, Curtis reiterated the importance of setting a good "normal" example for her children. The boundary between the glamorous star image and her "normal" private family life must be crossed, however, and involves body transformation. As soon as the photo shoot for the cover of *Redbook* is complete, she switches from Jamie Lee, the celebrity, into Jamie Lee, the mom, by changing from a fashionable off-the-shoulder white top and skintight pants—a look most busy mothers would find difficult, if not impossible to attain—into her comfortable jeans and running shoes.[37]

That same year, Curtis turned forty. She appeared in a "40 and Fabulous" feature in *People*, showcasing the celebrities who had reached the milestone but were still sex symbols. Curtis indicated, however, that she might give up the "glam life." She stated: "I'll back off when I can't do my work because it's hard to photograph me well." She declared that she wants to be an active mom and that she stays fit by keeping up with her two children.[38] Curtis's star image was reinvented around motherhood over the course of the 1990s. She not only emphasized motherhood in interviews and played mothers in her films, but she also began writing children's books, using themes and issues inspired by her personal life. Her first book, *When I Was Little: A Four-Year-Old's Memoir of Her Youth*, was published in 1993. It was about her daughter's boasting about "the good old days" when she was four years old.[39]

From True Lies to "True Thighs": The *More* Photo Shoot

The publication of the photograph of the "real" Jamie Lee Curtis in the September 2002 issue of *More* magazine was timed to coincide with the release of her fifth children's book, *I'm Gonna Like Me: Letting Off a Little Self-Esteem*.[40] She requested that, in addition to the picture of the "glamorous" Jamie Lee, the celebrity illusion, she be photographed as she really is without makeup, professionally styled hair, jewellery, and couture clothing. She was photographed using an unflattering full-body camera angle and a straightforward stance, wearing only a black sports bra and briefs. Curtis stated: "There's a reality to the way I look without my clothes on…. I don't have great thighs. I have very big breasts and a soft, fatty little tummy. And I've got back fat. People assume that I'm walking around in little spaghetti-strap dresses. It's insidious—Glam Jamie, the Perfect Jamie, the great figure, blah, blah, blah. And I don't want the unsuspecting forty-year-old women of the world to think that I've got it going on. It's such a fraud. And I'm the one perpetuating it."[41] She admitted that she participated in the creation of the myth of the "perfect Jamie" through her roles in movies like *Perfect*, *Trading Places*, and *True Lies*, and that the image of her lean, toned, and sexy body had made some women feel that they don't measure up. Exposing the fraud of her perfect body in the pages of *More* was part of Curtis's recovery from addictions to alcohol and painkillers, where "they talk about peeling an onion, exposing more layers." For Curtis, this involved self-acceptance and coming to terms with the feelings of inadequacy that had plagued her all her life as the daughter of film stars Janet Leigh and Tony Curtis.[42] This too was the message of the children's book she was promoting: the final line of the book reads, "I'm gonna like me 'cause I'm loved and I know it, and liking myself is the best way to show it."[43] Curtis revealed also that she had had some cosmetic surgery, liposuction, and Botox injections, but none of it had worked.

Amy Wallace, who interviewed Curtis for *More*, wrote: "In youth-obsessed Hollywood, where the dearth of good roles for women over 28 is a constant lament, it's a ballsy move to admit your age at all—let alone revel in it."[44] Curtis created a media frenzy with her photographs in *More*. The popular feminist magazine *Ms.* selected Curtis as one of its 2002 Women of the Year, "for humor, humanity, and courage in trading the beauty myth for the shared reality of unique and vulnerable human bodies."[45] Curtis and *More* editor-in-chief Susan Crandell gave interviews on all the morning television talk shows. Campbell Brown, interviewer at NBC's *Today*, seemed shocked, however, that Curtis wanted to be photographed as she really is and stated that there was no way she would sit down for a photo shoot "with no makeup, no control tops, no wonder bra."[46] In the *Today* interview, Susan Crandell indicated that it was no risk at all for *More* to print a photograph that does not show the ideal feminine body. Crandell suggested that in your forties and fifties, "you're comfortable in your skin. You feel good about your accomplishments and achievements and—and you put everything in perspective."[47] Crandell's comments are opposite to the message that communications scholar Carolyn Kitch found in *More*. Kitch argues that through editorial and advertising messages promising eternal youth, *More* communicates "a profoundly commercial vision based on the fear of aging rather than its celebration."[48]

Journalists in North America and abroad either applauded Curtis for championing the cause of women over 40 or criticized her for revealing her real body as they tried to sort out the meaning of Curtis's gesture, often drawing on the discourses of feminist body politics. In an interview for CBS's *The Early Show*, Lesley Jane Seymour, editor-in-chief of *Marie Claire* magazine, which targets women between the ages of eighteen and thirty-four, suggested that most women want the fantasy of the celebrity body. Seymour stated: "I want to see fat women, I want to see women just like me." But, she continued, "You put them on the cover, the magazine doesn't sell.... They want to see life just a little bit improved. Better than reality. Better than the girl next door."[49] On the other hand, *Chicago Sun-Times* columnist Cindy Richards praised Curtis "for keeping it real" for 40-something women and for admitting "that without the personal trainer, makeup professional and full-body girdle she isn't quite perfect." Curtis represents a new generation of women, the baby boomers in their forties and fifties for whom getting older is increasingly about "keeping it real," also known as the "makeunder" as opposed to the "makeover" that relies on a team of professional stylists, makeup, personal trainers, and oftentimes, cosmetic surgery.[50] In a similar vein, Laura Dempsey of the Dayton, Ohio, *Daily News*, praised Curtis for her actions. She pronounced the photograph of the real Jamie Lee "unbelievable" and "wonderful." Dempsey writes: "There's very little flab, mind you, but it's unmistakably flab on an unmistakable movie star." While acknowledging that this is hardly a sea change, Dempsey suggests that it is a start that couldn't come at a better time for young women. She used the discourses of social psychology, which attributes the increase in anorexia nervosa and other eating disorders among young women to the unrealistic images of women presented in the media.[51]

Muriel Gray, of the British newspaper *The Guardian,* raised the question of whether Jamie Lee Curtis was making the feminist statement that women over 40 have been waiting for. According to Gray, the article in *More* assumes that Curtis's body shape and fitness "has been one of western womanhood's primary concerns," when "the truth is that most of us don't give a damn." "Yes, Jamie," Gray writes, "I am certain that the women at the heart of the Middle Eastern conflict, the female farm workers of Botswana who are about to starve, the rural Indian woman carrying a bundle of sticks on her head for three kilometres to light a fire, are all deeply grateful to you for telling them it is OK to show off their fat." She describes Curtis's revelations as a "sad piece of therapeutic exhibitionism" being held up as a feminist statement; it is merely her "self-obsession masquerading as a new-found unselfconsciousness." Gray remarks: "It is difficult to take Curtis's crusade—trying to make women over 40 feel good about themselves—at face value, because she is a troubled Hollywood princess, as far removed from the real world as money and fame can buy." She further notes that while youth has always had a cult of beauty, there is evidence to suggest that the beauty of celebrities in their forties and fifties, and beyond—including Susan Sarandon, Sigourney Weaver, Frances McDormand, and Dame Judi Dench—is still appreciated.[52]

A discourse of feminist body politics was integrated into Joan Ryan's editorial published in the *San Francisco Chronicle.* Ryan begins with the question, why has Curtis's true-life photograph created such a press buzz? She explains: "Because in 2002, more than three decades into the women's movement, it is still a radical act for a woman to accept her body as it is." According to Ryan, the impossible ideal of the perfect body has been etched into women's psyche since childhood with our first Barbie. Curtis's photograph, Ryan argues, is a reminder of where the women's movement has fallen short. She concludes: "As we were getting the world to accept us for who we are, we never figured out how to accept ourselves."[53] A post-feminist generation of women, raised to reject artifice, is still betrayed by their own bodies, and self-worth is still about conformity to a feminine body ideal that is impossible for most women to measure up to.

In trying to sort out what Curtis's gesture really "meant," British journalist Kathryn Hughes presented another interpretation. She writes, "With Botox available on the high street and personal trainers advertising in newsagent windows, it was inevitable that the smart money would need to find some other way to distinguish itself." We need to look at the power dynamics that lie behind the photographs of any actress looking anything but perfect. Curtis was in control of the "makeunder" photo shoot, and she knew exactly what image she was trying to project. Hughes sought out the opinion of an academic, Angela McRobbie, an expert in feminist cultural studies, who cautioned against hailing photographs of middle-aged actresses as a breakthrough: "To 'come out' in this way, as though showing an imperfect face or body is an act of courage, is to perpetuate the values the gesture appears to challenge."[54]

One year later, in September 2003, Curtis appeared again on the cover of *More*, this time in the issue commemorating the magazine's fifth anniversary. Drawing on the tradition in women's magazine publishing of manufacturing a tone of intimacy and community around the theme of self-improvement, author and journalist Anne Taylor Fleming organized a reader roundtable with Curtis and four other women to discuss aging and self-esteem. The four women were representative of the magazine's target readership: they were in their forties and fifties, had successful careers, were either married or divorced, and were raising, or had raised, children. Predictably, given that the roundtable was for the same magazine that had published the photographs of the "real" Jamie Lee, the women lauded Curtis's actions as courageous and newsworthy. The women were at a time in their lives "when it's against the law to age," particularly for a woman film star like Curtis, "who was not supposed to age and not get fat and not be real." While Curtis was still talking about body acceptance as building self-esteem, the text of the roundtable suggests that the women were still struggling with their body issues. While they talked about the body acceptance that comes with aging, one of the women, Maia Danziger, mentioned that she had to lose five pounds before her upcoming vacation in Hawaii but that she hated that she was worrying about it. The women concurred that as teenagers, they were influenced by the ultra-thin fashion models in fashion magazines like *Seventeen*. Another participant in the roundtable, Leslie Steadman, who was twice divorced, indicated that issues of self-esteem were still problematic for her since there is no husband to come home to. Curtis responded: "I think the body issues are harder for single women, because they're still out there trying to attract. I've made a living off my body, and now I'm able to out that body for its reality. But I can do that because I have stability. I'm married."[55] Rather than a message of self-esteem and body acceptance, the text suggests that a woman must still rely on a man for self-worth and continue what would always be an elusive struggle for the perfect body.

In the 2003 article in *More*, Curtis stated, "What I did in *More* was never intended to become the sort of *Norma Rae* union movement for body image .... It was really a personal liberation."[56] The notoriety of the *More* photographs helped to revitalize her film career when she was cast in a starring role in the remake of Disney's *Freaky Friday*, released in the summer of 2003.[57] Ironically, while Curtis's objective was to minimize the emphasis on the feminine body ideal in popular culture, *Freaky Friday* is a classic Hollywood body-switch film. The films (the original and the remake) were based on Mary Rodger's book of the same title, intended for girls age eight and up, which appeared in the early 1970s, alongside the contemporary women's movement. The book focuses primarily on the daughter's experience of becoming her mother. The 1976 film, starring Jodie Foster as the thirteen-year-old Annabel and Barbara Harris as the mother who switches bodies with her daughter, gives equal time to both generations. In both the book and the 1976 film, the mother does not work outside the home. The 1976 film was a farce, and the daughter-as-mother has to improvise her way through a day of disastrous encounters with a washing machine, a stove, and a tipsy cleaning lady. All the while, she calls her husband a male chauvinist pig. Meanwhile, the mother in the teen's body discovers that schoolwork is not as easy to master as she had previously assured her daughter it was.

In the 2003 remake of *Freaky Friday*, the circumstances of the mother and daughter characters were altered. The remake is a fable rather than a farce grounded in the real-life situations of contemporary teenage girls and mature women. While the daughter in the 1976 film wants less from her mother, the daughter in the 2003 film desires more of her mother, and the daughter and mother are also much more involved in each other's lives. Curtis plays widow and psychotherapist Tess Coleman, who is about to remarry and is constantly at odds with Anna, her sixteen-year-old garage-band-guitarist daughter, played by Lindsay Lohan. During dinner at a Chinese restaurant, the mother and daughter quarrel when Anna asks to be excused from the wedding rehearsal dinner the following evening to attend a band audition at the House of Blues. The magic plot device comes in the form of a worn Hollywood racial stereotype: the meddling Chinese grandmother of the restaurant proprietor serves up a potion in fortune cookies given to the mother and daughter. When they wake up the next morning, Tess and Anna occupy each other's bodies. The premise of the movie is that they must find a way to understand each other by living in the other's body before they can switch back.

The body-swap narrative has been played out in a number of contexts in Hollywood films, including physical doubles changing places with one another and cross-dressing class, sexual, and national identities. The body-swap narrative in the 2003 remake of *Freaky Friday* is, as film critic Philippa Hawker states, "a swap with a lot"—it is about gender expectations, sexuality, self-awareness, aging, and feminine body ideals.[58] The sequences of transformation enact "visually as well as narratively a process of 'becoming something other' that is conducted through/over the star body."[59] Upon awakening the next morning, Anna in Tess's body (Curtis) looks in the mirror and discovers that she is trapped in a body that has its share of sags and wrinkles. She shrieks, "Oh, no, I'm old! I'm like the crypt-keeper." Curtis wonderfully replicates the body language of a teenage girl—the slouch, the rolled eyes at adults, and the pouting. In another sequence, represented through montage and upbeat music, Anna-as-Tess (Lohan) uses her mother's credit cards and buys a new hip wardrobe and a new haircut, and gets her ears pierced. Meanwhile, Tess in Anna's body wears her hair up and dresses maturely as she prepares for a day at high school.

Film reviewers made connections between Curtis's role in the movie and her efforts to debunk the myth of her perfect body and, in the process, bolster her self-esteem by making her public persona "real." References were made to her 2002 photo shoot in *More*. In interviews promoting the film, Curtis emphasized motherhood once again. She stated that she dresses appropriately for a mother in her mid-40s and that she believes in "age-appropriate" relationships. Curtis insisted, "Parents ... should be parents, not their kids' 'pals.'" She stated, "You have to let them go at some point in order for them to establish the chance to make good choices." At Curtis's insistence, the credo "make good choices" was incorporated into the script of the film.[60]

In the 2003 version, the female body is more sexualized than in the original film. Anna is attracted to a boy at school, Jake, a blond motorcycle rider of whom her mother would never approve. Anna's amazingly hip mother enraptures Jake. The film lingers on this mistaken-identity attraction. Although what the audience sees on the screen is a teenage boy pursuing a woman in her 40s, we are also offered the vicarious spectacle of an older-woman–younger-man relationship. Anna, inhabiting her mother's body, is shocked to discover that a teenage boy could desire Tess's body. The film, as Hawker suggests, explores female ambivalence about the body. "We see Anna-as-Tess, slightly horrified by the sag and overflow and excess that she now possesses, and we're aware that this is Tess's forty-something body, desiring and being desirable, even if that's not the way things are supposed to be at her age and in her situation."[61] Sexual desire does not work the other way, however. When Tess's fiancé, Ryan, attempts to kiss his future bride, Anna-as-Tess is repulsed.

Curtis appeared on the cover of *More* again in September 2006, this time wearing a navy blue halter dress adorned with a string of pearls, her silver hair styled in a short pixie cut, with hands on hips emphasizing her voluptuous body. Curtis discussed the impact of her decision to take on the issue of body image with journalist Amy Wallace, who had conducted the 2002 interview for *More*. Curtis expressed her complete surprise at public reaction to the 2002 photo shoot: "It turns out it will probably be the single biggest contribution I ever make as a public figure"—this despite her emphasis that the 2002 photo shoot was really about personal liberation. Moreover, Curtis was quick to add, "By the way, I do Pilates, I do yoga, I exercise, I eat very carefully. I'm not saying obesity or lack of exercise is fine." "I'm saying," she continued, "this is what I look like *and* I do that."[62]

Conclusion

The star image of film actresses, as this chapter on Jamie Lee Curtis illustrates, focuses on the feminine body as a cultural construct that requires a broader historical perspective to fully understand its meanings. In the 1980s, Curtis's star image was shaped in the political context of Reagan's America, where individualism centred on maintaining a healthy body was promoted. The feminine body ideal was one that was lean, toned, healthy, and large-breasted, and the terrain was primarily of white, middle-class women who were able to afford health-club memberships and cosmetic procedures necessary to attain the feminine body ideal. This was the feminine body ideal against which all other women were measured, and most often fell short. Curtis's star image was built around her ability to display the "perfect" body in her films. Yet she could also manipulate the publicity machine to control her career and her star image.

In 2002 Curtis, herself a baby boomer, reached out to the women of her generation when she exposed the illusion of the celebrity body by posing for *More* magazine in her underwear, staged with unforgiving lighting and without makeup or designer clothing. Film scholar Pam Cook writes that some female performers have resisted the roles assigned to them and suggests, "Perhaps this is where star quality resides."[63] In Hollywood, where young, thin, white actresses are valued, Curtis presented her "real" body. Although she used the media to her advantage, her photograph in *More* helped to renew feminist debate about women's bodies. Rather than body acceptance, it seems that for baby boomers, particularly women, the aging process was made even more difficult. Some critics have raised the question of whether the image of Curtis's plump and sagging star body has stimulated a fear of aging that has served to promote the consumption of anti-wrinkle creams and cellulite-firming products. Curtis, however, continues to speak out on television talk shows against the use of Botox, liposuction, and cosmetic surgery in Hollywood. Curtis's photograph in *More* has also been cited as an inspiration for "Dove's Campaign for Real Beauty," which uses so-called real women to advertise its skin-care products. This has sparked media debate as to whether body acceptance is actually being encouraged among women, when most women cannot measure up to the "real" women in the Dove advertisements or Curtis's so-called real woman photographs in *More*, thereby dooming most women to failure.

Curtis's ongoing public confrontations with her body image were revealed in the July 2007 issue of *Ladies' Home Journal* and in her fourth *More* cover and feature article in July 2008. Curtis appears on the covers as trim—some would say thin. She is described in *Ladies' Home Journal* as "glowing with the healthy good looks of someone who works out and eats smart." In the interviews, she commented on the 2002 photo spread in *More*. At the time, Curtis revealed, she had been only two years sober and had put on all the weight snacking on crackers or something to compensate for all the sugar she didn't get without consuming alcohol. Also she had just adopted her son and didn't have the free time for a lot of physical activity. Curtis was disturbed that some women interpreted the photos as meaning "Love yourself no matter what." A problem occurs, Curtis explained, "if what you're doing is unhealthy." In her case, she had not only gained weight but her cholesterol levels were elevated. By "making healthy choices," she had lost the weight. At age fifty, her goals are freedom from her addictions and comparisons with other people, and to be "fit and focused."

In *Ladies' Home Journal*, she reiterated that she felt badly that she has perpetuated the national obsession with people's bodies with the focus on her body that developed early in her career. Yet, while the article contends that Curtis decided to put her family first, get healthy again, and live by her own rules, she is still ambivalent about her image as a "star body." Curtis revealed that a friend of her mother had praised her for her weight loss, whispering: "You look like you again." Curtis stated: "I didn't know what to say. Because the problem is that's what I traded my life on. That's what I get everywhere I go. Everywhere I go. Am I nothing but a body? Am I nothing but someone who *talks* about her frickin' body?"[64] For Curtis the woman's remarks created some confusion; she was grateful for the compliment about her healthy body but disgusted that so much emphasis has been placed on her body over her other talents and contributions to society.

The body politics surrounding Jamie Lee Curtis's star image suggest that feminism must develop a new politics of the body. As Sandra Bartky suggests, these new "styles of the flesh" will require altered modes of sexual desire, the disappearance of mandatory gender markers, and the overthrow of white patriarchal dominance of the image. Only then will body acceptance be possible for all women.[65]

Notes

1   Amy Wallace, "True Thighs," *More* (September 2002): 90–5.
2   Jamie Lee Curtis and Laura Cornell, *I'm Gonna Like Me: Letting Off a Little Self-Esteem* (New York: Harper Collins, 2002).
3   Susan Faludi, *Backlash: The Undeclared War against American Women* (New York: Doubleday, 1991); Naomi Wolf, *The Beauty Myth* (Toronto: Random House, 1990).
4   Sandra Lee Bartky, *Femininity and Domination: Studies in the Phenomenology of Oppression* (New York: Routledge, 1990), pp. 39–40.
5   Judith Butler, *Gender Trouble: Feminism and the Subversion of Identity* (London: Routledge, 1990), p. 139.
6   Elizabeth Grosz, *Volatile Bodies: Toward Corporeal Feminism* (Bloomington: Indiana University Press, 1994), p. 19; Anne Balsamo, *Technologies of the Gendered Body: Reading Cyborg Women* (Durham: Duke University Press, 1996), pp. 162–3.
7   Richard Dyer, *Heavenly Bodies: Film Stars and Society* (London: Macmillan Educational Press, 1986); Richard Dyer, *Stars* (London: British Film Institute, 1998).
8   Dyer, *Heavenly Bodies*, pp. 2–3.
9   See, for example, Rebecca Feasey, "Stardom and Sharon Stone: Power as Masquerade," *Quarterly Review of Film and Video* 21.3 (July–September 2004): 199–207.
10   Dyer, *Heavenly Bodies*, pp. 19–59.
11   Richard de Cordova, *Picture Personalities: The Emergence of the Star System in America* (Urbana: University of Illinois Press, 1990).
12   P. David Marshall, *Celebrity and Power: Fame in Contemporary Culture* (Minneapolis: University of Minnesota Press, 1997), pp. 95–9.
13   Alan Nadel, *Flatlining on the Field of Dreams: Cultural Narratives in the Films of President Reagan's America* (New Brunswick, NJ: Rutgers University Press, 1997), pp. 3–11; Susan Jeffords, *Hard Bodies: Hollywood Masculinity in the Regan Era* (New Brunswick, NJ: Rutgers University Press, 1994), pp. 1–23; Clayton R. Koppes, "The Power, the Glitter, the Muscles: Movie Masculinities in the Age of Reagan," *Reviews in American History* 23.3 (1995): 528–34; Cheryl L. Cole, "Addiction, Exercise, and Cyborgs: Technologies of Deviant Bodies," in Geneviève Rail, ed., *Sport and Postmodern Times* (Albany: SUNY Press, 1998), pp. 261–76.
14   Cole, "Addiction, Exercise," p. 262.
15   Nadel, *Flatlining on the Field of Dreams*, pp. 86–101.
16   Yvonne Tasker, *Working Girls: Gender and Sexuality in Popular Cinema* (London: Routledge, 1998), p. 6.

17 Aaron Latham, "Looking for Mr. Goodbody," *Rolling Stone* 9 (June 1983): 20–6, 59, 61–2.

18 Laurie Schultz, "On the Muscle," in Jane Gaines and Charlotte Herzog, eds., *Fabrications: Costume and the Female Body* (New York: Routledge, 1990), pp. 59–78.

19 Jennifer Ellison, "Let Me Hear Your Body Talk: Aerobics for Fat Women Only, 1981–1985," in this volume.

20 Margaret Morse, "Artemis Aging: Exercise and the Female Body on Video," *Discourse* 10.1 (Fall/Winter 1987–88): 32–3.

21 *Perfect* soundtrack, Arista Records, 1985. Curtis also played the aerobics instructor in Jermaine Jackson's music video for the title song, thereby tying the film into other media.

22 Morse, "Artemis Aging," p. 37.

23 Rebecca Feasey uses Sharon Stone's manipulation of her star image in *Basic Instinct* to illustrate how the actress uses notions of distortion and performance to manipulate her environment and control her career. See Feasey, "Stardom and Sharon Stone."

24 Charlene Krista, "Jamie Lee Curtis: An Interview," *Films in Review* 35 (August/September 1985): 390.

25 "The Best Body in Movies: Jamie Lee Curtis," *Harper's Bazaar* (May 1985): 182–3, 212; "America's 10 Best Bodies," *McCall's* (May 1985): 104–9, 148, 150.

26 "Best Body in Movies," pp. 183, 212.

27 Gary Kinder, "Has Jamie Lee Curtis Finally Found Herself? God Knows," *Esquire* (July 1985): 66–73.

28 "Jamie Lee Curtis," *Vogue* (June 1985): 245, 312.

29 "Jamie Lee Curtis," p. 312.

30 Scott Haller, "Forget What the Song Says—Don't Call Jamie Lee Curtis the Closest Thing to Perfect," *People* (24 June 1985): 93.

31 *San Francisco Chronicle* (15 April 1985).

32 Krista, "Jamie Lee Curtis: An Interview," p. 391.

33 Tasker, *Working Girls*, p. 77.

34 Antonia Zerbisias, "*True Lies* Denigrates Women and Arabs," *Toronto Star* (12 August 1994), http://global.factiva.com (accessed 19 June 2006); Peter Bart, "Explosive Summer Action: Debating Truth about 'Lies,'" http://www.variety.com (accessed 3 September 2006).

35 Paula Chin, "Making a Splash," *People* (22 August 1994), http://global.factiva.com (accessed 23 October 2005).

36 Dyer, *Stars*, pp. 48–9.

37 Jim Calio, "Jamie Lee's Special Gift," *Redbook* (1 April 1998), http://global.factiva.com (accessed 29 November 2005).

38 Samatha Miller, "40 and Fabulous," *People* (31 August 1998), http://vnweb.hwwilsonweb.com (accessed 29 November 2005).

39 Curtis's children's books have also been part of the refashioning of her celebrity image, as the crossover project has become a necessary component of celebrity culture in recent years. Madonna, Jerry Seinfeld, John Lithgow, Katie Couric, Julie Andrews, and Maria Shriver are among the celebrities who have produced children's books. See Kate Taylor, "Entertainment," *Globe and Mail* (17 September 2003), http://global.factiva.com (accessed 28 November 2005).

40 Curtis and Cornell, *I'm Gonna Like Me.*

41 Amy Wallace, "True Thighs," *More* (September 2002): 92.

42 Wallace, "True Thighs," p. 92.

43 Curtis and Cornell, *I'm Gonna Like Me*.

44 Wallace, "True Thighs," p. 92.

45 "2002 Women of the Year," *Ms. Magazine* (December 2002), http://msmagazine.com/dec02/womenoftheyear.asp (accessed 26 October 2005).

46 NBC News, *Today* (21 August 2002), http://global.factiva.com (accessed 21 October 2005).

47 *Today* (21 August 2002).

48 Carolyn Kitch, "Selling the 'Boomer Babes': *More* and the 'New' Middle Age," *Journal of Magazine and New Media Research* 5.2 (Spring 2003), http://www.bse.edu/web/aejmcmagzine/journal/srchive/Spring_2003/Kitch.htm (accessed 25 October 2003).

49 CBS News, *The Early Show* (21 August 2002), http://global.factiva.com (accessed 21 October 2005).

50 Cindy Richards, "Thanks, Jamie, for Keeping It Real," *Chicago Sun-Times* (29 January 2003), http://global.factiva.com (accessed 17 November 2005). See also "Flab and All," *Globe and Mail* (7 September 2002).

51 Laura Dempsey, "The Reading Life: Honesty Fits Curtis Perfectly," *Dayton Daily News* (24 August 2002), http://global.factiva.com (accessed 21 October 2005).

52 Muriel Gray, "Is This a Feminist Statement?" *The Guardian* (22 August 2002), http://global.factiva.com (accessed 21 October 2005).

53 Joan Ryan, "Jamie Lee Curtis Has Nothing to Hide," *San Francisco Chronicle* (27 August 2002), http://global.factiva.com (accessed 21 October 2005).

54 Kathryn Hughes, "Body Politics—A Weight off Your Mind," *The Observer* (25 August 2002), http://global.factiva.com (accessed 16 December 2005).

55 "Keeping It Real: Jamie Lee and *More* Readers Sound Off," *More* (September 2003): 94–7.

56 "Jamie's Big Year," *More* (September 2003): 93.

57 *More* (September 2003): 92–7.

58 Philippa Hawker, "The Body Swap Politic," *The Age* (1 November 2003), http://global.factiva.com (accessed 28 December 2005).

59 Tasker, *Working Girls*, p. 27.

60 Tiffany Rose, "The Interview: Jamie Lee Curtis," *Independent on Sunday* (7 December 2003), http://global.factiva.com (accessed 29 November 2005); Jeff Strickler, "Acting Her Age," *Globe and Mail* (2 August 2003), http://global.factiva.com (accessed 18 November 2005); Jan Janssen, "Interview: Jamie Lee Curtis—Jamie Lee Freaks Out," *Daily Mirror* (19 December 2003), http://global.factiva.com (accessed 29 November 2005).

61 Hawker, "Body Swap Politic."

62 Amy Wallace, "How Jamie Grows," *More* (September 2006): 136–4, 212.

63 Pam Cook, "Border Crossings: Women and Film in Context," in Pam Cook and Philip Dodd, eds., *Women and Film: A Sight and Sound Reader* (Philadelphia: Temple University Press, 1995), p. xv.

64 Jeanne Marie Laskas, "Sunny, Side, Up," *Ladies' Home Journal* (July 2007): 118–26.

65 Sandra Lee Bartky, "Body Politics," in Alison M. Jaggar and Iris Marion Young, eds., *A Companion to Feminist Philosophy* (Oxford, UK: Oxford University Press, 2000), p. 329.

"Every Generation Has Its War": Representations of Gay Men with Aids and Their Parents in the United States, 1983–1993

Heather Murray

W hen the AIDS activist group ACT UP (AIDS Coalition to Unleash Power) staged street theatre-oriented protests in the late 1980s, one of its iconographic Ronald Reagan posters asked the question: "What If Your Son Gets Sick?" (fig. 1).[1] The question was deliberately provocative, of course, part of the ongoing needling about the president's son's sexuality that was present in both gay activist and gay humour sources, but it also had a more sombre underlying intention: gay men dying with AIDS were indeed sons who would be mourned by their parents, even in traditional families.[2] In a society that increasingly reinforced polarities between the so-called innocent victims of the disease and the presumably immoral ones, the simple idea that those dying with AIDS were family members was a poignant one.

When AIDS first became known in the early 1980s, it was deemed purely a gay disease. Doctors at the UCLA Medical Center and in New York City were puzzled that young gay men in their twenties and thirties were dying with pneumocystis pneumonia (PCP), an infection normally only seen in transplant or cancer patients. Some were suffering with a particularly virulent strain of Kaposi's sarcoma, a disfiguring skin cancer characterized by purple and brown lesions, previously only seen in aging Mediterranean men and even then considered not to be life threatening.[3] These patients all showed a lowering of their immune function, their bodies unable to ward off even typically harmless infections. Doctors first referred to these symptoms as GRID, or gay-related immune disorder, and only called the condition AIDS, or

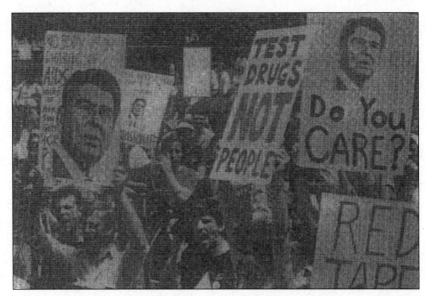

Figure 1   AIDS activists demonstrate in front of the White House, June 1, 1987, at the time of the Third International Conference on AIDS. Photo by Jane Rosett, from Douglas Crimp, ed., *AIDS: Cultural Analysis/Cultural Activism* (Cambridge, MA: MIT Press, 1988), p. 153. Reprinted courtesy of The MIT Press.

acquired immunodeficiency syndrome, after the Centers for Disease Control renamed the epidemic in 1982. Before human immunodeficiency virus (HIV) transmission became understood in 1984, early theories about the disease suggested that gay men contracted it through an immune overload that was the consequence of spending sleepless nights at gay bars and discotheques, inhaling poppers, and having promiscuous sex.[4] Early media reports followed suit by calling the disease the "gay plague."[5]

AIDS casualties multiplied rapidly throughout the 1980s: in 1981 the number of AIDS-related deaths was 225, jumping to 1,400 by 1983, 15,000 by 1985, 40,000 by 1987, and more than 100,000 by 1990.[6] The great majority of these deaths were young men between twenty-five and forty-four.[7] The disease spread rapidly within urban centres, most notably New York City, San Francisco, and Los Angeles. By the mid-1980s, however, the disease had made its way to other North American cities and rural areas.[8]

Throughout the 1980s, AIDS became a potent part of the politics and sensibility of the culture wars, the acrimonious divisions between social conservatives and traditionalists, on the one hand, and social liberals and pluralists, on the other, in late-twentieth-century United States. The body was often the site of these conflicts; controversy surrounded not just gay sexuality, but also abortion, pornography, and sex education.[9] Within the public imagination, AIDS added the dimension of a frightening, visible disease to an already entrenched New Right notion that homosexuality was unnatural.[10] As the Reagan-era Surgeon General C. Everett Koop noted, the disease was marked by mystery, fear, and the unknown. Those gay men who contracted it, especially during the early part of the decade, were seen as abstract or alien figures who suffered, as a 1985 *Newsweek* article suggested, "Miles from Home with No Place to Die."[11] In fact, many social observers, including American health care workers, harboured a notion of orphanhood when they conceived of gay men with AIDS, as though every AIDS sufferer had necessarily faced family excommunication.[12]

Many observers of the AIDS epidemic have thus characterized the disease as one that united gay men and lesbians as peers within volunteer care networks, bringing the notion of chosen families—of partners and friends—to the forefront, a kinship strategy that sociologist Kath Weston has suggested is a particularly poignant one for gay men and lesbians in the face of biological family rejection.[13] Yet this disease highlighted a more traditional kinship strategy, one often presumed to be unimaginable for gays, in that AIDS also overlapped the social lives, experiences, and cultures of gay men and their heterosexual parents. The family emerged in metaphors and images within gay activist rhetoric, figured in health advertising and gay fiction, and appeared in personal testimonies and memoirs by both gay men and their parents. Throughout the 1980s, gay men who suffered with this disease, and their families alike, often felt a powerful sense of isolation; they may have felt abandoned by indifferent politicians, alienated by callous images in visual and print media sources, and discriminated against by a fearful health care system. Added to this was the plain recognition that AIDS was a unique disease from the standpoint of the late twentieth century in that it was unrecoverable; not so unique historically was that it was a disease, as syphilis and leprosy were before it, fraught with connotations of moral waywardness that could induce family shame. As with syphilis, it was easy for social observers and commentators to denounce a disease morally when it was transmitted sexually.[14] As with delirium tremens, seen as an undesirable outcome of a chosen kind of socializing, AIDS could be seen as the equally disgraceful but more horrific consequence of a gay "lifestyle." Yet representations of the family relationship in both gay and mainstream culture show that AIDS also prompted a yearning for the basic acts of material care and nurturance that the family of origin seemed to embody. This magnified the presence and the fantasy of family life within gay consciousness and shaped a view of caring as a boon rather than a burden, a sensibility that would shape gay culture in the late twentieth century.

Morally Neutral vs. Morally Fraught Diseases

That AIDS was first named gay-related immune disorder indicates the extent to which it was perceived—at first by the medical community and then more broadly, including by parents—as a disease inherently related to gay sexuality, which in turn was conceived strictly as anal sex.[15] AIDS in the family brought gay sexuality and gay existence—real and imaginary—to the forefront. Portraits of parents at times highlighted a more general male voyeurism and queasiness about gay sex, one that seemed to suggest, as playwright Tony Kushner said, that gay men deserved to die simply for having sex with each other.[16] Paul Reed created a father who embodies this perspective in his 1984 book, *Facing It*, one of the first AIDS novels in North America. This father already considered his gay son, Andy, "his greatest disappointment." He could not abide his wife's mentioning his son's "disgusting illness," but on the other hand, "[h]e wasn't surprised; he knew the sorts of vile things that queers did—fucking strangers in alleys, sucking every cock that comes along, in bus stations, public parks, anywhere they could satisfy their groping lusts for men's flesh. And there was worse, he knew.... [I]t was no wonder Andy was sick. The whole subject made him nauseous."[17] The uneasiness here seemed to go beyond gay sex and to reach into a revulsion about sexuality and bodies in general, one that was grafted onto his gay son and his imagined sexual practices. This character blamed his son not simply for getting sick but for a failure to achieve a specific kind of masculinity, a pressure not only present in antebellum America but also thriving in late-twentieth-century America, and particularly poignant when homosexuality had become emblematic of and a repository for effeminate behaviours and emotions.

This gay writer's creation of a homophobic father evoked a condemnation of sodomy that saw a wider circulation during the 1980s. Supreme Court judges reinforced the idea of sodomy as unnatural in the 1986 *Bowers v. Hardwick* case by upholding the Georgia Sodomy Statute, one of the many state statutes prohibiting sodomy that were still on the books then and were not overturned until 2003.[18] Michael Hardwick had been arrested for having sex with another man in his own bedroom; the Supreme Court justified this invasion of privacy for an act of consensual sodomy on the grounds that not all private acts at home between family members could be protected, placing sodomy on the same plane as crimes such as murder and incest. Upholding Hardwick's conviction, the Supreme Court ruling said that this sexual behaviour had been denounced by "millenia [*sic*] of moral teaching." Was this idea of sodomy informed by AIDS, as well as these millennia of moral teaching? Sodomy restrictions notably were not applied to heterosexual sex.[19]

The connotations of anal sex and promiscuity discomfited some parents and seemed to taint the unqualified sympathy they might have offered had the disease been "just" cancer, or another more morally neutral disease. As Susan Sontag has pointed out, however, even cancer has been a disease fraught with interpretations of negligence; at times, individuals with cancer have been seen as self-indulgent and irresponsible about their health, perhaps reflecting a distinctly American view of health as an individual rather than a collective or state responsibility.[20] AIDS was especially vulnerable to the charge of individual neglect or irresponsibility. By the mid-1980s, mainstream American media sources and political culture had started distinguishing between "innocent" victims of the disease, such as newborns and the recipients of HIV-contaminated blood transfusions, and supposedly wilful perpetrators of the disease, such as gay men or drug users.[21] Media portraits of the innocents—especially hemophiliacs and children—were careful to show them as ingenuous, asexual beings. By contrast, portraits of gay men and drug users often showed them in urban settings, clustered together anonymously in bars, as if they had no daily life outside of promiscuity and certainly no family life.[22]

Mysterious Diseases for Mysterious Sons

These interpretations of the disease's sufferers also pervaded family life and were apparent in the desire to understand the origins of illness within a gay son. Postulating the cause of disease was not, of course, unique to AIDS, and this might have been particularly the case during the 1980s, when North American exercise and nutrition habits came under a sharper scrutiny.[23] However, AIDS seemed to demand of parents that they defend their sons from the taint of promiscuity.

For some parents, the notion of individual responsibility was not irrelevant, even in the face of their own children dying. The desire to attribute blame to their sons' perceived promiscuity did not preclude sympathy for their sickness, though it certainly precipitated a re-evaluation of the sexual revolution. Memoirs by mothers about their sons with AIDS constitute an intriguing body of sources in which to witness an internal dialogue about the causes of disease because it is here that mothers, in creating their own life story narratives, also construct narratives about disease and impute meaning to it.[24] One mother, Beverly Barbo, points out in the first page of her memoir about her son Tim: "Why is my son dying? Because he made some bad choices a few years ago, one of which resulted in the disease AIDS, and AIDS related cancer, Kaposi's Sarcoma, is killing him." Barbo believed that when her son first moved to California, he must have experienced the culture shock of gay acceptance and it was in this situation that she felt "sexual excesses do occur."[25] It is not clear, though, if her son had in fact been excessive or if he simply had had unprotected sex in a time of risk. Another mother memoirist, Ardath H. Rodale, seems haunted by how her son's AIDS death could have been avoided. Like Barbo, she notes that her son, David, grew up amidst an ethos that seemed to say, "Enjoy sex to the fullest.... People were encouraged to experiment with the latest ideas. There were suggested positions for having sex that I never heard of before—never even imagined! People throughout the media winked an eye at, even openly approved of, multiple partners." Careful to set herself apart from these sensibilities, she notes that she was brought up with more "Victorian attitudes" and that having sex in her day was not "a function of getting acquainted as it often is nowadays!" In her view, these more liberal sexual mores had led the younger generation "into anguish."[26] This perception had its adherents in the gay world as well.[27]

Though Rodale makes oblique references to her son's sexual partners as the probable cause of his death, she does not blame a perceived gay lifestyle. Instead, most of the book is devoted to memories of his innocence. Perhaps another function of memoirs is the stylization of certain memories in this way, and her stylization is quite striking because the picture to emerge is similar to the icon of the innocent victim. She writes that David had been a "good little boy, with a deep, wonderful chuckle," who wrote plays, was gentle with animals, and was "peace loving."[28] Her reminiscence keeps him young and perhaps consciously asexual. Rodale even appears to conceive of her son as a cultural type or a separate category of person: her dedication is to "all the Davids, and those who love them."

These representations gave gay sons an abstract quality as eternally loving and affable family members, even as they acknowledged, albeit haltingly, a sexuality that made their difference from parents striking. Yet for their parents, gay men with AIDS also represented and inhabited an unseen and unknown world of viruses and, especially during the epidemic's early years, uncertain means of transmission. Gay cartoonist Howard Cruse, who was noted for combining both satire and brutal realism in his comic strips, evoked these early AIDS fears in his six-page stream-of-consciousness story called "Safe Sex." The panels here depict many different scenarios of AIDS in American life, including one in which a mother serves her son at a holiday

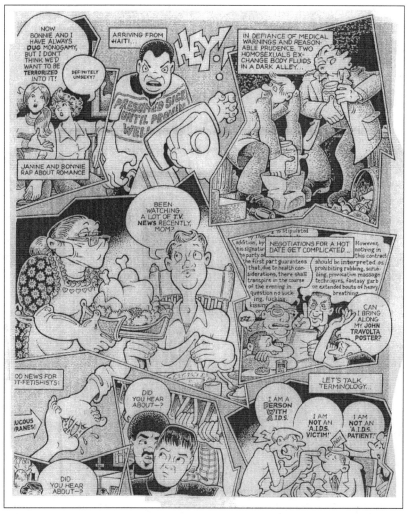

Figure 2 Drawing by Howard Cruse, from *Christopher Street* 79 (vol. 7, no. 9, 1983). 5. Reprinted with the permission of the artist.

dinner wearing long rubber gloves and a surgical mask, and her son asks her, "Been watching a lot of TV recently, Mom?" (fig. 2).[29]

Especially during the early 1980s, the hospital experience itself quite commonly reinforced the idea that AIDS might be contagious, amplifying the idea of plague, which, as Susan Sontag famously noted, had become AIDS's central metaphor.[30] Before it was widely known that the disease was virus based, hospitals confined AIDS patients to isolation zones, hospital workers refused to clean their rooms, and funeral workers refused to embalm their bodies.[31] These realities compounded the already deeply ingrained social prejudices against gays and shaped parental interactions with their dying sons. In her memoir, Barbara Peabody recounts how distressed she was when she had to visit her son at New York's St. Vincent's hospital in an isolation room. When she and her husband left this zone, they took off their "masks and gloves and stuffed them into the bag labeled 'Infectious Waste.' The yellow gowns go into 'Infectious Linens.'" Her experiences are reminiscent of one major artistic response to AIDS: choreographer Bill T. Jones's ballet *Absence*, in which the dancers were wrapped in bedclothes borrowed from Jones's dead partner and his current partner's hospital robes, as if to save these fragments of loved ones that otherwise would have been destroyed.[32] Such hospital precautions, even when in place to protect the person with AIDS as much as the parents, made Mrs. Peabody feel that she was visiting a leper.[33]

These reminiscences show that families were often placed in the complicated circumstance of fearing contamination and the physicality of the disease and yet wishing to show their loved ones compassion. Perhaps these fears attest to the success of public health advertising campaigns throughout the twentieth century, which, as historian Nancy Tomes says, were so successful in evoking an invisible world of germs that individuals grew constantly wary.[34] It would indeed be hard for family members not to pay heed to the place AIDS held in the public imagination as potentially more deadly than scientists had imagined. The visual and news media did little to dispel these thoughts, particularly when magazines, newspapers, radio, and television began reporting on AIDS more regularly after 1983.[35]

Basic acts of caring for someone with AIDS, then, could be fraught with fear. This was true for Marie Blackwell's family, who cared for her brother, Chet. Blackwell wrote up her family's story for the African American women's general interest magazine, *Essence*, in 1985. Here she makes it clear that Chet's gayness was firmly a part of their family lore and was never questioned. Chet "never had the pressure of having to 'break it to the family' [because] his being gay or acting sort of feminine" was what they considered a fundamental part of his personality. Mrs. Blackwell even told her son, "If you have to mess around with men, then go and find yourself a rich one." Chet was diagnosed with AIDS in 1983, a time when his family felt "totally ignorant about the extent of AIDS contagiousness." Thus, when they brought him home to care for him, Chet was not allowed in the family kitchen, and they were wary of touching any food that they had left for him in his room. Blackwell often turned him down "with the excuse of being on a diet. He always looked very disappointed when I didn't eat his offerings." She became desperate to find ways to make her brother feel less contaminated and yet still care for him in a way that necessitated intimate contact and gestures.

In this family, fears about AIDS and its prognosis also reflected a degree of mistrust of the medical profession. When Chet would have moments of feeling somewhat better, his mother would say, as if to convince herself, that he was "getting better. I knew those stupid-ass doctors didn't know what they were talking about.... All you have to do is eat a lot of food and be around people who love you. Those doctors just want to experiment."[36] The idea of hospitals as alien institutions was becoming quite engrained in late-twentieth-century United States and was one that prompted theologian Paul Ramsey to ask that doctors treat "the patient as person" in his 1970 book titled with that phrase.[37] A notion of doctor distrust, however, was particularly prevalent for African American families, owing to the greater public awareness during this period of a history of medical experimentation on African Americans, most notably the legacy of the Tuskegee experiments during the U.S. Public Health Service Syphilis Study in the 1930s and 1940s. This medical history specific to African Americans compounded a more general shift in public consciousness that regarded doctors with suspicion.[38]

The physicality of AIDS went far beyond connotations and hints of contamination, however. Those with full-blown AIDS became shockingly disfigured. They suffered from violent fevers, coughing, incontinence, and dementia, looks and smells and ailments that were well beyond the world of unseen germs. As would be true in Blackwell's family, many family members felt devastated by the emaciation the disease caused, by how waxen and sallow and skeletal their family members had become. The faces of those suffering with AIDS, too, could be ravaged by the purple-brown lesions of Kaposi's sarcoma, as though gay men with AIDS carried the visual lacerations and markings of a perceived non-ascetic life. Even an experienced physician such as Elisabeth Kübler-Ross—who had worked previously with African patients with syphilis, a disease whose ulcerations could terribly disfigure the face— found it trying to behold an AIDS patient scarred with Kaposi's sarcoma lesions. These physical symptoms were understandably shocking and painful for family members to behold in their loved ones. Kübler-Ross wrote of a young man with AIDS who had been estranged from his family, seeking one last visit home before he died. He confided to Ross that he had wondered, upon seeing his mother come out to greet him from the front porch, "what would happen if she really saw the purple lesions on his face? [Would she] stop and hesitate? [Would she] put her arms down and stop a few feet before they would hug each other?"[39] Though in this case the man's mother did not respond as he had feared, the anxiety about appearing grotesque was salient for many gay men within their families.

There is some universal character to observing a loved one with disease, of course, because the observers are always in some sense on the periphery, outside of the prolonged and painful suffering. Yet what was specific to this crisis was that the family members of gay men with AIDS were already somewhat peripheral to gay sons. Gay sexuality was often hidden from parents at least for some portion of time. In the words of memoirist Betty Clare Moffatt, reflecting on her then-estranged son Michael, the disease

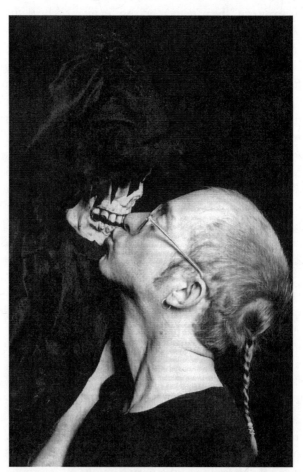

Figure 3   Bill Bytsura, "Tigger" (gelatin silver photo, 1992), in Ted Gott, ed., *Don't Leave Me This Way: Art in the Age of AIDS* (Canberra: National Gallery of Australia, 1994), p. 58. Courtesy Bill Bytsura and the Fales Library, New York University.

"had combined with the hiddenness of his life, the aloneness, too."[40] Her feeling resonated with media portraits that reinforced the idea of mysterious diseases for mysterious sons.[41] In one sense, the universal aspects of disease and suffering seemed to make their gay sons more familiar and knowable to parents, or at least more concrete. Yet in another sense, AIDS seemed to mark gay sons with another layer of abstraction, reinforcing the sense that parents were only the observers of their sons' veiled and obscure gay lives. Though her son did not develop AIDS until 1989, Bobbie Stasey recalls in her memoir that when her son came out to her in 1981, she became preoccupied with thoughts of a gay disease. Interspersed through her son's coming-out conversation as she recounts it is her stream of consciousness: "*A disease is killing homosexuals. / A mysterious disease killing homosexuals.*"[42] Just as gay men throughout the 1980s were starting to perceive and represent an interconnection between gay sex and death, as is illustrated in Bill Bytsura's photograph of a man kissing a hooded skeleton, parents appeared to be doing the same (fig. 3).[43]

At times, parents took note of a larger cultural phenomenon, of families finessing their son's illnesses so that their children did not die of this mysterious disease associated almost solely with homosexuals but instead died of Hodgkin's disease, or meningitis, or an unspecified lengthy illness. This misrepresentation of their children's illnesses seemed necessary in some cases to protect the family.[44] Even AIDS funerals had become the sites of anti-gay protests: mourners were spat upon, derided, and reminded of biblical condemnations of gays during the services.[45] There was even violence against the "innocent" victims of the disease.[46] The fabricated illnesses need to be considered in this context of profound stigma and even physical violence that was especially devastating for gays; Surgeon General C. Everett Koop said a new word needed to be coined for homophobia during these years because homophobia was simply not strong enough to capture the hatred he had witnessed.[47] Thus, discretion about children's illnesses could reflect a basic desire for dignity and protection in addition to, or perhaps even rather than, parental shame.

Community of Suffering

This discretion, however, added a layer of isolation to parents' grief. Jean Baker, who lost her son to AIDS, sought acknowledgement of her grief from a community of family sufferers. A central theme of her memoir is witnessing suffering, and the act of memoir writing itself could be seen as a call for witnesses in writing for a public audience. In a sense, she was doing what the hallucination sufferer of the nineteenth century did: abandoning a particular "culturally informed perception of reality" and searching for "an alternate reality" in which her specific grief could be recognized.[48] She recalls that after her son died she developed a preoccupation with reading obituaries, hoping for some connection to those who had endured the same sorrow she had. She would take note of the "death of a man, particularly between the ages of about twenty-five and forty or possibly even older, who was unmarried; whose survivors included parents, siblings, nieces, and nephews, but no spouse and no children; whose death was unexplained; and who was often involved in some creative field."[49] As she aptly observes, AIDS had a particularly devastating impact on the North American artistic community: gone were artists Keith Haring, David Wojnarowicz, and Robert Mapplethorpe, and writers Craig Harris and Essex Hemphill, among others.[50] This kind of obituary would "immediately alert me to think that maybe this unknown person was gay, like my son, and maybe this person had died from AIDS, like my son."[51]

The community of fellow sufferers was at times so elusive that family members of sons dying with AIDS sought community through identifying with collective sufferings of the past. For Barbara Peabody, AIDS was a genocide rather than a randomly cruel biological phenomenon; thus, she felt some affinity for witnesses to the Holocaust. After having seen a placard at a demonstration declaring AIDS "God's pest control," Peabody realized that some "sincere Christians" felt that AIDS was a "'final solution,' as the gas chambers were for the Jews."[52] It was not a coincidence that AIDS activists took up metaphors of war to describe what was happening to gay people during this period.[53] Some perceived the striking physical similarities between AIDS bodies and concentration camp victims. In the words of Peabody, who makes this comparison, both were "gaunt, knobby, emaciated … weak from malnourishment." What really struck her was what she calls "an AIDS face." An AIDS face was "prematurely aged. Men of 30 appear years older, the skin stretched tight over skin and jawbone…. The eyes are torturous, sunk deep into their bone-ridged hollows."[54] These World War II analogies were also common in artistic responses to AIDS. In his print "Prophylaxis: Blind Admonition," Michael Tidmus juxtaposes an image of a baby doll and a little boy against a mushroom cloud, with Hitler's face hovering in the background, inscribed with the words "AIDS Baby: (Born 1951)."[55] AIDS babies were, of course, deemed innocent victims of the disease; in Tidmus's photo, however, the innocents were adult gay men born soon after the Second World War. AIDS was producing a culture of suffering inflected with Holocaust imagery;

looking to the Holocaust for a verification of suffering was not unlike Jean Baker's motivation in scanning the obituaries.

In late-twentieth-century North America, however, the dying often were hidden, or at least removed from public view, placed within clinical atmospheres of hospitals and quickly disposed of in morgues and graves.[56] Reticence about the dying, moreover, is not unique to AIDS. Yet this particular historical moment of the experience of death could be said to have collided with a collective gay craving for family acknowledgement and care. This longing was a theme in philosopher/photographer Duane Michals's haunting AIDS photograph and narrative poem, "The Father Prepares His Dead Son for Burial" (1991). Lying on a mattress on the floor, the son in the photo appears too perfectly poised to be sleeping; on the other hand, he appears too robust to be dead. The room appears somewhat filthy, with spattered walls, dirty carpets, and scraps on the floor, yet the son lies sheathed in a white, translucent sheet, his face and body form apparent, prepared for burial by his father. The father had washed his son's body "slowly, deliberately, looking hard at him / for the last time. / He touches him with oil, carefully as if not to awaken him." In a scene of squalor, the father has cleansed his son most meticulously for his death. But in performing this loving ritual the father "begins to quiver with grief" and this escalates into a "terrible shout of anguish."[57] The odd juxtaposition of both alive and dead here suggests a yearning for parental caring rituals expressed throughout a child's lifetime: sleeping and dreaming, as opposed to oblivious and dead.

Activist Responses

Organizations responding to the AIDS crisis took into account this kind of longing and insisted that a son's dying could become a moment of profound family intimacy, which was so elusive in this photo. But both organizations and families had to contend with the acute hostility to gays and individuals with AIDS, hostility that continued throughout the 1980s and became an explicit part of the New Right view of moral problems in contemporary life. The slow responses of both the Reagan and Bush administrations to the AIDS crisis appeared to condone the suffering of individuals with AIDS and their families.[58] Moreover, the cost of drugs such as AZT (azidothymidine), particularly when the drug first began its testing in 1986 and 1987, was most exorbitant. At $10,000 a year, it was out of reach of those without medical insurance or Medicaid, and its side effects could be ghastly.[59] Not until 1987 did Congress, in response to protests about the high costs of AZT, give money to states to offset costs.[60]

Given this at times hopeless tenor of treatment of individuals with AIDS, gay activism experienced a rejuvenation, and one of its animating forces was the plain fact that individuals with AIDS were family members; the activist pleas were for recognition as much as for support or assistance. Drawing on an idea of participatory democracy and on activist street theatre and art, Larry Kramer founded ACT UP in New York City in 1987. Other groups soon appeared in Los Angeles and many other American cities, as well as in Canadian cities such as Vancouver. Taking up the artistic and advertising skills of its members, the group began to stage imaginative, dramatic, militant demonstrations.[61] ACT UP's first political funeral took place on election day in 1992, when 250 members carried the emaciated corpse of Mark Lowe Fisher, a New York architect, to the Bush–Quayle campaign headquarters in New York City's midtown. Protestors held up a banner that read, "Mark Lowe Fisher, 1953–92, Murder by George Bush," while chanting, "George Bush, you can't hide, we charge you with genocide."[62] Before he died, Mark Lowe Fisher had issued a statement about his prospective public funeral which became an ACT UP advertisement entitled "Bury Me Furiously." Acknowledging that his funeral was going to "shock people," he wanted, nevertheless, "to show the reality of my death, to display my body in public; I want the public to bear witness. We are not just spiraling statistics; we are people who have lives, who have purpose, who have lovers, friends, and families."[63] Did it take this kind of grisly, shocking protest simply to underscore the reality of AIDS sufferers and the basic claim that they, too, had loved ones?

"Every Generation Has Its War"

There was a kind of surreal, nightmarish quality about living with and caring for a loved one with AIDS in the context of a broader culture that scarcely acknowledged the mass grief that the epidemic had produced, preferring to focus instead on its risks or on the prurient aspects of gay sex. Family members and partners of gay men with AIDS seemed to be part of a war that nobody else recognized or experienced as a part of their daily lives. In an article in *Christopher Street* on AIDS writing, Michael Denneny wrote that his life had become a "surrealistic series of medical disasters, hospital vigils, and memorial services [while] everyday life went on as if nothing were happening." He wrote of Annie Dillard's advice to writers in a recent issue of the *New York Times Book Review*, to write as if you were dying "for an audience consisting solely of terminal patients." Yet she had not "imagine[d] that a whole generation of writers" was already living out this metaphor.[64]

Horrific and isolating as the disease was, portraits of gay men and their parents show that it also had the potential to offer sons and their parents a unique parallel experience. A generation of gay baby boomers was now witnessing the kind of mass deaths normally reserved for those in old age. In a letter to his aging father when his partner was dying, Robert John Florence wrote, "I sure know what it's like to be surrounded by people who are sick & dying, as you mentioned in your letter about the mobile home park. Several friends have died recently & my intimate friend of five years has been in the hospital eight times so far this year."[65] AIDS also could put sons closer to the calamities that their parents had seen in their own time. Writer James Edwin Parker's mother scarcely mentioned her son's involvement with men or sexuality, though she did know about it. He noted in a memoir piece that she must have been "somewhat aghast to think of the number of sexual partners I had, especially with people dropping dead of pneumonia and KS and other AIDS related diseases." Still, she appeared to feel a kinship with her son, seen through the lens of her past grief. When her son found out a friend was dying with AIDS, she offered: "I went through a similar thing, you know, with the war … the end result was the same: young men dying. Every generation has its war. You have to fight them when they happen."[66]

This cross-generational affinity encompassed a prospect of parents witnessing their sons' deaths in the family home. *Farm Journal* commented on this phenomenon in 1991 with its feature article "Back to the Farm to Die: Rural America Is about to be Blindsided by the AIDS Epidemic."[67] Yet even if a potential for a new-found human connection between parents and children existed through this disease, an ambivalence about the relationship also surfaced, one made more urgent by the prospect of returning home to die. The 1991 movie *Our Sons* evokes this theme of the domesticity of dying and a desire to represent a reconciliation between parents and children. This story is of two mothers who both had some emotional distance from their gay sons. One of the mother characters, who disowned her son for being gay when he was seventeen years old, reaches some sort of rapprochement with him on his deathbed. After her son dies, this mother takes her son's coffin home from San Diego to Arkansas, even though she has not been present in her son's life for years and yelled at him in the hospital that he had brought the disease on himself and was dying from "what he is."[68] There is a forced sense of reconciliation here, a suggestion that no matter how horribly parents had treated their gay children, they nonetheless had the right to their children in their dying moments and had ownership over their children's bodies and memories. Such portrayals could be said to affirm a connection between gays and tragedy and to deny the nuances of the family relationship, giving parents a primacy in their children's lives that perhaps the parents neither felt nor deserved. Yet this claim to family and home was also one that gay men made and represented, even if cautiously and haltingly. Rosalind Solomon captured this ambivalence about the home and parents in an arresting photograph that became part of her series "Portraits in the Time of AIDS." Here a son and parents pose in a backyard with a fence, shrubs, and garden. In the foreground, the son appears somewhat defiant or fed up, with arms folded and a resigned yet daring expression. His parents, hovering behind him, seem hardly posed at all but almost awkwardly placed in the photograph, standing outside in their backyard, as if momentarily in the way of the picture. Not only are they distant from their son, but they look aged, tired, old-fashioned, and detached from the scene, looking away from both their son and the photograph. The overall impression of the photograph is one of disjuncture and a feeling of disorientation. Yet the son's resolute stance suggests a need or perhaps a right to be rooted in families.[69]

One of the pulls that drew gay sons home was the care and nurturing offered there—or the memory, prospect, or hope of it. AIDS suggested a potential for intimacy that was not defined by knowing children's inner worlds or understanding their feelings but perhaps by a more basic kind of family love and the material aspects of care and nurturing qualities marked by domesticity. These expectations of nurturing might have been higher for mothers, and memoir writing by mothers reinforces this sense. Obviously, mother memoirs are not simply "true" bodies of evidence, but they suggest a desire for a collective identity of bereft mothers whose caring roles, as they pertained to this disease specifically, were not always acknowledged by the broader society. In her book on AIDS, Elisabeth Kübler-Ross describes mothers who, she feels, took on the most difficult physical duties of caring, bringing their sons home, cleaning up after them, providing their medication, and being on call all through their sons' sleepless, feverish nights, having little reprieve from their caring obligations. Kübler-Ross sees these tasks as particular to the feminine domestic sphere.[70] Perhaps they were seen as such by gays as well; one billboard advertisement in Los Angeles, for example, produced by the L.A. Gay and Lesbian Community Services Center and shown throughout the mid- and late 1980s, featured actress Zelda Rubinstein as a matronly looking woman flanked by a shirtless gay man. The slogan read: "Play Safely. L.A. Cares ... Like a Mother" (fig. 4).[71]

This is not to deny the existence of peer care between gay men (and between lesbians and gay men) within their own structures and organizations.

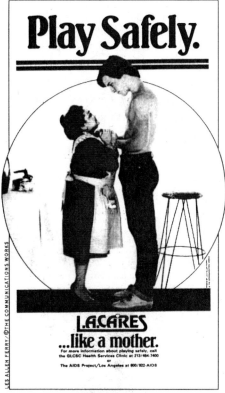

Play Safely.

L.A.CARES
...like a mother.

For more information about playing safely, call
the GLCSC Health Services Clinic at 213/464-7400
or
The AIDS Project/Los Angeles at 800/922-AIDS

LES ALLEN FERRY /©THE COMMUNICATIONS WORKS

Figure 4   From Scott Haller, "Fear and AIDS in
Hollywood," *People* magazine, September 23, 1985,
p. 33.

Yet even these gay caring cultures were inflected with a sense of the family, as the Community Services Center's ad shows.[72] In fact, for some parents, the re-embrace of the caring role could also become a re-evaluation of gay sexuality or their perceptions of gays. When Jean Baker reflected on the death of her son, she could not quite imagine that she had ever experienced her son's gayness as remotely tragic; she issued a poignant challenge to an interpretation of a child's homosexuality as a family tragedy and used the memoir as a forum of repentance, in a sense. "How strangely insignificant [now] seemed the fact of his gayness," she writes. "How difficult to believe I had ever thought his being gay was a tragedy. Being gay is not the tragedy; what is tragic is that any parent can reject a child simply because the child is gay. And, of course, the death of one's child is the ultimate tragedy."[73]

Conclusion

As Jean Baker's testimony suggests, AIDS changed how gay sons and their parents imagined each other. Even as AIDS made gay sexuality more vivid and highlighted a chasm between gays and heterosexuals, the disease nonetheless emphasized the importance of familial care and shaped an often conflicted but nonetheless mutual gay and parental fantasy of family intimacy in the face of death. Moreover, care, inflected with a sense of family domesticity, came to be viewed as an essential, even spiritual, act of witnessing that intensified the fantasy of family love. In gay culture and the culture of parents observing their sons, a new relationship to family and domesticity took form.

Notes

1 See the picture graphics in Douglas Crimp, ed., AIDS: Cultural Analysis, Cultural Activism (Cambridge, MA: MIT Press, 1988).

2 On Reagan's son, see Gay Comix 6 (Winter 1985): back cover.

3 Neil Miller, Out of the Past: Gay and Lesbian History from 1869 to the Present (New York: Vintage, 1995), p. 439.

4 James Curran, "The CDC and the Investigation of the Epidemiology of AIDS," in Victoria A. Harden and John Parascandola, eds., AIDS and the Public Debate: Historical and Contemporary Perspectives (Amsterdam: IOS Press, 1995), p. 23.

5 See Dennis Altman, AIDS in the Mind of America (Garden City, NY: Doubleday, 1986), p. 17.

6 John D'Emilio and Estelle Freedman, Intimate Matters: A History of Sexuality in America (1988; University of Chicago Press, 1997), p. 354; 1990 statistic from Eric Marcus, Making History: The Struggle for Gay and Lesbian Equal Rights, 1945–90: An Oral History (New York: HarperCollins, 1992), p. 405.

7 Ronald Bayer and Gerald Oppenheimer, AIDS Doctors: Voices from the Epidemic (New York: Oxford University Press, 2000), p. 171.

8 See Jacques Bourque, "AIDS: Where's It Left Us?" Angles, Vancouver (May 1986): 11.

9 See James Davison Hunter, Before the Shooting Begins: Searching for Democracy in America's Culture War (New York: Free Press, 1994), p. 3.

10 See Jennifer Terry, An American Obsession: Science, Medicine, and Homosexuality in Modern Society (Chicago: University of Chicago Press, 1999).

11 See C. Everett Koop, "The Early Days of AIDS as I Remember Them," in Harden and Parascandola, eds., AIDS and the Public Debate, p. 18. See also Jean Seligmann and Nikki Finke Greenburg, "Only Months to Live and No Place to Die: The Tragic Odyssey of a Victim Turned Pariah," Newsweek (12 August 1985): 26.

12 One 1995 study of American health care providers who worked with AIDS patients concluded that the majority of health providers believed people with AIDS simply did not have families. See Nina Glick Schiller, "The Invisible Women: Caregiving and AIDS," in Karen V. Hansen and Ilta Garey, eds., Families in the United States: Kinship and Domestic Politics (Philadelphia: Temple University Press, 1998), p. 554.

13 Kath Weston, Families We Choose: Lesbians, Gays, and Kinship (New York: Columbia University Press, 1991), p. 35.

14 On this, see Susan Sontag, *AIDS and Its Metaphors* (New York: Farrar, Straus & Giroux, 1988), p. 56.

15 See Anthony S. Fauci, "AIDS: Reflections on the Past, Considerations for the Future," in Harden and Parascandola, eds., *AIDS and the Public Debate*, p. 68.

16 Patrick Pacheco, "Tony Kushner Speaks out on AIDS, Angels, Activism and Sex in the 90s," in Tony Kushner, *Angels in America: Part 1: Millennium Approaches* (New York: Theatre Communications Group, 1992), p. 22.

17 Paul Reed, *Facing It: A Novel of AIDS* (San Francisco: Gay Sunshine Press, 1984), pp. 153 and 154.

18 See David B. Goodstein, "Our Sweet 16th: Remembering 1967," *The Advocate* 377 (29 September 1983): 30.

19 For an analysis of privacy as a concept in this case, see Jed Rubenfeld, "The Right to Privacy," *Harvard Law Review* 102 (February 1989): 747–8.

20 Sontag, *AIDS and Its Metaphors*, p. 25. On the theme of individual versus collective responsibility, see Dennis Altman, "Legitimation through Disaster: AIDS and the Gay Movement," in Elizabeth Fee and Daniel Fox, eds., *AIDS: The Burdens of History* (Berkeley: University of California Press, 1988), p. 336.

21 Dennis Altman attributes this division to *New York Times* journalist Robin Henig in an article she wrote about "innocent bystanders": "AIDS: A New Disease's Deadly Odyssey," *New York Times Magazine* (6 February 1983): 36. See Altman, *AIDS in the Mind of America*, p. 74.

22 See Timothy E. Cook and David C. Colby, "The Mass-Mediated Epidemic: The Politics of AIDS on the Nightly Network News," in Elizabeth Fee and Daniel Fox, eds., *AIDS: The Making of a Chronic Disease* (Berkeley: University of California Press, 1992), 84–122.

23 See Antoine Prost and Gerard Vincent, eds., *Riddles of Identity in Modern Times*, trans. Arthur Goldhammer, vol. 5 of *A History of Private Life*, Philippe Ariès and Georges Duby, general eds. (Cambridge, MA: Harvard University Press, 1987), pp. 85f.

24 On the narrative dimension of memoirs, see Mary Jo Maynes, Jennifer L. Pierce, and Barbara Lasett, *Telling Stories: The Use of Personal Narratives in the Social Sciences and History* (Ithaca, NY: Cornell University Press, 2008), p. 2.

25 Beverly Barbo, *The Walking Wounded: A Mother's True Story of Her Son's Homosexuality and His Eventual AIDS Related Death* (Lindsborg, KS: Carlsons', P.O. Box 364, 1987), pp. 1, 73.

26 Ardath H. Rodale, *Climbing toward the Light: A Journey of Growth, Understanding, and Love* (Emmaus, PA: Good Spirit Press, 1989), pp. 180–1.

27 See Michael Callen, *Surviving AIDS* (New York: HarperCollins, 1990), p. 4. See also Dudley Clendinen and Adam Nagourney, *Out for Good: The Struggle to Build a Gay Rights Movement in America* (New York: Touchstone, 2001), pp. 515f.

28 Rodale, *Climbing toward the Light*, pp. 58–9.

29 Howard Cruse, "Safe Sex," *Christopher Street* 7.7, Issue 79 (1983): 5.

30 See Douglas A. Feldman and Julia Wang Miller, *The AIDS Crisis: A Documentary History* (Westport, CT: Greenwood Press, 1998), p. 135.

31 See Feldman and Miller, *AIDS Crisis*, p. 242; Daniel Fox, "AIDS and American Health Policy," in Fee and Fox, eds., *AIDS: The Burdens of History*, p. 335.

32 See Richard Golstein, "The Impact of AIDS on American Culture," in Harden and Parascandola, eds., *AIDS and the Public Debate*, p. 135.

33 Barbara Peabody, *The Screaming Room: A Mother's Journal of Her Son's Struggle with AIDS: A True Story of Love, Courage, and Dedication* (San Diego, CA: Oak Tree Publishers, 1986), p. 18.

34   Nancy Tomes, *The Gospel of Germs: Men, Women and the Microbe in American Life* (Cambridge, MA: Harvard University Press, 1998).

35   See Rodger Streitmatter, *Unspeakable: The Rise of the Gay and Lesbian Press in America* (Boston: Faber & Faber, 1995), p. 261.

36   Marie Blackwell, "AIDS in the Family," *Essence* (August 1985): 56, 106.

37   See Suzanne E. and James Hatty, *The Disordered Body: Epidemic Disease and Cultural Transformation* (Albany: SUNY Press, 1999), p. 15.

38   On Tuskegee, see Sander L. Gilman, "AIDS and Syphilis: The Iconography of Disease," in Crimp, ed., *AIDS: Cultural Analysis*, p. 100; and see James H. Jones, *Bad Blood: The Tuskegee Syphilis Experiment* (New York: Free Press, 1981).

39   Elisabeth Kübler-Ross, *AIDS: The Ultimate Challenge* (New York: Macmillan, 1987), p. 23.

40   Betty Clare Moffatt, *When Someone You Love Has AIDS: A Book of Hope for Family and Friends* (New York: Plume, 1986), p. 5.

41   See James Kinsella, *Covering the Plague: AIDS and the American Media* (New Brunswick, NJ: Rutgers University Press, 1989), pp. 76, 136.

42   Bobbie Stasey, *Just Hold Me While I Cry: A Mother's Life-Enriching Reflections on Her Family's Emotional Journey through AIDS* (Albuquerque: Elysian Hills, 1993), p. 12 (italics in original).

43   Bytsura's photograph is in Ted Gott, *Don't Leave Me This Way: Art in the Age of AIDS* (Canberra: National Gallery of Australia; New York: Thames and Hudson, 1994), p. 58. On the theme of gay sex and death, see Liz Grosz and Elspeth Probyn, eds., *Sexy Bodies: The Strange Carnalities of Feminism* (New York: Routledge, 1995), p. 297.

44   See Cindy Ruskin, "Taking Up Needles and Thread to Honor the Dead Helps AIDS Survivors Patch Up Their Lives," *People* (12 October 1987): 44, and *The Quilt: Stories from the NAMES Project* (New York: Pocket Books, 1988), p. 78.

45   See Paul Monette, *Last Watch of the Night: Essays Too Personal and Otherwise* (New York: Harcourt Brace, 1994), p. 109.

46   On violence against the Ray family, for example, see Gilman, "AIDS and Syphilis," p. 105. On violence against Ryan White, see Feldman and Miller, *AIDS Crisis*, p. 113, and Tomes, *Gospel of Germs*, p. 256.

47   See Koop, "The Early Days of AIDS," pp. 15–16.

48   Ric N. Caric, "Hideous Monsters before the Eye: Delirium Tremens and Manhood in Antebellum Philadelphia," in this volume.

49   Jean Baker, *Family Secrets: Gay Sons, A Mother's Story* (New York: Harrington Park Press, 1998), p. 5.

50   See Erika Doss, *Twentieth-Century American Art* (New York: Oxford University Press, 2002), p. 223.

51   Baker, *Family Secrets*, p. 5. See also Peter Nardi, "AIDS and Obituaries: The Perception of Stigma in the Press," in Michelle Cochrane, ed., *When AIDS Began: San Francisco and the Making of an Epidemic* (New York: Routledge, 2004), pp. 159–68.

52   Peabody, *Screaming Room*, p. 153.

53   See Michael S. Sherry, "The Language of War in AIDS Discourse," in Timothy F. Murphy and Suzanne Poirier, eds., *Writing AIDS: Gay Literature, Language, and Analysis* (New York: Columbia University Press, 1993), p. 40.

54   Peabody, *Screaming Room*, p. 154.

55   Michael Tidmus, "Prophylaxis: Blind Admonition," in "From a Life: Selections Gay and Grave" (1993), in Gott, *Don't Leave Me This Way*, p. 227.

56   See Philippe Aries, *Western Attitudes toward Death: From the Middle Ages to the Present* (Baltimore: Johns Hopkins University Press, 1974), p. 87. See also David Dempsey,

The Way We Die: An Investigation of Death and Dying in America Today (New York: Macmillan, 1975), pp. 124f.

57 Duane Michals, "The Father Prepares His Dead Son for Burial" (1991), reproduced in Gott, *Don't Leave Me This Way*, p. 130.

58 See Altman, *AIDS in the Mind of America*, p. 118. See also Ronald Bayer, *Private Acts, Social Consequences: AIDS and the Politics of Public Health* (New Brunswick, NJ: Rutgers University Press, 1989), p. 169.

59 See Peter Arno and Karyn Feiden, *Against the Odds: The Story of AIDS Drug Development, Politics, and Profits* (New York: HarperCollins, 1992), pp. 18, 84.

60 See Altman, *AIDS in the Mind of America*, p. 121; Fox, "AIDS and American Health Policy," p. 335.

61 See Clendinen and Nagourney, *Out for Good*, pp. 547f, and T.V. Reed, *The Art of Protest: Culture and Activism from the Civil Rights Movement to the Streets of Seattle* (Minneapolis: University of Minnesota Press, 2005), pp. 179–213.

62 See Timothy McDarrah, "An AIDS Victim Protests from Beyond Grave," *New York Times*, Obituaries (2 November 1992), and Sarah Wood, "Coffin Protest," *New York Newsday* (3 November 1992); both articles in Lesbian Herstory Archives, Collection # 91-1, ACT UP.

63 Mark Lowe Fisher, "Bury Me Furiously," in Lesbian Herstory Archives, Collection # 91-1, ACT UP.

64 Michael Denneny, "A Quilt of Many Colors: AIDS Writing and the Creation of Culture," *Christopher Street* 12.9, Issue 141 (1989): 16, 18.

65 Robert John Florence, "Coming In," *Out/Look* 2.6 (Fall 1989): 67.

66 James Edwin Parker, "Snakes, Trolls, and Drag Queens," in Dean Kostos and Eugene Grygo, eds., *Mama's Boy: Gay Men Write about Their Mothers* (New York: Painted Leaf Press, 2000), p. 106.

67 See Greg Lamp, "Back to the Farm to Die," *Farm Journal* (January 1991): 17–20.

68 *Our Sons*, dir. John Erman (1991).

69 See Rosalind Solomon, "Untitled," in *Portraits in the Time of AIDS*, exhibition catalog (New York: New York University, Grey Art Gallery, 1988), p. 11.

70 See Kübler-Ross, *AIDS: The Ultimate Challenge*, pp. 32–3, 35–7.

71 Cornell University, Division of Rare and Manuscript Collections, Collection #7615, Michael Ellis, box 2, file 22, *Time Magazine* (12 August 1985): 47; and Scott Haller, "Fear and AIDS in Hollywood," *People* (23 September 1985): 33.

72 See D'Emilio and Freedman, *Intimate Matters*, p. 356, and Altman, *AIDS in the Mind of America*, p. 83. See also Michael Henquist, "An Epidemic in the Family," *The Advocate* 404 (2 October 1984): 29, 56, and Gregory M. Herek and Beverly Greene, *AIDS, Identity, and Community: The HIV Epidemic and Lesbian and Gay Men* (Thousand Oaks, CA: Sage Publications, 1995), p. 4.

73 Baker, *Family Secrets*, p. 181.

Bibliography

Primary Sources: Archives

ACT UP, Brooklyn, New York

Fisher, Mark Lowe. "Bury Me Furiously." Lesbian Herstory Archives, Collection #91-1.

McDarrah, Timothy. "An AIDS Victim Protests from Beyond Grave." *New York Times*, Obituaries (2 November 1992). Lesbian Herstory Archives, Collection, #91-1.

Wood, Sarah. "Coffin Protest." *New York Newsday* (3 November 1992). Lesbian Herstory Archives, Collection, #91-1.

Canadian Women's Movement Archives, Ottawa, Canada.

The Bolster, Vancouver (August 1981 to May 1983).

City Archives of Philadelphia

"Men's Register" and "Women's Register," Alms House.

Cornell University, Ithaca, New York

Cornell University, Division of Rare and Manuscript Collections. Collection #7615, Michael Ellis, box 2, file 22.

Ellison, Jenny, Personal Collection

Cold Mountain Institute Vancouver Workshops, September–November 1979.

Cold Mountain Journal.

LaL Newsletter, Calgary 1.1 (January 1983).

Historical Society of Pennsylvania

Anonymous. "Observations on Mania a Potu." 1830.

Fire Company Collection.

Schell, Frank H. "Old Volunteer Fire Laddies, the Famous, Fast, Faithful, Fistic, Fire Fighters of Bygone Days." Frank H. Schell Papers. 1920.

Snowden, Isaac. "An Inaugural Essay on Delirium tremens." 1817.

Kotalik, J., Personal Collection

Kotalik, Dr. J. "A Case-Control Study of the Effectiveness of Cervical Cytology Screening in North-Western Ontario." Presentation notes found among Dr. Kotalik's personal collection of files, n.d.

Kotalik et al. "The Effectiveness of Cervical Cancer Screening in Northwestern Ontario." Draft of report from Dr. J. Kotalik's personal files gathered during his study in the late 1980s, p. 1.

London Borough of Hackney Archives

D/S/54/3 "NCCPC Newsletter – 1966."

National Archives for Black Women's History (NABWH), Mary McLeod Bethune Council House Historic Site.

National Council of Negro Women Records (NCNW) in the NABWH, "Estelle Obsorne, 80, Is Dead: Leader in Nursing Profession," *New York Times* (17 December 1981): D23.

NCNW Records in the NABWH, letter by Estelle Osborne to "Friends" (16 April 1963), series 10, box 19, folder 13.

NCNW Records, "Conquer Uterine Cancer: An American Cancer Society Project in cooperation with the National Council of Negro Women," series 10, box 19, folder 13.

National Archives of Canada

"Briefing Notes for the Minister – Cervical Cancer Screening." Page 2, RG 29, file 630-75-1.

Canada – Advisory Committee on Medical Research. RG 29, file 311-C1-31, vol. 1180.

Canada – Advisory Committee on Medical Research. RG 29, file 311-C1-31, vol. 1180. Canada. Fall 1978. Page 2, RG 29, file 6030-75-1.

"Cancer Conference – Ottawa." 1947. RG 29, file 311-C1-37, vol. 1183.

"Control of Cancer of the Uterine Cervix: A National Health Objective." Draft – Surveillance and Risk Assessment Divisions, Health and Welfare Canada. 1988. RG 29, file 6760-4-3.

Dr. Ernest Ayre. *National Research Council of Canada – Advisory Committee on Medical Research.* 1947–48. RG 29, file 311-C1-31, vol. 1180.

"Have You Had a Pap Test Recently?" Health and Welfare Canada. Fall 1978. RG 29, file 6030-75-1, p. 2.

Health and Welfare Canada. "Questionnaire on the Impact of the Walton Report on Cervical Cancer Screening Programs." RG 29-2, file 6030-75-1.

Health and Welfare Canada. "Questionnaire on the Impact of the Walton Report on Cervical Cancer Screening Programs." RG 29-1-4, file 6030-75-1.

"Health Objective." Draft – Surveillance and Risk Assessment Divisions, Health and Welfare Canada. 1988. RG 29, file 6760-4-3.

House of Commons Standing Committee on Health and Welfare. Minutes of Proceedings and Evidence. 3 October 1967.

"In Situ Cervical Cancer in Young Women." Ontario Medical Association Report to Council. 18–19 June 1984. Committee on Child Welfare. RG 29, file 6760-4-3, box 75.

National Cancer Institute of Canada. "Briefing Notes for the Minister – Cervical Cancer Screening." RG 29, file 311-C1-21, vol. 1180.

Powell, Marion. *Report on Therapeutic Abortion Services in Ontario: A Study Commissioned by the Ministry of Health.* 27 January 1987.

Report of the Royal Commission on the Status of Women. Ottawa: Information Canada, 1970.

"The Role of Mass Surveys in the Detection of Cancer." RG 29, file 311-C1-8.

National Cancer Institute (U.S.)

Miller, B.A., et al., eds. *Racial/Ethnic Patterns of Cancer in the United States 1988–1992, National Cancer Institute.* NIH Pub. No. 96-4104. Bethesda, MD, 1996.

National Cancer Institute. *El Papanicolaou: I Un Habíto Saludable, Para Toda La Vida!* Bethesda, MD: Oficina de Comunicación sobre el Cáncer, Instituto Nacional del Cáncer, 1998.

National Cancer Institute. "Pap Tests: A Healthy Habit for Life." National Institutes of Health, Public Health Service, NIH Publication No. 96-3213, updated July 2001.

Partridge, Kate, Personal Collection

The Bolster, Vancouver (August 1983 to November 1984).

Large as Life Newsletter, Calgary (January 1983 to October 1984).

YMCA Fitness Leadership Course. Vancouver YMCA, 1981.

Provincial Archives of Ontario

"Cancer Research – Pap Smear, 1964." RG 10, file 1-1-3.40.

"A Cytology Screening Programme for Cancer of the Cervix in the Province of Ontario, Draft 1965." RG 10, file 71-4-5.

"Ontario Cervical Screening Program: Strategic Plan." Division of Preventive Oncology Cancer Care Ontario, 1999, p. 1.

Personal letter addressed to Hon. J.W. Spooner from M.B. Dymond, Minister of Health. 23 December 1963. RG 10, file 1-1-3.40.

University of Pennsylvania Van Pelt-Dietrich Library

Burton, William. "Burton's Comic Songster." 1838.

Lea, Willis M. "An Essay on Mania a Potu." 1826.

Randolph, Charles. "An Essay upon Mania a Potu." 1825.

Thomas, Richard Henry. "An Inaugural Essay on Mania á Potu." 1827.

Washington, James. "An Inaugural Dissertation on Delirium tremens." 1827.

U.S Library of Congress

Fitch Correspondence. Peter Force Collection.

Wellcome Institute Archives

"Medical Women's Federation." F13-file SA-NWF-F13 – 1.

SA/MWF/F.13/3. Draft newsletter. 1965. "National Cervical Cancer Prevention Campaign – How the Campaign Began."

Women's Institute Archive

"History of the Cancer Detection Clinic." N4-Container 45.

"History of the Cancer Detection Clinic – Women's College Hospital." N4-Container 59-file 1.

Primary Sources: Books

Adair, F.L., ed. *Maternal Care: The Principles of Antepartum, Intrapartum, and Postpartum Care for the Practitioner of Obstetrics.* 2nd ed. Chicago: University of Chicago Press, 1941.

Albutt, H. Arthur. *The Wife's Handbook: How a Woman Should Order Herself during Pregnancy, in the Lying-in Room, and after Delivery.* Sydney: Modern Medical Publishing Co., 1890s.

Anonymous. "Spanking Jack and Other Songs." In "Songs, 1805." Philadelphia: Library Company of Philadelphia, 1805.

Arthur, T.S. *Six Nights with the Washingtonians.* Philadelphia, 1841.

Badgley, Robin F., Denyse Fortin Caron, and Marion G. Powell. *Committee on the Operation of the Abortion Law.* Ottawa: Minister of Supply and Services Canada, 1977.

Barbo, Beverly. *The Walking Wounded: A Mother's True Story of Her Son's Homosexuality and His Eventual AIDS-Related Death.* Lindsborg, KS: Carlsons', P.O. Box 364, 1987.

Bate, J.W. *The Book of Secrets and Private Medical Adviser.* Chicago, 1895.

Bell, Suzanne. "Fitness for Large Women." In Catrina Brown and Karin Jasper, eds., *Consuming Passions: Feminist Approaches to Weight Preoccupation and Eating Disorders.* Toronto: Second Story Press, 1993.

Benevolent Society of New South Wales. *Report of the Benevolent Society of New South Wales. For the year ending 31st December 1888.* Sydney: Benevolent Society of New South Wales, 1889.

Black, George. *Everybody's Medical Adviser and Consulting Family Physician.* Sydney: William Dobell & Co, n.d.

Boston Women's Health Course Collective. *Our Bodies, Ourselves.* Boston: New England Free Press, 1971.

Bowes, Nancy, Varda Burstyn, and Andrea Knight. *Access Granted: Too Often Denied: A Special Report to Celebrate the 10th Anniversary of the Decriminalization of Abortion.* Ottawa: CARAL, 1998.

Brewer, Gail Sforza, and Tom Brewer. *What Every Pregnant Woman Should Know: The Truth about Diet and Drugs in Pregnancy.* Rev. ed. New York: Penguin, 1977, 1984.

Burfoot, Annette. "The Fetal Voyager: Women in Modern Medical Visual Discourse." In Bernard Lightman and Ann Shteir, eds., *Figural Vocabularies of*

Gender in Science, Medicine, and Technology. Hanover, NH: University Press of New England, 2006. Pp. 337–56.

———. "Surprising Origins in Italian Horror: Florentine 18th-Century Wax Anatomical Models." In Anthony Tamburri, ed., *Italian Cultural Studies 2002*. Boca Raton: Bordighiera Press, 2006. Pp. 38–50.

Butler, Sandra, and Barbara Rosenblum. *Cancer in Two Voices*, 2nd ed. San Francisco: Spinsters Ink Books, 1996.

Carrington, William J. *Safe Convoy: The Expectant Mother's Handbook*. Philadelphia: J.B. Lippincott, 1944.

Castallo, Mario, and Audrey Walz. *Expectantly Yours: A Book for Expectant Mothers and Prospective Fathers*. New York: Macmillan, 1943.

Chavasse, P.H. *Man's Strength and Woman's Beauty. A Treatise on The Physical Life of Both Sexes*. Melbourne: Standard Publishing Co., 1879.

Childbirth by Choice Trust. *No Choice: Canadian Women Tell Their Stories of Illegal Abortion*. Toronto: Childbirth by Choice Trust, 1998.

Coghlan, T.A. *The Wealth and Progress of New South Wales, 1900–01*. Sydney: William Applegate Gullick, 1902.

Curtis, Jamie Lee, and Laura Cornell. *I'm Gonna Like Me: Letting Off a Little Self-Esteem*. New York: HarperCollins, 2002.

Cutter, Calvin. *First Book of Anatomy*. Philadelphia, 1854.

Danforth, William C. *A Woman's Health*. New York: Farrar & Rinehart, 1941.

De Lee, Sol T. *Safeguarding Motherhood*. Philadelphia: J.B. Lippincott, 1949.

Eisenberg, Arlene, Heidi Eisenberg Markoff, and Sandee Eisenberg Hathaway, *What to Expect When You're Expecting*. New York: Workman, 1984.

Ellis, John. *The Avoidable Causes of Disease, Insanity and Deformity*. New York, 1860.

Encyclopædia Anatomica. Köln, Germany: Taschen, 1999.

Fawcett, B. *Childbirth without Danger and Nearly Painless*. Sydney: F. Cunningham & Co. Printers, 1882.

Findlen, Paula. *Possessing Nature: Museums, Collecting and Scientific Culture in Early Modern Italy*. Berkeley: University of California Press, 1994.

Fitch, John. *The Autobiography of John Fitch*. Ed. Frank D. Praeger. Philadelphia: American Philosophical Society, 1976.

Fonda, Jane. *Jane Fonda's Workout Book*. New York: Simon & Schuster, 1981.

Foucault, Michel. *Madness and Civilization*. New York: Routledge, 2006.

Francis, Alexander. *Pregnancy and Normal Labour: A Practical Guide for the Use of Mothers and Nurses Living in the Bush*. Brisbane: Outridge & Co., 1891.

Fullerton, George. *The Family Medical Guide*. Sydney: William Maddock, 1884.

Gallup, George H. *The Gallup Poll: Public Opinion 1935–1971*. New York: Random House, 1972.

Genné, William H. *Husbands and Pregnancy: The Handbook for Expectant Fathers*. New York: Association Press, 1956.

Goodrich, Frederick W., Jr. *Natural Childbirth: A Manual for Expectant Parents.* Englewood Cliffs, NJ: Prentice-Hall, 1950.

Groll, Jeremy, and Lorie Groll. *Fertility Foods: Optimize Ovulation and Conception through Food Choices.* New York: Simon & Schuster, 2006.

Guttmacher, Herbert. *Into this Universe: The Story of Human Birth.* New York: Viking Press, 1937.

———. *Pregnancy, Birth, and Family Planning: A Guide for Expectant Parents in the 1970s.* New York: Viking Press, 1973.

History of the American Society for the Control of Cancer, 1913–1943. New York: New York City Cancer Committee, 1944.

Hope, Jackqueline. *Big, Bold and Beautiful.* Toronto: Macmillan Canada, 1996.

The Irish Journey: Women's Stories of Abortion. Dublin: Irish Family Planning Association, 2000.

Lodge, David. *A David Lodge Trilogy: Changing Places, Small World, Nice Work.* London: Penguin Books, 1993.

Lykke, Nina. "Feminist Cultural Studies of Technoscience." In Anneke Smelik and Nina Lykke, eds., *Bits of Life: Feminism at the Intersections of Media, Bioscience, and Technology.* Seattle: University of Washington Press, 2008.

Milinaire, Caterine. *Birth: Facts and Legends.* New York: Harmony Books, 1974.

Moffatt, Betty Clare. *When Someone You Love Has AIDS: A Book of Hope for Family and Friends.* New York: Plume, 1986.

Monette, Paul. *Last Watch of the Night: Essays Too Personal and Otherwise.* New York: Harcourt Brace, 1994.

Mosher, Clelia Duel. *The Mosher Survey: Sexual Attitudes of 45 Victorian Women.* Ed. James MaHood and Kristine Wenburg. Intro. Carl N. Degler. New York: Arno Press, 1980.

Muskett, Philip E. *The Illustrated Australian Medical Guide.* 2 vols. Sydney: William Brooks & Co., 1903.

Nathanielsz, Peter, and Christopher Vaughan. *The Prenatal Prescription.* New York: HarperCollins, 2001.

National Research Council, Committee on Maternal Nutrition. *Maternal Nutrition and the Course of Pregnancy.* Washington, DC: National Academy of Sciences, 1970.

The New Negro Forget-Me-Not Songster: Containing All the New Negro Songs Ever Published, with a Choice Collection of Ballad Songs, Now Sung in Concerts. Cincinnati: Stratton & Barnard, 1848.

O'Sullivan, M.U. *The Proclivity of Civilised Woman to Uterine Displacement: The Antidote. Also Other Contributions to Gynaecological Surgery.* Melbourne: Stillwell & Co. Printers, 1894.

Pancoast, S., and C.C. Vanderbeck. *The Ladies' New Medical Guide.* Rev. ed. Philadelphia: John E. Potter, 1890.

Papanicolaou, George N., and Herbert Frederick Traut. *Diagnosis of Uterine Cancer by the Vaginal Smear.* New York: Commonwealth Fund, 1943.

Paré, Ambroise. *On Monsters and Marvels*. Trans. Janis L. Pallister. 1571. Chicago: University of Chicago Press, 1995.

Parry, John B. "The Firemen's Songster." Philadelphia: Library Company of Philadelphia, 1855.

Peabody, Barbara. *The Screaming Room: A Mother's Journal of Her Son's Struggle with AIDS: A True Story of Love, Courage, and Dedication*. San Diego, CA: Oak Tree Publishers, 1986.

Pelrine, Eleanor Wright. *Abortion in Canada*. Toronto: New Press, 1972.

Powers, Doris. "Statement to the Abortion Caravan." In *Women Unite! An Anthology of the Canadian Women's Movement*. Toronto: Canadian Women's Educational Press, 1972.

Reed, Paul. *Facing It: A Novel of AIDS*. San Francisco: Gay Sunshine Press, 1984.

Richards, F.C., and S. Edin Eutalia. *Ladies Handbook of Home Treatment*. Melbourne: Signs Publishing Co., 1905.

Rodale, Ardath. *Climbing toward the Light: A Journey of Growth, Understanding, and Love*. Emmaus, PA: Good Spirit Press, 1989.

Rollin, Betty. *First, You Cry*. New York: Harper Paperbacks, 2000.

Ruskin, Cindy. *The Quilt: Stories from the NAMES Project*. New York: Pocket Books, 1988.

Schiebinger, Londa. "Skeletons in the Closet: The First Illustrations of the Female Skeleton in Eighteenth-Century Anatomy." In Londa Schiebinger, ed., *Feminism and the Body*. New York: Oxford University Press, 2000.

Schrader, Christian. *Popular Medical Guide*. Sydney: Direct Supply Company, 1887.

Schultz, Dodi. *Have Your Baby – and Your Figure, Too!* New York: Pyramid Books, 1970.

Sedgwick, Eve. *The Epistemology of the Closet*. Berkeley: University of California Press, 1990.

Shaw, Jessica. *Reality Check: A Close Look at Accessing Abortion Services in Canadian Hospitals*. Ottawa: Canadians for Choice, 2006.

Slemons, J. Morris. *The Nutrition of the Fetus*. New Haven, CT: Yale University Press, 1919.

———. *The Prospective Mother: A Handbook for Women during Pregnancy*. New York: D. Appleton & Co., 1919.

Stasey, Bobbie. *Just Hold Me While I Cry: A Mother's Life-Enriching Reflections on Her Family's Emotional Journey through AIDS*. Albuquerque: Elysian Hills, 1993.

Stevens, Anne E. *Maternity Handbook for Pregnant Mothers and Expectant Fathers by the Maternity Center Association, New York City*. New York: G.P. Putnam's Sons, 1932.

Temperance Lecturer and Almanac of the American Temperance Union. Philadelphia: Library Company of Philadelphia, 1844.

Temperance Monitor. Philadelphia: Library Company of Philadelphia, 1836, 1838.

Thompson, Rezin. *The Medical Adviser: Full and Plain Treatise on the Theory and Practice of Medicine Especially Adapted to Family Use*. Melbourne: Standard Publishing Co., 1884.

Thoms, Herbert, with Laurence G. Roth. *Understanding Natural Childbirth: A Book for the Expectant Mother*. New York: McGraw-Hill, 1950.

Trott, Lona L. *American Red Cross Home Nursing*. Philadelphia: Blakiston, 1942.

White, Phillip S. *Journal of the Proceedings of the National Division of the Sons of Temperance*. Philadelphia: Library Company of Philadelphia,1847.

Wright, Erna. *The New Childbirth*. New York: Hart Publishing, 1966.

Zabriskie, Louise. *Mother and Baby Care in Pictures*. 3rd ed. Philadelphia: J.P. Lippincott, 1946.

Primary Sources: Journal Articles, Newspapers, and Magazines

"16,000 Women." *Cancer News* 11.1 (1957): 2–9.

"2002 Women of the Year." *Ms. Magazine* (December 2002). http://msmagazine.com/dec02/womenoftheyear.asp (accessed 26 October 2005).

"Abortions up 25.6 percent." *Canadian News Facts* (16–30 November 1973): 1113.

Allegretti, Esther. "Dr. George N. Papanicolaou: Profile." *Cancer News* (Summer 1957): 13–15.

"America's 10 Best Bodies." *McCall's* (May 1985): 104–9, 148, 150.

Anderson, L.S. "The Mushroom Crowd: Social and Political Aspects of Population Pressure." *CMAJ* 91 (5 December 1964): 1213–22.

Anglin, Gerald. "The Pill That Could Shake the World." *Chatelaine* (October 1953): 16–17, 99–103.

Baldwin, W.F. "To the Editor: True Ovarian Failure?" *CMAJ* (18 March 1967): 681.

Balls-Headley, Dr. "Case of Porro's Operation on a Ricketty Dwarf – Recovery." *Australian Medical Journal (AMJ)* (15 December 1886).

Bart, Peter. "Explosive Summer Action: Debating Truth about 'Lies.'" http://www.variety.com (accessed 3 September 2006).

Bartel, Pauline. "Women at Large – Empathy Is Key to Helping 'Fluffy Ladies' Regain Esteem." *St. Petersburg Times* (5 April 1987): 6F.

Barton, Mary. "Review of the Sanitary Appliance with a Discussion on Intra-Vaginal Packs," *British Medical Journal* 1 (25 April 1942): 524–5.

Batten, Jack. "Is There a Male Conspiracy against the Pill?" *Chatelaine* (July 1969): 17, 40.

———. "Is This Operation Necessary?" *Chatelaine* (August 1975): 48, 56–8.

Beeston, Joseph L. "Obstetrical Statistics – A Record of 800 Cases of Midwifery with Analysis and Observations." *Australasian Medical Gazette (AMG)* (September 1891).

Bell, Suzanne. "Fat and Fit: Classes for Women." *Kinesis* (May 1984).

Benson, Ezra Taft, with Theodore Irwin. "American Nutrition Paradox: Want Amidst Plenty." *Today's Health* (May 1960): 23–5, 66–7.

Berzi, A., C. Cipriani, and M. Poggesi. "Florentine Science Museums." *Journal of the Society for the Bibliography of Natural History* 9.4 (1980): 423.

"The Best Body in Movies: Jamie Lee Curtis." *Harper's Bazaar* (May 1985): 182–3, 212.

Bird, F.D. "President's Address." *Intercolonial Medical Journal of Australia* 1 (January 1896).

Blackwell, Marie. "AIDS in the Family." *Essence* (August 1985): 56, 105–8.

Bliss, Betsy. "Do-It-Yourself Cervical Cancer Test." *Toronto Star* (20 June 1967): 46.

Bond, Tony. "Conception and Birth: Birth Control ... a Factual Survey ... Abortion." *Varsity: Review* (12 March 1965).

Bourque, Jacques. "AIDS: Where's It Left Us?" *Angles*, Vancouver (May 1986): 11.

Brody, Jane. "HPV Vaccine: Few Risks, Many Benefits." *New York Times* (15 May 2007): 7.

Byrne, William S. "Fevers of the Puerperal State." *AMG* (August 1890).

Calio, Jim. "Jamie Lee's Special Gift." *Redbook* (1 April 1998). http://global.factiva .com (accessed 29 November 2005).

"A Case of Caesarean Section." *AMG* (October 1886).

Cassels, Derek. "Now the Good news ... about Breast Cancer." *Chatelaine* (June 1973): 50.

Chernick, Beryl A. "Blood Pressure and Body Weight Changes during Oral Contraceptive Treatment." *CMAJ* (28 September 1968): 593–9.

Chin, Paula. "Making a Splash." *People* (22 August 1994). http://global.factiva.com (accessed 23 October 2005).

"The CMA Comments on the Food and Drug Committee Report 'Hazards of the Oral Contraceptive.'" Association News: Special Supplement. *CMAJ* (19 December 1970): 1417.

Cooley, Donald G. "Men Behind the Medical Miracles – Part II." *Today's Health* 37 (February 1959): 24–5, 66–7.

Coopersmith, B.I. "Dexedrine and Weight Control in Pregnancy." *American Journal of Obstetrics and Gynecology* 58.4 (1949): 664–72.

Corbin, T.W. "Case of Ectopic Gestation." *AMG* (December 1891).

———. "Midwifery Experiences." *AMG* (May 1892).

Cruse, Howard. "Safe Sex." *Christopher Street* 7.7, Issue 79 (1983): 5.

Cunningham, A.J. "Letters to the Journal: Physicians and Contraception." *CMAJ* (9 January 1965): 87.

Curtis, Lindsay. "Your Health." *Toronto Star* (5 September 1973): E4.

———. "Your Health." *Toronto Star* (25 January 1974): D2.

Dempsey, Laura. "The Reading Life: Honesty Fits Curtis Perfectly." *Dayton Daily News* (24 August 2002). http://global.factiva.com (accessed 21 October 2005).

Denneny, Michael. "A Quilt of Many Colors: AIDS Writing and the Creation of Culture." *Christopher Street* 12.9, Issue 141 (1989): 15–21.

Dickinson, J.H., and G.C. Smith, "A New and Practical Oral Contraceptive Agent: Norethindrone with Mestranol." *CMAJ* (10 August 1963): 242–5.

Dooren, Jennifer Corbett. "Merck Cervical-Cancer Vaccine Is Approved for Use in Women: Gardasil Could Sharply Cut Key Viruses Behind Disease." *Wall Street Journal* (9 June 2006): 16.

"Doubt U.S. Cancer Test Economical for Ontario." *Toronto Star* (21 October 1955): 62.

Dukelow, D.A. "School for Expectant Families." *Today's Health* (March 1950): 31, 53.

Dunlop, Marilyn. "Pioneer of the A-Bomb Now Making War on Cancer." *Toronto Star* (5 July 1971): 5.

———. "Men May Hold Virus That Causes Cancer in Women: Scientist." *Toronto Star* (5 April 1973): 49.

"The Editor Replies." *CMAJ* (9 January 1965): 88.

Editorial. "Psychopathology of the Pill." *CMAJ* (31 January 1970): 217.

Editorial. "Thromboembolic Disease and Oral Contraceptives." *CMAJ* (5 August 1967): 302.

Eggerston, Laura. "Adverse Events Reported for HPV Vaccine." *CMAJ* 177.10 (2007).

"Expect to Look Your Best." *Good Housekeeping* (January 1960): 66–73.

Fasten, Nathan. "The Myth of Prenatal Influence." *Today's Health* (October 1950): 27, 42.

Fisher, Douglas. "This Noise of Women Gags Voice of Reason." *Vancouver Sun* (19 May 1970).

Fitzgerald, T.N. "Presidential Address, Medical Society of Victoria." *AMJ* (15 January 1880).

"Flab and All." *Globe and Mail* (7 September 2002).

Florence, Robert John. "Coming In." *Out/Look* 2.6 (Fall 1989): 67.

Foreman, J. "Notes on Two Cases of Caesarean Section." *AMG* (20 September 1900).

Fortescue, George. "Case of Ovarian Disease." *AMG* (April 1884).

Galton, Lawrence. "What's New in Health: Who Forgets the Pill?" *Chatelaine* (May 1965): 16.

Garde, H.C. "A Case of Porro's Operation for Rachitis of the Pelvis." *AMG* (March 1888).

Gay Comix 6 (Winter 1985): back cover.

Gillen, Mollie. "Our New Abortion Law: Already Outdated?" *Chatelaine* (November 1969).

———. "Why Women Are Still Angry over Abortion." *Chatelaine* (October 1970).

Globe and Mail (7 September 2002, 2 August 2003, 17 September 2003).

Godson, Clement. "Porro's Operation." *British Medical Journal* (*BMJ*) 26 (January 1884).

Goodstein, David B. "Our Sweet 16th: Remembering 1967." *The Advocate* 377 (29 September 1983): 30.

Graham, Sir James. "Obstetric Nursing with Special Reference to Savage Races." *Australasian Nurses Journal* 2 (1904): 54.

Gray, Muriel. "Is This a Feminist Statement?" *The Guardian* (22 August 2002). http://global.factiva.com (accessed 21 October 2005).

The Guardian (22 August 2002).

Haller, Scott. "Forget What the Song Says – Don't Call Jamie Lee Curtis the Closest Thing to Perfect." *People* (24 June 1985): 93.

———. "Fear and AIDS in Hollywood." *People* (23 September 1985): 33.

Hamilton, J.A.G. "Midwifery Experiences." *AMG* (April 1892).

Hardie, David. "Case of Extra-Uterine Pregnancy – Operation at the Eighth Month." *AMG* (20 June 1896).

Harper's Bazaar (May 1985).

Harris, Gardiner. "Panel Unanimously Recommends Cervical Cancer Vaccine for Girls 11 and Up." *New York Times* (30 June 2006): A12.

Harrison, Mrs. D. "Letter to the Editor: 'Who Forgets the Pill?'" *Chatelaine* (August 1965): 68.

Haviland, Thomas N., and Lawrence Charles Parish. "A Brief Account of the Use of Wax Models in the Study of Medicine." *Journal of the History of Medicine* 1 (1970): 52–75.

Hawker, Philippa. "The Body Swap Politic." *The Age* (1 November 2003). http://global.factiva.com (accessed 28 December 2005).

Hawkins, John H.W. "Address of Mr. Hawkins, at Faneuil Hall, Boston." Eleventh Annual Report of the Maryland State Temperance Society, Baltimore, 1842.

Haynes, E.J.A. "Abdominal Extra-Uterine Foetation of Eight Months Duration – Operation." *AMG* (October 1892).

"Hazards of the Oral Contraceptive." Medical News: Special Supplement. *CMAJ* (30 May 1970): 1193.

"Health." *Chatelaine* (January 1972, May 1972).

Henig, Robin. "AIDS: A New Disease's Deadly Odyssey." *New York Times Magazine* (6 February 1983): 36.

Henquist, Michael. "An Epidemic in the Family." *The Advocate* 404 (2 October 1984): 29 and 56.

Higgans, Mrs. E.M. "Letter to the Editor." *Chatelaine* 35.2 (February 1962): 92.

Hilloowala, Rumy. "Illustrations from the Wellcome Institute Library: The Origin of the Wellcome Anatomical Waxes *albinus* and the Florentine Collection at *La Specola*." *Medical History* 28 (1984): 432–7.

Hooper, J.W. Dunbar. "Case of Pregnancy with Carcinoma of Cervix." *AMJ* (15 September 1889).

Hopkinson, Francis. "Account of the Federal Procession of July 4, 1788." *American Museum*, Philadelphia 8 (July 1788).

Horan, J.D., and J.J. Lederman. "To the Editor: Possible Asthmongenic Effect of Oral Contraceptives." *CMAJ* (20 July 1968): 130–1.

"How to Tell Your Daughter." *Parents Magazine* 22 (December 1947): 138.

Hughes, Kathryn. "Body Politics – A Weight off Your Mind." *The Observer* (25 August 2002). http://global.factiva.com (accessed 16 December 2005).

Jakins, W.V. "Ruptures of the Uterus." *AMJ* (15 November 1881).

"Jamie Lee Curtis." *Vogue* (June 1985).

Jamieson, James. "Puerperal Fever: Its Causes, Prevalence, and Prevention." *AMJ* (January 1879).

———. "The Present State of the Puerperal Fever Question." *AMJ* (15 June 1884).

———. "Recent Contributions to the Antiseptic Method." *AMJ* (15 July 1885).

Janssen, Jan. "Interview: Jamie Lee Curtis – Jamie Lee Freaks Out." *Daily Mirror* (19 December 2003). http://global.factiva.com (accessed 29 November 2005).

Jenkins, E.J. "Presidential Address, NSW Branch BMA." *AMG* (April 1896).

Jerome S. Peterson. "Cancer Facts for Women." *Hygeia* 24 (June 1964).

"Judy: Reaction to Book Surprised Her." *Vancouver Sun* (25 January 1969).

Kenyon, Ron. "The Pill Nobody Talks About." *Chatelaine* (November 1961): 31, 62, 64.

Kinder, Gary. "Has Jamie Lee Curtis Finally Found Herself? God Knows." *Esquire* (July 1985): 66–73.

Kingsbury, Donald. "We Send Her to the Butcher Shop." *McGill Daily* (30 October 1967).

Krista, Charlene. "Jamie Lee Curtis: An Interview." *Films in Review* 35 (August/ September 1985).

Ladies' Home Journal (July 2007).

Lamp, Greg. "Back to the Farm to Die." *Farm Journal* (January 1991): 17–20.

Lansberg, Michele. "Your Gynecologist: Show Me a Gynecologist and I'll Show You a Male Chauvinist (Even If She's a Woman)." *Chatelaine* (August 1973): 42, 64–6.

Laskas, Jeanne Marie. "Sunny, Side, Up." *Ladies' Home Journal* (July 2007): 118–26.

"The Last Word Is Yours." *Chatelaine* (August 1973): 134.

Latham, Aaron. "Looking for Mr. Goodbody." *Rolling Stone* 9 (June 1983): 20–6, 59, 61–2.

"Launch Drive to Wipe Out Uterine Cancer." *Today's Health* 39 (September 1961).

"Law's Choice – or Girls'?" Reprinted from *Toronto Star* in *Vancouver Sun* (26 May 1970).

Little, Dr. Speaker at the 16th General Meeting of the Medical Society of Queensland. *AMG* (May 1893).

Lorde, Audre. *The Cancer Journals*, special edition. San Francisco: Aunt Lute Books, 2007 [1980].

Macdonald, Ian. "House Told Money Governs Abortion." *Vancouver Sun* (28 January 1969).

Marks, C.F. "Address on Medicine as a Department of State – A Suggestion." *AMG* (20 February 1897).

Marten, R. Humphrey. "Reminiscences of the Late Lord Lister." *AMG* (23 March 1912).

Mattatall, Fiona. "A Very Real Art." *Canadian Medical Association Journal* 164.7 (2001): 1027–8.

McCall's (May 1985).

McCullough, John W.S. "The Prevention of Cancer." *Chatelaine* (November 1930): 15.

Mechanics Free Press (12 April 1828, 13 January 1830).

Meyer, Dr. President's Address, Vic Branch BMA. *AMG* (January 1895).

Miller, Samatha. "40 and Fabulous." *People* (31 August 1998). http://vnweb.hw -wilsonweb.com (accessed 29 November 2005).

More (September 2002, September 2003, September 2006).

Musgrove, J.E., and M.J. Tushig. "To the Editor: The Contraceptive Pill and Major Arterial Emboli in a Teen-Aged Girl." *CMAJ* (12 October 1968): 724–5.

Newman, Robert C. "Your Health." *Toronto Star* (27 July 1978): D8.

Nisbet, W.B. "The Education of Midwives." *AMG* (June 1891).

Nouch, Kathleen. "I Learned to Live with Cancer." *Chatelaine* (June 1959): 30, 85–8.

Nyulasy, Frank A. "Notes on a Case of Craniotomy – Subsequent Successful Induction of Premature Labour – Child Incubated." *AMG* (1898).

"Ontario Cervical Screening Program: Program Report 1997–2000." Toronto, ON: Cancer Care Ontario, n.d.

"Oral Contraceptives." *CMAJ* (10 August 1963): 270.

"Ottawa Drug Authorities Look for Better 'Pill.'" *CMAJ* (31 January 1970): 219.

Papanicolaou, George N. "Cancer That Can Be Cured." *Today's Health* (May 1958).

Pennsylvanian (8 August 1835, 29 March 1836).

People (24 June 1985, 22 August 1994, 31 August 1998).

Perkins, Gordon W. "To the Editor: Physicians and Contraception." *CMAJ* (29 March 1965): 631–2.

Perreaux, Les. "6-month Abortion Option in Wings." *Montreal Gazette* (11 September 2004).

Philadelphia Gazette (1841–42).

"Physicians and Contraception." *CMAJ* (10 October 1964): 820.

"Pills for Birth Control" *CMAJ* (28 January 1961): 227.

Port-Folio (23 February 1806).

Public Ledger (1841–48).

Radiance. 1984–2000. Available at the Nellie Langord Rowell Library, York University.

Read, George. "Letter to the Editor." *AMG* (November 1883).

Redbook. 1 April 1998.

"Review of *The Story of Menstruation*," *Journal of the American Medical Association* 133 (5 April 1947): 1033.

Richards, Cindy. "Thanks, Jamie, for Keeping It Real." *Chicago Sun-Times*
    (29 January 2003). http://global.factiva.com (accessed 17 November 2005).

Ringrose, Douglas C.A. "Current Concepts in Conception Control." *CMAJ*
    (10 August 1963): 246–48.

Rockett, Eve. "Five Days on a Fat Farm." *Chatelaine* (May 1980).

Rolling Stone. June 1983.

Rose, Tiffany. "The Interview: Jamie Lee Curtis." *Independent on Sunday*
    (7 December 2003). http://global.factiva.com (accessed 29 November 2005).

Ruben, Leon, and Arnold Rogers. "To the Editor: Neurological Symptoms and
    Oral Contraceptives." *CMAJ* (23 March 1968): 609.

Ryan, Joan. "Jamie Lee Curtis Has Nothing to Hide." *San Francisco Chronicle*
    (27 August 2002). http://global.factiva.com (accessed 21 October 2005).

San Francisco Chronicle. 15 April 1985, 27 August 2002.

Sangster, Dorothy. "I Faced Up to Cancer." *Chatelaine* (September 1954): 51.

Saunders, Adele. "Plain Talk about Cancer." *Chatelaine* (November 1945): 63.

Saunders, Vincent E. "A Memo to Negro Women: Uterine Cancer Can Be Re-
    duced." *Negro Digest* 10 (August 1961): 25–30.

Schmeck, Harold Jr. "Cancer Pioneer Nears Age of 75." *New York Times* (11 May
    1958).

Schwenger, Cope. "Abortion in Canada as a Public Health Problem and as a
    Community Health Measure." *Canadian Journal of Public Health* 64.3 (1973):
    223–30.

Seligmann, Jean, and Nikki Finke Greenburg. "Only Months to Live and No Place
    to Die: The Tragic Odyssey of a Victim Turned Pariah." *Newsweek* (12 August
    1985): 26.

Sellers, George Escol. "Memoirs." American Philosophical Society, 1898.

Sprigg, Peter. "A Promising Vaccine …" *Washington Times* (17 July 2006): A17.

Squire, Roberta. "I'm Married, Happy, and Went through Hell for a Legal Abor-
    tion." *Chatelaine* (October 1970).

Strickler, Jeff. "Acting Her Age." *Globe and Mail* (2 August 2003). http://global
    .factiva.com (accessed 18 November 2005).

Tabb, John Prosser. "Statistics of the Causes of Death in the Philadelphia Hospital,
    Blockley, during a Period of Twelve Years." *American Journal of Medical Sciences*
    8 (1844).

Tallin, G.P.R. "Legal Implications of the Non-Therapeutic Practices of Doctors."
    CMAJ (4 August 1962): 207–15.

Taylor, Kate. "Entertainment." *Globe and Mail* (17 September 2003). http://global
    .factiva.com (accessed 28 November 2005).

"Thousands of Canadian Women Have Been Needlessly Upset." The Association
    Speaks. *CMAJ* (14 February 1970): 227.

The Tickler (1807–10). Historical Society of Pennsylvania.

Tietze, Christopher, et al. "Teaching of Fertility Regulation in Medical Schools: A
    Survey in the United States and Canada, 1964." *CMAJ* (2 April 1966): 719.

"Toronto Mother Tells of Her Experiences in Having a Legal Abortion in London." *Toronto Star* (13 June 1969), reprinted in *Pro-Choice Forum* (September 1999): 8.

Toronto Star. 12 August 1994.

Trimble, George X. "To the Editor: Vascular Headaches and Oral Contraceptives." *CMAJ* (4 June 1966): 1241.

United States Gazette (28 October 1841).

Verco, J.C. "Should a Medical Man Practise Midwifery While in Charge of a Case of Puerperal Fever?" *AMG* (January 1889).

Walker, J. L. "Methyclothiazide in Excessive Weight Gain and Edema of Pregnancy." *Obstetrics and Gynecology* 27.2 (1966): 247–51.

"The Walton Report." *CMAJ* 114 (1976).

Waring, Gerald. "Report from Ottawa." *CMAJ* (28 February 1968): 419.

Warren, W. Edward. 'Notes upon Three Successful Craniotomy Operations, All in the Case of the Same Patient." *AMG* (August 1884).

Way, E.W. "Modern Research and Child-Bed Fever." *AMG* (15 August 1893).

Wearing, Morris P. "The Use of Norethindrone (2 Mg.) with Mestranol (0.1 Mg) in Fertility Control: A Preliminary Report." *CMAJ* (10 August 1963): 239–41.

Webb, Jean F. "Special Article: Canadian Thalidomide Experience." *CMAJ* (9 November 1963): 987.

"What Does a Girl Do If She's in the Middle of the School Year and Suddenly Discovers She's Pregnant?" *Varsity* (6 March 1968).

"What You Can Do about Birthmarks." *Good Housekeeping* (September 1960): 131.

White, W.L. "Killer of Women." *Ladies' Home Journal* 64 (November 1947).

Whyte, J.C. "To the Editor: Oral Contraception and Thromboembolic Disease." *CMAJ* (20 July 1968): 131.

"Women Declare War." *Pedestal* (March 1970).

"Women! You Need No Longer Die from Your No. 1 Cancer Killer." *Toronto Star* (31 March 1955): 38.

Wood, David A. "Looking ahead in Research." *Cancer News* (Winter 1957): 16.

Woodward, Elizabeth. "Do You Scare Her to Death?" *Parents* 24 (1949): 52.

Worrall, Ralph. "Ectopic Gestation Complicating Normal Pregnancy – Abdominal Section – Recovery." *AMG* (January 1893).

Zerbisias, Antonia. "*True Lies* Denigrates Women and Arabs." *Toronto Star* (12 August 1994). http://global.factiva.com (accessed 19 June 2006).

Zimm, Angela, and Justin Bloom. "FDA Approves Merck's Cervical Cancer Vaccine." *Boston Globe* (9 June 2006; accessed online 26 October 2009).

Primary Sources: Interviews

Bell, Suzanne. Interview by Jenny Ellison, digital recording. New Westminster, BC, 4 October 2005.

———. Follow-up interview by Jenny Ellison, digital recording. New Westminster, BC, 16 August 2006.

Booth, Evelyn. Interview by Jenny Ellison, digital recording. North Vancouver, BC, 11 October 2005.

Gillingham, Ruth. Interview by Jenny Ellison, digital recording. Prince Albert, SK, 27 July 2006.

Laue, Ingrid. Interview by Jenny Ellison, digital recording. North Vancouver, BC, 3 October 2005.

Low, James. Interview by Annette Burfoot at Museum of Health Care, Kingston, ON, 21 March 2002.

"Medical Edge: Ask the Mayo Clinic." *Seattle Post Intelligencer* (17 December 2007): F3.

O'Brien, Joan (Dal Santo). Interview by Jenny Ellison, digital recording. Sechelt, BC, 7 October 2005.

Partridge, Kate. Interview by Jenny Ellison, digital recording. Crediton, ON, 20 September 2005.

———. Follow-up interview by Jenny Ellison, digital recording. Exeter, ON, 16 April 2006.

———, and Joan Dal Santo. "Large as Life." Interview by Stan Peters and Ann Mitchell. *CBC Radio Noon* (Vancouver), 15 September 1981.

Peat, Carol. Interview by Jenny Ellison, digital recording. London, ON, 17 June 2006.

Sandler, Jody. Interview by Jenny Ellison, digital recording. North Vancouver, BC, 5 October 2005.

Tallman, Ellen. Interview by Jenny Ellison, digital recording. Vancouver, BC, 12 October 2005.

White, Susan. Interview by Jenny Ellison, digital recording. Winnipeg, MB, 11 July 2006.

Winslow, Marjorie. Interview by Rona Rustige, former curator of the Kingston Museum of Health Care, Belleville, ON, 13 July 1996.

Primary Sources: Media and Art

Cancer in Women. Produced by Cheryl Wright. NFB of Canada – Atlantic Region, 1974.

Girl Stuff. Churchill Films, 1982.

Gott, Ted. *Don't Leave Me This Way: Art in the Age of AIDS*. Canberra: National Gallery of Australia; New York: Thames and Hudson, 1994.

Growing Girls. Film Producers Guild, National Committee for Visual Aids in Education, 1949.

It's Wonderful Being a Girl. Johnson & Johnson, 1968.

Meigs, Joe V. *Time and Two Women.* Audio Productions, 1957. Distr. American Cancer Society.

Michals, Duane. "The Father Prepares His Dead Son for Burial" (1991). Reproduced in Ted Gott, *Don't Leave Me This Way: Art in the Age of AIDS.* Canberra: National Gallery of Australia; New York: Thames and Hudson, 1994.

Naturally a Girl. Johnson & Johnson, 1973.

Our Sons. Dir. John Erman, 1991.

Perfect Soundtrack. Arista Records, 1985.

Personal Health for Girls. Coronet Instructional Films, 1972.

Solomon, Rosalind. "Untitled," in *Portraits in the Time of AIDS*, exhibition catalog (New York: New York University, Grey Art Gallery, 1988), p. 11.

Tidmus, Michael. "Prophylaxis: Blind Admonition." In "From a Life: Selections Gay and Grave" (1993), in Ted Gott, *Don't Leave Me This Way: Art in the Age of AIDS.* Canberra: National Gallery of Australia; New York: Thames and Hudson, 1994.

Primary Sources: Pamphlets and Booklets

Birth Control Handbook. Montreal: Student's Society of McGill University, 1969.

CARAL. *Protecting Abortion Rights in Canada: A Special Report to Celebrate the 15th Anniversary of the Decriminalization of Abortion.* Ottawa: CARAL, 2003.

Cherniak, Donna, and Allan Feingold, eds. *Birth Control Handbook.* September 1969.

"Effectiveness of Strategies to Increase Cervical Cancer Screening." *Public Health Research, Education, and Development Program.* Published by Ontario Ministry of Health. P. 1.

Giller, Doris. "Abortion in Montreal." Reprinted from the *Montreal Star* in Donna Cherniak and Allan Feingold, eds., *Birth Control Handbook.* Montreal: Student's Society of McGill University, January 1969. P. 34.

Gunther von Hagens' Body Worlds: The Anatomical Exhibition of Real Human Bodies. 7th printing. Exhibition catalogue. Heidelberg: Verlagsgesellschaft, 2005.

Kingsbury, Donald. "Pregnancy and Social Action." In Donna Cherniak and Allan Feingold, eds., *Birth Control Handbook.* January 1969. Pp. 33–4.

"Ontario Is Taking Shape." CCO Newsletter (Fall 1997).

The Story of Menstruation, Walt Disney Productions, with Kimberly-Clark Corporation (1946).

Suggested Material for Teaching Mothers' Classes. Brooklyn: Maternity Center Division of the Visiting Nurse Association of Brooklyn, 1941.

Primary Sources: Websites

Burfoot, Annette. "Surprising Origins: Florentine 18th-Century Wax Anatomical Models as Inspiration for Italian Horror." *Kinoeye* 2.9 (13 May 2002). http://www.kinoeye.org/02/09/burfoot09.html (accessed 7 September 2010).

Canadian Cancer Society. http://www.cancer.ca/ccs/internet/standard/0,2939,3172_14980_langId-en,00.html (accessed February 2002).

CBS News. *The Early Show.* 21 August 2002. http://global.factiva.com (accessed 21 October 2005).

"Closing In on Cancer: The National Cancer Institute Is Founded, 1930–1950." http://press2.nci.nih.gov/sciencebehind/cioc/nci/nci.htm (official government site for NCI).

Don't Spread Germs, directed by John Krish. UK: Central Office of Information for Ministry of Health, 1948. http://www.archive.org/details/dont_spread_germs_TNA (accessed 1 August 2007).

"FDA Licenses New Vaccine for Prevention of Cervical Cancer and Other Diseases in Females Caused by Human Papillomavirus." Press release (8 June 2006). http://www.fda.gov/bbs/topics/news/2006/new01385.html (accessed 26 October 2009).

"Glory of Woman: An Introduction to Prescriptive Literature." Rare Book, Manuscript, and Special Collections Library, Duke University. http://library.duke.edu/specialcollections/bingham/guides/glory/index.html (accessed 2 June 2010).

"Growing Up and Liking It." Milltown, NJ: Personal Products Corporation, 1944. Located at Museum of Menstruation, Menarche Education Booklets. http://www158.pair.com/hfinley/guli44a.htm (accessed 6 November 2000).

"How Many Women Get Cancer of the Cervix?" American Cancer Society website. http://www.cancer.org (accessed 11 April 2009).

"HPV and Cervical Cancer." British Columbia Cancer Agency. http://www.bccancer.bc.ca/PPI/Prevention/infection/HPV.htm (accessed July 2010).

National Cancer Institute of Canada. http://www.ncic.cancer.ca (accessed August 2008).

NBC News. *Today* (21 August 2002). http://global.factiva.com (accessed 21 October 2005).

Prelinger Collection and Prelinger Archives. http://www.archive.org/details/prelinger (accessed 27 August 2007).

The Spirit of '43. A Walt Disney Donald Duck Technicolor Film. 1943. YouTube. http://www.youtube.com/watch?v=WaVTc-Ur89Q (accessed 28 August 2007).

"Swedish Tourism Fears Grow as Sweden Fights for Late Term Abortion." http://swenglishrantings.com/entry/?tag=stockholm (accessed 22 August 2008).

"TV Commercial for GARDASIL [Quadrivalent Human Papillomavirus (Types 6, 11, 16, 18) Recombinant Vaccine]." http://www.gardasil.com/tv-commercial-for-gardasil.html (accessed 15 January 2009).

"Women over 50 Still Need Pap Tests." *Ontario Cancer Facts.* October 2001.
http://www.cancercare.on.ca/reports_211.htm (accessed January 2004).

Secondary Sources: Articles

Akrich, Madeline. "The De-Scription of Technical Objects." In Wiebe E. Bijker
and John Law, eds., *Shaping Technology/Building Society: Studies in Sociotechnical Change.* Cambridge: MIT Press, 1992. Pp. 205–24.

Altman, Dennis. "Legitimation through Disaster: AIDS and the Gay Movement."
In Elizabeth Fee and Daniel Fox, eds., *AIDS: The Burdens of History.* Berkeley:
University of California Press, 1988.

Anderson, C.M., and J.G. Thornton. "Screening for Cervical Cancer Graphs May
Mislead." *BMJ* 309 (8 October 1994): 953–4.

Armstrong, David. "The Doctor–Patient Relationship: 1930–80." In Peter Wright
and Andrew Treacher, eds., *The Problem of Medical Knowledge: Examining the
Social Construction of Medicine.* Edinburgh: Edinburgh University Press, 1982.
Pp. 109–22.

Armstrong, Elizabeth M. "Lessons in Control: Prenatal Education in the Hospital." *Social Problems* 47.4 (2000): 583–605.

Backhouse, Constance. "The Celebrated Abortion Trial of Dr. Emily Stowe, Toronto, 1879." *Canadian Bulletin of Medical History/Bulletin canadien d'histoire
de la médecine* 8 (1991): 159–87.

Barker, Kristin. "Birthing and Bureaucratic Women: Needs Talk and the Definitional Legacy of the Sheppard–Towner Act." *Feminist Studies* 29.2 (Summer
2003): 344.

Barlow, Tani, et. al. "The Modern Girl around the World: A Research Agenda and
Preliminary Findings." *Gender and History* 17.2 (August 2005): 245–94.

Bartky, Sandra Lee. "Body Politics." In Alison M. Jaggar and Iris Marion Young,
eds., *A Companion to Feminist Philosophy.* Oxford, UK: Oxford University Press,
2000.

Best, Alyssa. "Abortion Rights along the Irish–English Border and the Liminality
of Women's Experiences." *Dialectical Anthropology* 29 (2005): 423–37.

Bordo, Susan. "Anorexia Nervosa: Psychopathology as the Crystallization of
Culture." In Irene Diamond and Lee Quinby, eds., *Feminism and Foucault: Reflections on Resistance.* Boston: Northeastern University Press, 1988.

Boutelier, Mary, and Lucinda SanGiovanni. "Politics, Public Policy and Title IX."
In Susan Birrell, ed., *Women, Sport and Culture.* Champaign: Human Kinetics,
1994.

Brumberg, Joan Jacobs. "'Something Happens to Girls': Menarche and the Emergence of the Modern American Hygienic Imperative." *Journal of the History of
Sexuality* 4.1 (July 1993): 99–127.

Caric, Ric. "Blustering Brags, Dueling Inventors, and Corn-Square Geniuses:
Artisan Leisure in Philadelphia, 1785–1825." *American Journal of Semiotics* 12
(1995 [1998]): 323–41.

———. "'To Drown the Ills That Discompose the Mind': Care, Leisure, and Identity among Philadelphia Artisans and Workers, 1785–1840." *Pennsylvania History* 64 (1997): 465–89.

———. "Displays of Degradation: The Washingtonian Temperance Movement in Philadelphia, 1841–1845." *Ohio Valley History Association* (25 October 2002).

———. "To the Convivial Grave and Back: John Fitch as a Case Study in Cultural Failure, 1785–1792." *Pennsylvania Magazine of History and Biography* 126.4 (October 2002).

———. "From Ordered Buckets to Honored Felons: Fire Companies and Cultural Transformation in Philadelphia, 1785–1850." *Pennsylvania History* 72 (Spring 2005): 117–58.

Casper, Monica J., and Adele E. Clarke. "Making the Pap Smear into the 'Right Tool' for the Job: Cervical Cancer Screening in the USA, circa 1940–95." *Social Studies of Science* 28.2 (1998): 255–90.

Chuppa-Cornell, Kim. "Filling a Vacuum: Women's Health Information in Good Housekeeping's Articles and Advertisements, 1920–1965." *The Historian* 67.3 (2005): 454–73.

Cole, Cheryl L. "Addiction, Exercise, and Cyborgs: Technologies of Deviant Bodies." In Geneviève Rail, ed., *Sport and Postmodern Times*. Albany, NY: SUNY Press, 1998. Pp. 261–76.

Collins, Leslea Haravon. "Working out the Contradictions: Feminism and Aerobics." *Journal of Sport and Social Issues* 26.1 (February 2002): 91.

Comeau, Pauline. "Debate Begins over Public Funding for HPV Vaccine." *CMAJ* 176.7 (2007): 913.

Cook, Pam. "Border Crossings: Women and Film in Context." In Pam Cook and Philip Dodd, eds., *Women and Film: A Sight and Sound Reader*. Philadelphia: Temple University Press, 1995.

Cook, Timothy E., and David C. Colby. "The Mass-Mediated Epidemic: The Politics of AIDS on the Nightly Network News." In Elizabeth Fee and Daniel Fox, eds., *AIDS: The Making of a Chronic Disease*. Berkeley: University of California Press, 1992. Pp. 84–122.

Cossey, Dilys. "Britain." In Ann Furedi, ed., *The Abortion Law in Northern Ireland: Human Rights and Reproductive Choice*. Belfast: Irish Family Planning Association Northern Ireland, 1995. Pp. 56–62.

Costos, Daryl, Ruthie Ackerman, and Lisa Paradis. "Recollections of Menarche: Communication between Mothers and Daughters Regarding Menstruation." *Sex Roles* 46.1–2 (January 2002): 49–59.

Craig, C. "The Egregious Dr. Beaney of the Beaney Scholarships." *Medical Journal of Australia* 1 (1950): 593–98.

Craig, Lee A., Barry Goodwin, and Thomas Grennes. "The Effect of Mechanical Refrigeration on Nutrition in the United States." *Social Science History* 28.2 (2004): 325–36.

Crosman, Robert. "Do Readers Make Meaning?" In Susan R. Suleiman and Inge Crosman, eds., *The Reader in the Text: Essays on Audience and Interpretation.* Princeton, NJ: Princeton University Press, 1980. Pp. 149–64.

Curran, James. "The CDC and the Investigation of the Epidemiology of AIDS." In Victoria A. Harden and John Parascandola, eds., *AIDS and the Public Debate: Historical and Contemporary Perspectives.* Amsterdam: IOS Press, 1995.

Curtis, Bruce. "Rural Idiocy or Agrarian Virtue? Schooling and Political Subjection in Lower Canada." Paper presented at "The Liberal Order in Canadian History," 3 March 2006, Montreal, McGill University Institute for the Study of Canada.

Davis, Nanette J. "The Abortion Consumer: Making It through the Network." *Urban Life and Culture* 2.4 (January 1974): 432–59.

Davis, Susan. "'Making Night Hideous': Christmas Revelry and Public Disorder in Nineteenth-Century Philadelphia." *American Quarterly* 34 (1982).

Davison, Graeme. "The Exodists: Miles Franklin, Jill Roe and the 'Drift to the Metropolis.'" *History Australia* 2.2 (June 2005): 35–42.

Deem, Rosemary. "Unleisured Lives: Sport in the Context of Women's Leisure." *Women's Studies International Forum* 10.4 (1987): 423–32.

Ditz, Toby L. "Shipwrecked; or, Masculinity Imperiled: Mercantile Representations of Failure and the Gendered Self in Eighteenth-Century Philadelphia." *Journal of American History* 81 (1994).

Douglas, Susan. "Narcissism as Liberation." In Jennifer Scanlon, ed., *The Gender and Consumer Culture Reader.* New York: New York University Press, 2000.

"Effectiveness of Strategies to Increase Cervical Cancer Screening in Clinic-Based Settings." *Public Health Research, Education, and Development Program.* Toronto: Ontario Ministry of Health, December 2000.

Ellison, Jenny. "'Stop Postponing Your Life until You Lose Weight and Start Living Now': Vancouver's Large as Life Action Group, 1979–1985." *Journal of the Canadian Historical Association* 18.1 (2007): 254.

———. "Aerobics for Fat Women Only." In Sondra Solovay and Esther Rothblum, eds., *The Fat Studies Reader.* New York: New York University Press, 2009.

Fauci, Anthony S. "AIDS: Reflections on the Past, Considerations for the Future." In Victoria A. Harden and John Parascandola, eds., *AIDS and the Public Debate: Historical and Contemporary Perspectives.* Amsterdam: IOS Press, 1995.

Feasey, Rebecca. "Stardom and Sharon Stone: Power as Masquerade." *Quarterly Review of Film and Video* 21.3 (July–September 2004): 199–207.

Featherstone, Lisa. "The Kindest Cut? The Origins of the Caesarean Section in Australia." In Marie Porter, Patricia Short and Andrea O'Reilly, eds., *Mother Power? Contemporary Feminist Voices.* Toronto: Women's Press, 2005. Pp. 25–40.

———. "Imagining the Black Body: Race, Gender and Gynaecology in Late Colonial Australia." *Lilith* 15 (2006): 86–96.

Feldberg, Georgina, Molly Ladd-Taylor, Allison Li, and Kathryn McPherson. "Comparative Perspectives on Canadian and American Women's Health Care since 1945." In Georgina Feldberg, Molly Ladd-Taylor, and Kathryn McPherson, eds., *Women, Health and Nation*. Montreal and Kingston: McGill-Queen's University Press, 2001.

Flamiano, Dolores. "Covering Contraception: Discourses of Gender, Motherhood and Sexuality in Women's Magazines, 1938–1969." *American Journalism* (Summer 2000).

Fletcher, Ruth. "'Pro-life' Absolutes, Feminist Challenges: The Fundamentalist Narrative of Irish Abortion Law 1986–1992." *Osgoode Hall Law Journal* 36.1 (Spring 1998): 1–62.

Fox, Daniel. "AIDS and American Health Policy." In Elizabeth Fee and Daniel Fox, eds., *AIDS: The Making of a Chronic Disease*. Berkeley: University of California Press, 1992.

Freud, Sigmund. "Psychoanalytic Notes upon an Autobiographical Account of a Case of Paranoia (Dementia Paranoides)." In Phillip Rieff, ed., *Three Case Histories*. New York: Collier, 1963.

Gandevia, Bryan. "Some Aspects of the Life and Work of James George Beaney." *Medical Journal of Australia* 1 (1953): 614–19.

———. "Beaney, James George." *Australian Dictionary of Biography, 1851–1890*. Melbourne: Melbourne University Press, 1966. Pp. 124–6.

Gardner-Thorpe, Christopher. "The Land They Left Behind." In John Pearne, ed., *Pioneer Medicine in Australia*. Brisbane: Amphion Press, 1988.

Gilman, Sander L. "AIDS and Syphilis: The Iconography of Disease." In Douglas Crimp, ed., *AIDS: Cultural Analysis, Cultural Activism*. Cambridge, MA: MIT Press, 1988.

Gold, Rachel Benson. "Lessons from before Roe: Will Past Be Prologue?" *The Guttmacher Report* 6.1 (March 2003). http://www.guttmacher.org/pubs/tgr/06/1/gr060108.html (accessed 12 July 2006).

Golstein, Richard. "The Impact of AIDS on American Culture." In Victoria A. Harden and John Parascandola, eds., *AIDS and the Public Debate: Historical and Contemporary Perspectives*. Amsterdam: IOS Press, 1995.

Hall, Stuart. "The Rediscovery of Ideology: The Return of the Repressed in Media Studies." In John Storey, ed., *Cultural Theory and Popular Culture: An Introduction*. 4th ed. London: Pearson Education, 2006.

Hartley, Cecilia. "Letting Ourselves Go: Making Room for the Fat Body in Feminist Scholarship." In *Bodies out of Bounds: Fatness and Transgression*. Berkeley: University of California Press, 2001). Pp. 60–73.

Hayter, Charles. "Cancer: The Worst Scourge of Civilized Mankind." *Canadian Bulletin of Medical History* 2.2 (2003): 260.

Heamen, Elspeth. "Revisiting the Origins of the Liberal Order Framework." Paper presented at "The Liberal Order in Canadian History," 3 March 2006, Montreal, McGill University Institute for the Study of Canada.

Henshaw, Stanley K. "The Accessibility of Abortion Services in the United States." *Family Planning Perspectives* 23.6 (1991): 246–52.

"The HPV Vaccine." *Washington Post* (12 January 2007).

Jewell, R. Todd, and Robert W. Brown. "An Economic Analysis of Abortion: The Effect of Travel Cost on Teenagers." *Social Sciences Journal* 37.1 (2000): 113–24.

Kassirer, Eve. "Impact of the Walton Report on Cervical Cancer Screening Programs in Canada." *Canadian Medical Association Journal* 122 (1980): 419.

Kennard, Margot. "Producing Sponsored Films on Menstruation: The Struggle over Meaning." In Elizabeth Ann Ellsworth and Marianne Whatley, eds. *Ideology of Images in Educational Media: Hidden Curriculums in the Classroom*. New York: Teachers College Press, 1990.

Kissling, Elizabeth Arveda. "On the Rag on Screen: Menarche in Film and Television." *Sex Roles* 46.12 (2002): 5–12.

Kitch, Carolyn. "Selling the 'Boomer Babes': *More* and the 'New' Middle Age." *Journal of Magazine and New Media Research* 5.2 (Spring 2003). http://www.bse.edu/web/aejmcmagzine/journal/srchive/Spring_2003/Kitch.htm (accessed 25 October 2003).

Kline, Ronald. "Construing 'Technology' as 'Applied Science': Public Rhetoric of Scientists and Engineers in the United States, 1880–1945." *Isis* 86.2 (1995): 194–221.

Koop, C. Everett. "The Early Days of AIDS as I Remember Them." In Victoria A. Harden and John Parascandola, eds., *AIDS and the Public Debate: Historical and Contemporary Perspectives*. Amsterdam: IOS Press, 1995.

Koppes, Clayton R. "The Power, the Glitter, the Muscles: Movie Masculinities in the Age of Reagan." *Reviews in American History* 23.3 (1995): 528–34.

Laclau, Ernesto. "Discourse." In R.E. Goodin and P. Pettit, eds., *A Companion to Contemporary Political Philosophy*. London: Blackwell, 1993.

Lee, Simon. "Abortion Law in Northern Ireland: The Twilight Zone." In Ann Furedi, ed., *The Abortion Law in Northern Ireland: Human Rights and Reproductive Choice*. Belfast: Irish Family Planning Association Northern Ireland, 1995. Pp. 16–26.

Lenskyj, Helen. "Good Sports: Feminists Organizing on Sport Issues in the 1970s and 1980s." *Resources for Feminist Research* 20.2/4 (1991): 130–35.

Levine, Susan, and Hamil R. Harris. "Wave of Support for HPV Vaccination of Girls." *Washington Post* (12 January 2007).

Lloyd, Mona. "Feminism, Aerobics and the Politics of the Body." *Body & Society* 2.2 (June 1996): 79–98.

Loudon, Irvine. "Deaths in Childbed from the Eighteenth Century to 1935." *Medical History* 30 (1986): 1–41.

Maguire, Joseph, and Louise Mansfield. "'Nobody's Perfect': Women, Aerobics, and the Body Beautiful." *Sociology of Sport Journal* 15 (1998): 125.

Markula, Pirkko. "Firm but Shapely, Fit but Sexy, Strong but Thin: The Postmodern Aerobicizing Female Bodies." *Sociology of Sport Journal* 12.4 (1995): 434.

Martin, Michelle H. "Postmodern Periods: Menstruation Media in the 1990s." *The Lion and the Unicorn* 23.3 (September 1999): 395–414.

———. "'No One Will Ever Know Your Secret!' Commercial Puberty Pamphlets for Girls from the 1940s to the 1990s." In Claudia Nelson and Michelle H. Martin, eds., *Sexual Pedagogies: Sex Education in Britain, Australia, and America, 1879–2000.* New York: Palgrave, 2003.

Marx, Karl. "The Eighteenth Brumaire of Louis Bonaparte." In Robert C. Tucker, *The Marx—Engels Reader.* New York: Norton, 1978.

McKay, Ian. "The Liberal Order Framework: A Prospectus for a Reconnaissance of Canadian History." *Canadian Historical Review* 81.4 (2000): 617–45.

McLaren, Angus. "Sexual Revolution? The Pill, Permissiveness and Politics." In *Twentieth-Century Sexuality: A History.* Oxford: Blackwell Publishers, 1999. Pp. 166–92.

Merskin, Debra. "Adolescence, Advertising and the Ideology of Menstruation." *Sex Roles* 40.1 (June 1999): 941–57.

Morantz, Regina. "The Lady and Her Physician." In Mary S. Hartman and Lois Banner, eds., *Clio's Consciousness Raised: New Perspectives on the History of Women.* New York: Harper Torchbooks, 1974. Pp. 38–53.

Morse, Margaret. "Artemis Aging: Exercise and the Female Body on Video." *Discourse* 10.1 (Fall/Winter 1987–88): 32–3.

Mullally, Siobhan. "The Abortion Debate in Ireland: Repartitioning the State." In Vijay Andrew, ed., *Women's Health, Women's Rights: Perspectives on Global Health Issues.* Toronto: York University Centre for Feminist Research, 2003. Pp. 27–49.

Nardi, Peter. "AIDS and Obituaries: The Perception of Stigma in the Press." In Michelle Cochrane, ed., *When AIDS Began: San Francisco and the Making of an Epidemic.* New York: Routledge, 2004. Pp. 159–68.

Nathan, Debbie. "Abortion Stories on the Border." In Maxine Baca Zinn, Pierrette Hondagneu-Satelo, and Michael Messner, eds., *Gender through the Prism of Difference.* 2nd ed. Needham Heights, MA: Allyn and Bacon, 2000. Pp. 123–5.

Nestel, Sheryl. "Delivering Subjects: Race, Space and the Emergence of Legalized Midwifery in Ontario." In Sherene H. Razack, ed., *Race, Space and the Law: Unmapping a White Settler Society.* Toronto: Between the Lines Press, 2002. Pp. 233–55.

Oikawa, Mona. "Cartographies of Violence: Women, Memory, and the Subject(s) of the 'Internment.'" In Sherene H. Razack, ed., *Race, Space and the Law: Unmapping a White Settler Society.* Toronto: Between the Lines Press, 2002. Pp. 73–98.

Oldenziel, Ruth. "Why Masculine Technologies Matter." In Nina E. Lerman, Ruth Oldenziel, and Arwen P. Mohun, eds., *Gender and Technology: A Reader.* Baltimore: Johns Hopkins University Press, 2003. Pp. 37–71.

Pacheco, Patrick. "Tony Kushner Speaks Out on AIDS, Angels, Activism and Sex in the 90s." In Tony Kushner, *Angels in America: Part 1: Millennium Approaches.* New York: Theatre Communications Group, 1992. Pp. 15–26.

Parker, James Edwin. "Snakes, Trolls, and Drag Queens." In Dean Kostos and Eugene Grygo, eds. *Mama's Boy: Gay Men Write about Their Mothers.* New York: Painted Leaf Press, 2000. Pp. 99–109.

Pheterson, Gail, and Yamila Azize. "Abortion Practice in the Northeast Caribbean: 'Just Write Down Stomach Pain.'" *Reproductive Health Matters* 13.26 (2005): 44–53.

Phizacklea, Annie. "Women, Migration and the State." In Kum-Kum Bhavnani, ed., *Feminism and "Race."* Oxford: Oxford University Press, 2001. Pp. 319–30.

The Proceedings of Cancer 2000, April 1992. A Report on the Work of a National Task Force, Cancer 2000: Strategies for Cancer Control in Canada. Toronto: Smithkline Breecham Pharma, 1992.

Prost, Antoine. "Public and Private Spheres in France." In Antoine Prost and Gerard Vincent, eds., *Riddles of Identity in Modern Times.* Vol. 5 of *A History of Private Life.* General eds. Arthur Goldhammer Philippe Aries and Georges Duby. Cambridge: Harvard University Press, 1987.

Quinn, Mike, Penny Babb, Jennifer Jones, and Elizabeth Allen. "Effect of Screening on Incidence of and Mortality from Cancer of Cervix in England: Evaluation Based on Routinely Collected Statistics." *British Medical Journal* 318 (3 April 1999): 904.

Reagan, Leslie J. "Crossing the Border for Abortions: California Activists, Mexican Clinics, and the Creation of a Feminist Health Agency in the 1960s." In Georgina Feldberg, Molly Ladd-Taylor, Alison Li, and Kathryn McPherson, eds., *Women, Health, and Nation: Canada and the United States since 1945.* Montreal and Kingston: McGill-Queen's University Press, 2003. Pp. 355–78.

Revie, Linda. "More Than Just Boots! The Eugenic and Commercial Concerns behind A.R. Kaufman's Birth Controlling Activities." *Canadian Bulletin of Medical History* 23.1 (2006): 119–43.

Rimke, Heidi Marie. "Governing Citizens through Self-Help Literature." *Cultural Studies* 14.1 (January 2000): 62.

Rochat, Roger W. "Pap Smear Screening: Has It Lowered Cervical Cancer Mortality among Black Americans?" *Phylon* 38.4 (1977): 429–47.

Rodgers, Sanda. "Abortion Denied: Bearing the Limits of the Law." In Cynthia Flood, ed., *Just Medicare: What's In, What's Out, How We Decide.* Toronto: University of Toronto Press, 2006. Pp. 107–36.

Rubenfeld, Jed. "The Right to Privacy." *Harvard Law Review* 102 (February 1989): 737–807.

Rubinstein, Annette. "Subtle Poison: The Puerperal Fever Controversy in Victorian Britain." *Historical Studies* 20 (1983): 420–38.

Ruskin, Cindy. "Taking Up Needles and Thread to Honor the Dead Helps AIDS Survivors Patch Up Their Lives." *People* (12 October 1987): 42–49.

Saunders, Kay, and Katie Spearritt. "Is There Life after Birth: Childbirth, Death and Danger for Settler Women in Colonial Queensland." *Journal of Australian Studies* 29 (June 1991): 64–79.

Schiller, Nina Glick. "The Invisible Women: Caregiving and AIDS." In Karen V. Hansen and Ilta Garey, eds., *Families in the United States: Kinship and Domestic Politics*. Philadelphia: Temple University Press, 1998.

Schlesinger, E.R. "The Sheppard-Towner Era: A Prototype Case Study in Federal-State Relationships." *American Journal of Public Health* 57.6 (1967): 1034–40.

Schultz, Laurie. "On the Muscle." In Jane Gaines and Charlotte Herzog, eds., *Fabrications: Costume and the Female Body*. New York: Routledge, 1990. Pp. 59–78.

Sethna, Christabelle. "The Cold War and the Sexual Chill: Freezing Girls out of Sex Education." *Canadian Woman Studies/les cahiers de la femme* 17 (1998): 57–61.

———. "The University of Toronto Health Service, Oral Contraception and Student Demand for Birth Control, 1960–1970." *Historical Studies in Education/ Revue d'histoire de l'éducation* 17.2 (2005): 265–92.

———. "The Evolution of the *Birth Control Handbook*: From Student Peer-Education Manual to Feminist Self-Empowerment Text, 1968–1975." *Canadian Bulletin of Medical History/Bulletin canadien d'histoire de la médecine* 23.1 (2006): 89–118.

———, and Marion Doull. "Far From Home? A Pilot Study Tracking Women's Journeys to a Canadian Abortion Clinic." *Journal of Obstetrics and Gynaecology Canada* (August 2007): 640–47.

Shelton, James D., Edward A. Brann, and Kenneth F. Schulz. "Abortion Utilization: Does Travel Distance Matter?" *Family Planning Perspectives* 8.6 (1976): 260–62.

Sherry, Michael S. "The Language of War in AIDS Discourse." In Timothy F. Murphy and Suzanne Poirier, eds., *Writing AIDS: Gay Literature, Language, and Analysis*. New York: Columbia University Press, 1993. Pp. 39–53.

Smith, Tom. "The Polls – A Report: Sexual Revolution?" *Public Opinion Quarterly* 54.3 (1990): 415–35.

Smith-Rosenberg, Carroll, and Charles Rosenberg. "The Female Animal: Medical and Biological Views of Woman and Her Role in Nineteenth-Century America." *Journal of American History* 60 (1973–74): 332–56.

Sterling, Abigail-Mary E.W. "The European Union and Abortion Tourism: Liberalizing Ireland's Abortion Law." *Boston College International and Comparative Law Review* 20.2 (Summer 1997): 385–406.

Thearle, M.J., and Helen Gregory. "Childbirth by Choice – Midwifery in Queensland from Pre-history to the 1930s." *Fourth Biennial Conference of the National Midwives Association*. Brisbane, 1985.

Treichler, Paula A. "Feminism, Medicine, and the Meaning of Childbirth." In Mary Jacobus, Evelyn Fox Keller, and Sally Shuttleworth, eds., *Body/Politics: Women and the Discourses of Science*. New York: Routledge, 1990. Pp. 113–38.

Warsh, Cheryl Krasnick. "Vim, Vigour and Vitality: Power Foods for Kids in Canadian Popular Magazines." In Marlene Epp, Franca Iacovetta, and Valerie Korinek, eds., *Edible Histories, Cultural Politics: Towards a Canadian Food History*. Toronto: University of Toronto Press, 2010.

Zivi, Karen D. "Who Is the Guilty Party? Rights, Motherhood, and the Problem of Prenatal Drug Exposure." *Law and Society Review* 34.1 (2000): 237–58.

Secondary Sources: Books

Allyn, David. *Make Love Not War: The Sexual Revolution: An Unfettered History.* New York: Little, Brown, 2000.

Altman, Dennis. *AIDS in the Mind of America.* Garden City, NY: Doubleday, 1986.

America's Culture War. New York: Free Press, 1994.

Apple, Rima. *Vitamania: Vitamins in American Culture.* New Brunswick, NJ: Rutgers University Press, 1996.

———. *Perfect Motherhood: Science and Childrearing in America.* New Brunswick, NJ: Rutgers University Press, 2006.

Appleby, Brenda Margaret. *Responsible Parenthood: Decriminalizing Contraception in Canada.* Toronto: University of Toronto Press, 1999.

Aries, Philippe. *Western Attitudes toward Death: From the Middle Ages to the Present.* Baltimore, MD: Johns Hopkins University Press, 1974.

Armstrong, Elizabeth M. *Conceiving Risk, Bearing Responsibility: Fetal Alcohol Syndrome and the Diagnosis of Moral Disorder.* Baltimore: Johns Hopkins University Press, 2003.

Arno, Peter, and Karyn Feiden. *Against the Odds: The Story of AIDS Drug Development, Politics, and Profits.* New York: HarperCollins, 1992.

Arnup, Katherine. *Education for Motherhood.* Toronto: University of Toronto Press, 1994.

Asbell, Bernard. *The Pill: A Biography of the Drug That Changed the World.* New York: Random House, 1995.

Baker, Jean. *Family Secrets: Gay Sons, A Mother's Story.* New York: Harrington Park Press, 1998.

Balsamo, Anne. *Technologies of the Gendered Body: Reading Cyborg Women.* Durham: Duke University Press, 1996.

Bartky, Sandra Lee. *Femininity and Domination: Studies in the Phenomenology of Oppression.* New York: Routledge, 1990.

Bashford, Alison. *Purity and Pollution: Gender, Embodiment and Victorian Medicine.* New York: St. Martin's Press, 1998.

Bayer, Ronald. *Private Acts, Social Consequences: AIDS and the Politics of Public Health.* New Brunswick, NJ: Rutgers University Press, 1989.

———, and Gerald Oppenheimer. *AIDS Doctors: Voices from the Epidemic.* New York: Oxford University Press, 2000.

Berridge, Virginia, and Kelly Loughlin, eds. *Medicine, the Market and the Mass Media: Producing Health in the Twentieth Century.* London: Routledge, 2005.

Big, Bold and Beautiful. Toronto: Macmillan Canada, 1996.

Blumberg, Leonard, with William L. Pittman. *Beware the First Drink: The Washington Temperance Movement and Alcoholics Anonymous.* Seattle: Glen Abbey Books, 1991.

Bordo, Susan. *Unbearable Weight*. Berkeley: University of California Press, 1993.

Boston Women's Health Book Collective. *Our Bodies, Ourselves: A Book By and For Women*. New York: Simon & Schuster, 1971.

Bourdieu, Pierre. *Outline of a Theory of Practice*. Cambridge: Cambridge University Press, 1977.

Brandt, Allan M., and Paul Rozin. *Morality and Health*. New York: Routledge, 1997.

Branson, Susan. *These Fiery Frenchified Dames: Women and Political Culture in Early National Philadelphia*. Philadelphia: University of Pennsylvania Press, 2001.

Breitenberg, Mark. *Anxious Masculinity in Early Modern England*. Cambridge: Cambridge University Press, 1996.

Brodie, Janine, Shelley A.M. Gavigan, and Jane Jenson. *The Politics of Abortion*. Toronto: Oxford University Press, 1992.

Brown, Catrina, and Karin Jasper, eds. *Consuming Passions: Feminist Approaches to Weight Preoccupation and Eating Disorders*. Toronto: Second Story Press, 1993.

Brumberg, Joan Jacobs. *The Body Project: An Intimate History of American Girls*. New York: Random House, 1997.

———. *Fasting Girls: The History of Anorexia Nervosa*. New York: Vintage, 2000.

Bushman, Richard L. *The Refinement of America: Persons, Houses, Cities*. New York: Knopf, 1992.

Butler, Judith. *Gender Trouble: Feminism and the Subversion of Identity*. London: Routledge, 1990.

Callen, Michael. *Surviving AIDS*. New York: HarperCollins, 1990.

Carnes, Mark C. *Secret Ritual and Manhood in Victorian America*. New Haven, CT: Yale University Press, 1991.

———, and Clyde Griffen. *Meanings for Manhood*. Chicago: University of Chicago Press, 1990.

Chernin, Kim. *The Obsession: Reflections on the Tyranny of Slenderness*. New York: Harper & Row Perennial Library, 1981.

Clendinen, Dudley, and Nagourney, Adam. *Out for Good: The Struggle to Build a Gay Rights Movement in America*. New York: Touchstone, 2001.

Clow, Barbara. *Negotiating Disease: Power and Cancer Care, 1900–1950*. Montreal and Kingston: McGill-Queen's University Press, 2001.

Connell, R.W. *Masculinities*. 2nd ed. Berkeley: University of California Press, 2005.

Conroy, David W. *In Public Houses: Drink and the Revolution of Authority in Colonial Massachusetts*. Chapel Hill: University of North Carolina Press, 1995.

Cosentino, Frank, and Maxwell Howell. *A History of Physical Education in Canada*. Toronto: General Publishing, 1971.

Craig, Maxine Leeds. *Ain't I a Beauty Queen: Black Women, Beauty, and the Politics of Race*. New York: Oxford University Press, 2002.

Crimp, Douglas, ed. *AIDS: Cultural Analysis, Cultural Activism*. Cambridge, MA: MIT Press, 1988.

Davis, Susan G. *Parades and Power: Street Theatre in Nineteenth-Century Philadelphia*. Philadelphia: Temple University Press, 1986.

de Cordova, Richard. *Picture Personalities: The Emergence of the Star System in America*. Urbana: University of Illinois Press, 1990.

Delaney, Janice, Mary Jane Lupton, and Emily Toth. *The Curse: A Cultural History of Menstruation*. 2nd ed. Champaign: University of Illinois Press, 1988.

D'Emilio, John, and Estelle Freedman. *Intimate Matters: A History of Sexuality in America*. Chicago: University of Chicago Press, 1997.

Dempsey, David. *The Way We Die: An Investigation of Death and Dying America Today*. New York: Macmillan, 1975.

Dorsey, Bruce. *Reforming Men and Women: Gender in the Antebellum City*. Ithaca, NY: Cornell University Press, 2002.

Doss, Erika. *Twentieth-Century American Art*. New York: Oxford University Press, 2002.

Dreyfus, Hubert L., and Paul Rabinow. *Michel Foucault: Beyond Structuralism and Hermeneutics*. Chicago: University of Chicago Press, 1983.

Dunphy, Catherine. *Morgentaler: A Difficult Hero*. Toronto: Random House of Canada, 1996.

Dyer, Richard. *Heavenly Bodies: Film Stars and Society*. London: Macmillan Educational Press, 1986.

———. *Stars*. London: British Film Institute, 1998.

Eberwein, Robert. *Sex Ed: Film, Video and the Framework of Desire*. New Brunswick, NJ: Rutgers University Press, 2000.

Ehrenreich, Barbara, and Deirdre English. *For Her Own Good: 150 Years of the Experts' Advice to Women*. London: Pluto Press, 1979.

———, and Deirdre English. *For Her Own Good: Two Centuries of the Experts' Advice to Women*. Rev. ed. New York: Anchor Books, 1978, 2005.

Fallon, Patricia, and Melanie Katzman. *Feminist Perspectives on Eating Disorders*. New York: Guilford Press, 1994.

Faludi, Susan. *Backlash: The Undeclared War against American Women*. New York: Doubleday, 1991.

Fee, Elizabeth, and Daniel Fox. *AIDS: The Burdens of History*. Berkeley, CA: University of California Press, 1988.

Feldberg, Georgina, Molly Ladd-Taylor, and Kathryn McPherson, eds. *Women, Health, and Nation: Canada and the United States since 1945*. Montreal and Kingston: McGill-Queen's University Press, 2003.

Feldman, Douglas A., and Julia Wang Miller. *The AIDS Crisis: A Documentary History*. Westport, CT: Greenwood Press, 1998.

Ford, Edward. *Bibliography of Australian Medicine, 1790–1900*. Sydney: Sydney University Press, 1976.

Foucault, Michel. *Technologies of the Self: A Seminar with Michel Foucault*. Ed. Luther H. Martin, Huck Gutman, and Patrick H. Hutton. Amherst: University of Massachusetts Press, 1988.

———. *The History of Sexuality: An Introduction*. Trans. Robert Hurley. New York: Random House, 1990 [1978].

———. *Discipline and Punish: The Birth of the Prison*. Trans. Alan Sheridan. New York: Vintage Books, 1995 [1977].

Friedan, Betty. *The Feminine Mystique*. New York: Dell, 1963.

Gaines, Jane, and Charlotte Herzog, eds. *Fabrications: Costume and the Female Body*. New York: Routledge, 1990.

Gardner, Kirsten E. *Early Detection: Women, Cancer, and Awareness Campaigns in the Twentieth-Century United States*. Chapel Hill: University of North Carolina Press, 2006.

Ginsburg, Faye D. *Contested Lives: The Abortion Debate in the American Community*. Berkeley: University of California Press, 1989.

Golden, Janet, Richard Alan Meckel, and Heather Munro Prescott. *Children and Youth in Sickness and Health: A Handbook and Guide*. New York: Greenwood Press, 2004.

Gorn, Elliott. *The Manly Art: Bare-Knuckle Prize Fighting in America*. Ithaca, NY: Cornell University Press, 1989.

Grant, Julia. *Raising Baby by the Book: The Education of American Mothers*. New Haven, CT: Yale University Press, 1998.

Grant, Nicole J. *The Selling of Contraception: The Dalkon Shield Case, Sexuality, and Women's Autonomy*. Columbus: Ohio State University Press, 1992.

Greenberg, Amy. *Cause for Alarm: The Volunteer Fire Department in the Nineteenth-Century City*. Princeton: Princeton University Press, 1998.

———. *Manifest Manhood and the Antebellum American Empire*. New York: Cambridge University Press, 2005.

Grescoe, Taras. *The End of Elsewhere: Travels among the Tourists*. Toronto: McFarlane Walter & Ross, 2003.

Grosz, Elizabeth. *Volatile Bodies: Toward Corporeal Feminism*. Bloomington: Indiana University Press, 1994.

———, and Elspeth Probyn, eds. *Sexy Bodies: The Strange Carnalities of Feminism*. New York: Routledge, 1995.

Grover, Kathryn. *Fitness in American Culture: Images of Health, Sport and the Body, 1830–1940*. Baltimore, MD: Johns Hopkins University Press, 1974.

Hall, M. Ann. *Feminism and Sporting Bodies*. Windsor: Human Kinetics, 1996.

———. *The Girl and the Game: A History of Women's Sport in Canada*. Peterborough: Broadview Press, 2004.

Harden, Victoria A., and John Parascandola, eds. *AIDS and the Public Debate: Historical and Contemporary Perspectives*. Amsterdam: IOS Press, 1995.

Harrison, Julia. *Being a Tourist: Finding Meaning in Pleasure Travel*. Vancouver: UBC Press, 2003.

Hartmann, Maren, Thomas Berker, Yves Punie, and Katie Ward. *Domestication of Media and Technology*. Berkshire, UK: Open University Press, 2005.

Hatty, Suzanne E., and James Hatty. *The Disordered Body: Epidemic Disease and Cultural Transformation*. Albany: SUNY Press, 1999.

Height, Dorothy I. *Open Wide the Freedom Gates: A Memoir*. New York: Public Affairs, 2003.

Herek, Gregory M., and Beverly Greene. *AIDS, Identity, and Community: The HIV Epidemic and Lesbian and Gay Men*. Thousand Oaks, CA: Sage Publications, 1995.

Hill, Daniel. *Advertising to the American Woman, 1900–1999*. Columbus, OH: Ohio State University Press, 2002.

Hopwood, Nick. *Embryos in Wax: Models from the Ziegler Studio*. Cambridge: Whipple Museum of the History of Science, 2002.

Howell, Maxwell, and Reet A. Howell. *History of Sport in Canada*. Champaign, IL: Stipes, 1981.

Hunter, James Davison. *Before the Shooting Begins: Searching for Democracy in America's Culture War*. New York: Free Press, 1994.

Inglis, Brian. *A History of Medicine*. London: Weidenfeld and Nicolson, 1965.

Insight Team of the Sunday Times of London. *Suffer the Children: The Story of Thalidomide*. New York: Viking Press, 1979.

Jacobus, Mary, and Evelyn Keller. *Body/Politics: Women and the Discourses of Science*. New York: Routledge, 1990.

Jagger, Alison M., and Iris Marion Young, eds. *A Companion to Feminist Philosophy*. Oxford: Oxford University Press, 2000.

Jasen, Patricia. *Wild Things: Nature, Culture, and Tourism in Ontario 1870–1914*. Toronto: University of Toronto Press, 1995.

Jeffords, Susan. *Hard Bodies: Hollywood Masculinity in the Reagan Era*. New Brunswick, NJ: Rutgers University Press, 1994.

Jeffreys, Sheila. *Anti-Climax: A Feminist Perspective on the Sexual Revolution*. London: Woman's Press, 1990.

Jenson, Jane. "Getting to Morgentaler: From One Representation to Another." In Janine Brodie, Shelley A.M. Gavigan, and Jane Jenson, *The Politics of Abortion*. Toronto: Oxford University Press, 1992. Pp. 24–25.

Jones, James H. *Bad Blood: The Tuskegee Syphilis Experiment*. New York: Free Press, 1981.

Kanfer, Stefan. *Serious Business: The Art and Commerce of Animation in America from Betty Boop to Toy Story*. New York: Da Capo, 2000.

Kaur, Raminder, and John Hutnyk, eds. *Travel Worlds: Journeys in Contemporary Cultural Politics*. London: Zed Books, 1999.

Kellough, Gail. *Aborting Law: An Exploration of the Politics of Motherhood and Medicine*. Toronto: University of Toronto Press, 1996.

Kidd, Bruce. *The Struggle for Canadian Sport*. Toronto: University of Toronto Press, 1996.

Kimmel, Michael. *Manhood in America: A Cultural History*. 2nd ed. New York: Oxford, 2006.

Kinsella, James. *Covering the Plague: AIDS and the American Media*. New Brunswick, NJ: Rutgers University Press, 1989.

Klepp, Susan, and Billy Smith. *The Importunate: The Voyage and Adventures of William Moraley, an Indentured Servant*. State College, PA: Pennsylvania State University Press, 1992.

Korinek, Valerie J. *Roughing It in the Suburbs: Reading Chatelaine Magazine in the Fifties and Sixties*. Toronto: University of Toronto Press, 2000.

Kübler-Ross, Elizabeth. *AIDS: The Ultimate Challenge*. New York: Macmillan, 1987.

Kushner, Rose. *Breast Cancer: A Personal History and an Investigative Report*. New York: Harcourt Brace Jovanovich, 1975.

Laurie, Bruce. *Working People of Philadelphia, 1800–1850*. Philadelphia: Temple University Press, 1980.

———. *Artisans into Workers: Labor in Nineteenth-Century America*. Urbana: University of Illinois Press, 1989.

Leavitt, Judith. *Typhoid Mary: Captive to the Public's Health*. Boston: Beacon Press, 1996.

Lenskyj, Helen. *Out of Bounds: Women, Sport and Sexuality*. Toronto: Women's Press, 1986.

Levine, Lawrence W. *The Unpredictable Past: Explorations in American Cultural History*. New York: Oxford University Press, 1993.

Lott, Eric. *Love and Theft: Blackface Minstrelsy and the American Working Class*. New York: Oxford University Press, 1995.

Luker, Kristen. Abortion and the Politics of Motherhood. Berkeley: University of California Press, 1985.

Lyons, Pat, and Debbie Burgard. *Great Shape: The First Exercise Guide for Large Women*. New York: Arbor House–William Morrow, 1988.

Marchessault, Janine, and Kim Sawchuk, eds. *Wild Science: Reading Feminism, Medicine, and the Media*. London: Routledge, 2000.

Marcus, Eric. *Making History: The Struggle for Gay and Lesbian Equal Rights, 1945–90: An Oral History*. New York: HarperCollins, 1992.

Marks, Lara V. *Sexual Chemistry: A History of the Contraceptive Pill*. New Haven, CT: Yale University Press, 2003.

Marrett, Loraine D., et al. *Cervical Cancer in Ontario: 1971–1996*. Cancer Care Ontario – Surveillance Unit and the Ontario Screening Program Division of Preventive Oncology, 1999.

Marshall, David P. *Celebrity and Power: Fame in Contemporary Culture*. Minneapolis: University of Minnesota Press, 1997.

Maynes, Mary Jo, Jennifer L. Pierce, and Barbara Lasett. *Telling Stories: The Use of Personal Narratives in the Social Sciences and History*. Ithaca, NY: Cornell University Press, 2008.

McCalman, Janet. *Sex and Suffering. Women's Health and a Woman's Hospital: The Royal Women's Hospital, Melbourne 1856–1996.* Melbourne: Melbourne University Press, 1998.

McCann, Carole R. *Birth Control Politics in the United States, 1916–1945.* Ithaca, NY: Cornell University Press, 1994.

McLaren, Angus. *Our Own Master Race: Eugenics in Canada, 1885–1945.* Toronto: McClelland and Stewart, 1990.

———, and Arlene Tigar McLaren. *The Bedroom and the State: The Changing Practices and Politics of Contraception and Abortion in Canada, 1880–1980.* Toronto: McClelland and Stewart, 1986.

———. *The Bedroom and the State: The Changing Practices and Politics of Contraception and Abortion in Canada, 1880–1997.* 2nd ed. Toronto: Oxford University Press, 1997.

Meigs, Joe Vincent. *Surgical Treatment of Cancer of the Cervix.* New York: Grune & Stratton, 1954.

———, and Somers H. Sturgis, eds. *Progress in Gynecology.* 4 vols. New York: Grune & Stratton, 1947.

Meranze, Michael. *Laboratories of Virtue: Punishment, Revolution, and Authority in Philadelphia, 1760–1835.* Chapel Hill: University of North Carolina Press, 1996.

Merleau-Ponty, Maurice. *The Phenomenology of Perception.* New York: Routledge, Kegan & Paul, 1962.

Messbarger, Rebecca. *The Century of Women: Representations of Women in Eighteenth-Century Italian Public Discourse.* Toronto: University of Toronto Press, 2002.

Meyerowitz, Joanne, ed. *Not June Cleaver: Women and Gender in Postwar America, 1945–1960s.* Philadelphia: Temple University Press, 1994.

Miller, Neil. *Out of the Past: Gay and Lesbian History from 1869 to the Present.* New York: Vintage, 1995.

Mitchinson, Wendy. *Giving Birth in Canada, 1900–1950.* Toronto: University of Toronto Press, 2002.

Moran, Jeffrey. *Teaching Sex: The Shaping of Adolescence in the 20th Century.* Cambridge: Harvard University Press, 2000.

Morantz-Sanchez, Regina. *Sympathy and Science: Women Physicians in American Medicine.* New York: Oxford University Press, 1985.

———. *Conduct Unbecoming a Woman: Medicine on Trial in Turn-of-the-Century Brooklyn.* New York: Oxford University Press, 1999.

Moscucci, Ornella. *The Science of Woman: Gynaecology and Gender in England, 1800–1929.* Cambridge: Cambridge University Press, 1990.

Muldoon, Maureen. *The Abortion Debate in the United States and Canada: A Sourcebook.* New York: Garland Publishing, 1991.

Murphy-Lawless, Jo. *Reading Birth and Death: A History of Obstetric Thinking.* Cork, Ireland: Cork University Press, 1998.

Myrsiades, Lynda S. *Splitting the Baby: The Culture of Abortion in Literature and Law, Rhetoric and Cartoons*. New York: Peter Lang, 2002.

Nadel, Alan. *Flatlining on the Field of Dreams: Cultural Narratives in the Films of President Reagan's America*. New Brunswick, NJ: Rutgers University Press, 1997.

Nash, Ilana. *American Sweethearts: Teenage Girls in Twentieth-Century Popular Culture*. Bloomington: Indiana University Press, 2006.

Newman, Simon. *Parades and the Politics of the Street: Festive Culture in the Early American Republic*. Philadelphia: University of Pennsylvania Press, 2000.

———. *Embodied History: The Lives of the Poor in Early Philadelphia*. Philadelphia: University of Pennsylvania Press, 2003.

Oakley, Ann. *Women Confined: Towards a Sociology of Childbirth*. Oxford: Martin Robertson, 1980.

Orbach, Susie. *Fat Is a Feminist Issue: A Self-Help Guide for Compulsive Overeaters*. New York: Berkley Books, 1979.

Otter, William. *History of My Own Times*. Ed. Richard B. Stott. Ithaca, NY: Cornell University Press, 1995.

Oudshoorn, Nelly. *Beyond the Natural Body: Archaeology of Sex Hormones*. New York: Routledge, 1994.

Owram, Douglas. *Born at the Right Time: A History of the Baby Boom Generation*. Toronto: University of Toronto Press, 1996.

Parascandola, John, and Victoria A. Harden, eds. *AIDS and the Public Debate: Historical and Contemporary Perspectives*. Amsterdam: IOS Press, 1995.

Patterson, James T. *The Dread Disease: Cancer and Modern American Culture*. Cambridge: Harvard University Press, 1987.

Petherbridge, Deanna, and Ludmilla Jordanova. *The Quick and the Dead: Artists and Anatomy*. Berkeley: University of California Press, 1997.

Poovey, Mary. *Uneven Developments: The Ideological Work of Gender in Mid-Victorian England*. Chicago: University of Chicago Press, 1995.

Prost, Antoine, and Gerard Vincent, eds. *Riddles of Identity in Modern Times*. Vol. 5 of *A History of Private Life*. General eds. Arthur Goldhammer Philippe Aries and Georges Duby. Cambridge: Harvard University Press, 1987.

Rail, Geneviève, ed. *Sport and Postmodern Times*. Albany, NY: SUNY Press, 1998.

Reagan, Leslie J. *When Abortion Was a Crime: Women, Medicine, and the Law in the United States, 1867–1973*. Berkeley: University of California Press, 1997.

———, Nancy Tomes, and Paula Treichler, eds. *Medicine's Moving Pictures: Medicine, Health and Bodies in American Film and Television*. Rochester: University of Rochester Press, 2007.

Reed, T.V. *The Art of Protest: Culture and Activism from the Civil Rights Movement to the Streets of Seattle*. Minneapolis: University of Minnesota Press, 2005.

Remer, Rosalind. *Printers and Men of Capital: Philadelphia Book Publishers in the New Republic*. Philadelphia: University of Pennsylvania Press, 1996.

Rilling, Donna. *Making Houses, Crafting Capitalism: Master Builders in Early Philadelphia, 1790–1850*. Philadelphia: University of Pennsylvania Press, 2000.

Roach, Catherine M. *Mother/Nature: Popular Culture and Environmental Ethics.* Bloomington: Indiana University Press, 2003.

Robertson, Thomas, et al. *Televised Medicine Advertising and Children.* New York: Praeger, 1979.

Roediger, David. *The Wages of Whiteness: Race and the Making of the American Working Class.* London: Verso, 1991.

Rogers, Naomi. *Dirt and Disease: Polio before FDR.* New Brunswick, NJ: Rutgers University Press, 1992.

Rolston, Bill, and Anna Eggert, eds. *Abortion in the New Europe: A Comparative Handbook.* Westport, CT: Greenwood Press, 1994.

Rorabaugh, W.J. *The Alcoholic Republic: An American Tradition.* Oxford: Oxford University Press, 1979.

Rose, Nikolas. *Governing the Soul: The Shaping of the Private Self.* London: Routledge, 1989.

Rotundo, E. Anthony. *American Manhood: Transformations in Masculinity from the Revolution to the Modern Era.* New York: Basic, 1994.

Salinger, Sharon. *Taverns and Drinking in Early America.* Baltimore: Johns Hopkins University Press, 2004.

Sammand, Nicholas. *Babes in Tomorrowland: Walt Disney and the Making of the American Child, 1930–1960.* Durham, NC: Duke University Press, 2005.

Sarker, Sonita, and Esha Niyogi De, eds. *Trans-Status Subjects: Gender in the Globalization of South and Southeast Asia.* Durham: Duke University Press, 2002.

Savage-Smith, Emilie. *Islamic Culture and the Medical Arts.* Bethesda, MD: National Library of Medicine, 1994.

Schaefer, Eric. *Bold! Daring! Shocking! True! A History of Exploitation Films, 1919–1959.* Durham: Duke University Press, 1999.

Scharf, John, and Thompson Westcott. *A History of Philadelphia, 1609–1884.* Philadelphia: L. Ewarts, 1884.

Schenken, Suzanne O'Dea. *From Suffrage to the Senate: An Encyclopedia of American Women in Politics.* Santa Barbara, CA: ABC-CLIO, 1999.

Schrum, Kelly. *Some Wore Bobby Sox: The Emergence of Teenage Girls' Culture, 1920–1945.* New York: Palgrave, 2004.

Schultz, Ronald. *The Republic of Labor: Philadelphia Artisans and the Politics of Class, 1720–1830.* New York: Oxford University Press, 1993.

Scranton, Phillip. *Proprietary Capitalism: The Textile Manufacture at Philadelphia, 1800–1885.* Cambridge: Cambridge University Press, 1983.

Seale, Clive. *Health and the Media.* Oxford: Blackwell, 2004.

Seid, Roberta Pollack. *Never Too Thin: Why Women Are at War with Their Bodies.* New York: Prentice Hall Press, 1989.

Sellers, Charles. *The Market Revolution: Jacksonian America, 1815–1846.* New York: Oxford University Press, 1994.

Shelton, Cynthia J. *The Mills of Manayunk: Industrialization and Social Conflict in the Philadelphia Region, 1787–1837.* Baltimore: Johns Hopkins University Press, 1986.

Silverstone, Roger. *Consuming Technologies: Media and Information in Domestic Spaces*. London: Routledge, 1992.

Sloane, David, and Beverlie Sloane. *Medicine Moves to the Mall*. Baltimore: Johns Hopkins University Press, 2003.

Smith, Billy G. *The "Lower Sort": Philadelphia's Laboring People, 1750–1800*. Ithaca, NY: Cornell University Press, 1990.

Smith, Pamela H., and Paula Findlen, eds. *Merchants and Marvels: Commerce, Science and Art in Early Modern Europe*. New York: Routledge, 2002.

Sontag, Susan. *AIDS and Its Metaphors*. New York: Farrar, Straus & Giroux, 1988.

Speert, Harold. *Obstetric and Gynecologic Milestones: Essays in Eponymy*. New York: Macmillan, 1958.

Stafford, Barbara Maria. *Body Criticism: Imaging the Unseen in Enlightenment Art and Medicine*. Cambridge, MA: MIT Press, 1994.

Stage, Sarah. *Female Complaints: Lydia Pinkham and the Business of Women's Medicine*. New York: W.W. Norton, 1979.

Storey, John. *Cultural Theory and Popular Culture: An Introduction*. 4th ed. Harlow, UK: Pearson, 2006.

Streitmatter, Rodger. *Unspeakable: The Rise of the Gay and Lesbian Press in America*. Boston: Faber & Faber, 1995.

Strong-Boag, Veronica. *The New Day Recalled*. Toronto: Copp Clark Pitman, 1988.

Tasker, Yvonne. *Working Girls: Gender and Sexuality in Popular Cinema*. London: Routledge 1998.

Terry, Jennifer. *An American Obsession: Science, Medicine, and Homosexuality in Modern Society*. Chicago: University of Chicago Press, 1999.

Thalidomide Task Force. *Report of the Thalidomide Task Force*. Vol. 1. Ottawa: War Amputation of Canada, 1989.

Thomson, Ann. *Winning Choice on Abortion: How British Columbian and Canadian Feminists Won the Battles of the 1970s and 1980s*. Victoria, BC: Trafford, 2004.

Thompson, Peter. *Rum Punch and Revolution: Taverngoing and Public Life in Eighteenth-Century Philadelphia*. Philadelphia: University of Pennsylvania Press, 1998.

Tomes, Nancy. *The Gospel of Germs: Men, Women, and the Microbe in American Life*. Cambridge, MA: Harvard University Press, 1998.

Tone, Andrea. *Devices and Desires: A History of Contraceptives in America*. New York: Hill & Wang, 2001.

Urry, John. *The Tourist Gaze: Leisure and Travel in Contemporary Societies*. London: Sage Publications, 1990.

Vinikas, Vincent. *Soft Soap, Hard Sell: American Hygiene in an Age of Advertisement*. Ames, IA: Iowa State University Press, 1992.

Vostral, Sharra. *Under Wraps: A History of Menstrual Hygiene and Technologies of Passing*. Lanham, MD: Rowman & Littlefield, 2008.

Waldstreicher, David. *In the Midst of Perpetual Fetes: The Making of American Nationalism, 1776–1820*. Chapel Hill: University of North Carolina Press, 1997.

Warsh, Cheryl Krasnick, and Veronica Strong-Boag, eds. *Children's Health Issues in Historical Perspective*. Waterloo, ON: Wilfrid Laurier University Press, 2005.

Watkins, Elizabeth Siegel. *On the Pill: A Social History of Oral Contraceptives 1950–1970*. Baltimore: Johns Hopkins University Press, 1998.

Watts, Steven. *The Magic Kingdom: Walt Disney and the American Way of Life*. Boston: Houghton Mifflin, 1997.

Wertz, Richard W., and Dorothy C. Wertz. *Lying-in: A History of Childbirth in America*. New Haven: Yale University Press, 1989.

Westcott, Thompson. *Life of John Fitch, Inventor of the Steamboat*. Philadelphia: Lippincott, 1857.

Weston, Kath. *Families We Choose: Lesbians, Gays, and Kinship*. New York: Columbia University Press, 1991.

Wilentz, Sean. *Chants Democratic: New York and the Making of the American Working Class, 1788–1850*. Oxford: Oxford University Press, 1984.

Williamson, Judith. *Decoding Advertisements*. London: Marion Boyars, 1978.

Willis, Evan. *Medical Dominance: The Division of Labour in Australian Health Care*. Sydney: George Allen and Unwin, 1983.

Willis, Susan. *A Primer for Daily Life*. London: Routledge, 1991.

Wolf, Naomi. *The Beauty Myth*. Toronto: Random House, 1990.

Secondary Sources: Dissertations

Bruce, Marny J. "Physical Activity, Physical Fitness and Health: Leisure-Time Physical Activity Trends in Canada from 1981 to 1998 and the Prospective Prediction of Health Status from Health-Related Physical Fitness." Unpublished MA thesis, York University, Toronto, Ontario, 2002.

Ellison, Jennifer. "Our Most Charming Girls: Female Athletes in Canadian Advertisements, 1928 to 2002." Unpublished MA thesis, Carleton University, 2002.

Friedenfelds, Lara. "Materializing the Modern, Middle-Class Body: Menstruation in the Twentieth-Century United States." Unpublished PhD dissertation, Harvard University, 2003.

Kennard, Margot. "The Corporation in the Classroom: The Struggles over Meanings of Menstrual Education in Sponsored Films, 1947–1983." Unpublished PhD dissertation, University of Wisconsin, 1989.

Swanson, Beth S. "A History of the Rise of Aerobic Dance in the United States through 1980." Unpublished MA thesis, San Jose State University, 1996.

Wasserlein, Frances Jane. "'An Arrow Aimed at the Heart': The Vancouver Women's Caucus and the Abortion Campaign, 1969–1971." Unpublished MA thesis, Simon Fraser University, 1990.

Contributors

Editor

Cheryl Krasnick Warsh is a professor of history at Vancouver Island University in Nanaimo, British Columbia. Her publications include *Prescribed Norms: Women and Health in Canada and the U.S. since 1800*; *Moments of Unreason: The Practice of Canadian Psychiatry and the Homewood Retreat, 1883–1923*; *Children's Health Issues in Historical Perspective* (co-edited with Veronica Strong-Boag); *Drink in Canada: Historical Essays*; *The Changing Face of Drink: Substance, Imagery and Behaviour* (co-edited with Jack S. Blocker, Jr.); and the forthcoming *Consuming Modernity: Changing Gendered Behaviours and Consumerism, 1919–1945* (co-edited with Dan Malleck). She is the former editor-in-chief of the *Canadian Bulletin of Medical History/Bulletin canadien d'histoire de la médecine*.

Chapter Authors

Annette Burfoot is an associate professor of sociology at Queen's University, teaching feminist science studies and visual culture. She edited *The Encyclopedia of Reproductive Technologies* and co-edited (with Susan Lord) *Killing Women: The Visual Culture of Gender and Violence*, and has numerous publications on gender and science, science fabulation, and the visual culture of medical science.

Christina Burr is an associate professor of history at the University of Windsor. Her publications include *Spreading the Light: Work and Labour Reform in Late-Nineteenth-Century Toronto* and *Canada's Victorian Oil Town: The Transformation of Petrolia from Resource Town into a Victorian*

Community. Her current research focuses on global beauty ideals and the body using the personal care products manufactured by the multinational corporation Unilever from the 1920s to the present.

Ric N. Caric is a professor of international and interdisciplinary studies at Morehead State University in Kentucky. His social theory and American history articles have appeared in *Philosophy in the Contemporary World*, *Pennsylvania History*, and other journals. Caric is finishing a book on popular culture in antebellum Philadelphia, and his political commentary can be found at his "Red State Impressions" blog.

Lisa Forman Cody is an associate professor of history and associate dean of the Faculty of History at Claremont McKenna College in Los Angeles. She is the author of *Birthing the Nation: Sex, Science, and the Conception of Eighteenth-Century Britons* (2005), which won the Berkshire Conference of Women Historians Best First Book of the Year Prize, the Phi Alpha Theta Best First Book Prize, and the Western Association of Women Historians Frances Keller Richardson-Sierra Prize. She is working on two books tentatively entitled *Divided We Stand: Divorce and Sexual Scandal in the Age of the American Revolution* and *Imaginary Values: Health, Wealth, and Human Labor in the British Imperial imagination, 1660–1840.*

Jenny Ellison recently received her doctorate in history from York University in Toronto. Her research on the fat-acceptance movement has appeared in the *Fat Studies Reader* (2009) as well as the *Journal of the Canadian Historical Association.* Her current research examines self-esteem as a women's health issue.

Lisa Featherstone is a lecturer in Australian history at the University of Newcastle, Australia. She has published in gender history, medical history, and the history of sexuality, and is currently writing a book entitled *Let's Talk about Sex: Histories of Sexuality in Australia from Federation to the Pill*, to be published by Cambridge Scholars Publishing in 2011.

Kirsten E. Gardner is an associate professor of history and women's studies at the University of Texas at San Antonio. She is the author of *Early Detection: Women, Cancer, and Awareness Campaigns in Twentieth-Century United States.*

Mandy Hadenko is a doctoral candidate in the Department of History, York University, Toronto. Her dissertation is entitled "Cervical Cancer and the Canadian Woman: Provincial Roles in Cancer Prevention."

Heather Molyneaux recently received her doctorate in history from the University of New Brunswick. Her dissertation examines the representation of women in the *Canadian Medical Association Journal* pharmaceutical advertisements. She has published in *Acadiensis* and has an article co-written with Linda Kealey in the *Journal of Canadian Studies*.

Heather Murray is an assistant professor in the Department of History, University of Ottawa. Her monograph, *Not in This Family: Gays and Their Parents in North America, 1945–1990s*, was published in 2010 by the University of Pennsylvania Press.

Christabelle Sethna is an associate professor at the Institute of Women's Studies and Faculty of Health Sciences, University of Ottawa. She has published numerous articles on sex education, contraception, and abortion history. She has completed a SSHRC-funded study on the impact of the birth control pill on single Canadian women between 1960 and 1980. She is currently working on another SSHRC-funded research project on the travel that Canadian women undertake to access abortion services, past and present.

Sharra L. Vostral is an associate professor, holding a joint appointment in the Department of Gender and Women's Studies and the Department of History at the University of Illinois, Urbana-Champaign. Her book, *Under Wraps: A History of Menstrual Hygiene Technology* (2008), examines the social and technological history of sanitary napkins and tampons, and the efforts to hide menstruation and menstrual artifacts, as well as the effects of technology upon women's experiences of menstruation. She co-edited *Feminist Technology* (2010), which explores feminist methods, theories, politics, and interventions in the design of artifacts. Her current research is a history of toxic shock syndrome and its relationship to tampon use during the early 1980s.

Index